FUNDAMENTALS OF

Periodontal Instrumentation

FUNDAMENTALS OF

Periodontal Instrumentation

Fourth Edition

JILL S. NIELD-GEHRIG, RDH, MA
Allied Health & Public Service Education
Asheville-Buncombe Technical Community College
Asheville, North Carolina

Editor: Lawrence McGrew
Associate Managing Editor: Angela Heubeck
Marketing Manager: Debby Hartman
Production Editor: Jennifer D. Weir

530 Walnut Street
Philadelphia, Pennsylvania 19106

351 West Camden Street
Baltimore, Maryland 21201-2436 USA

The author and publisher are not responsible (as a matter of product liability, negligence, or otherwise) for any injury resulting from any material contained herein. This publication contains information relating to general principles for the delivery of dental treatment and should not be construed as specific instructions for individual clinicians or patients. Not all recommendations for positioning and instrumentation are suitable for all clinicians and patients.

Printed in the United States of America.

Library of Congress Cataloging-in-Publication Data

Nield-Gehrig, Jill S. (Jill Shiffer)
   Fundamentals of periodontal instrumentation / Jill S. Nield-Gehrig.—4th ed.
      p. ; cm.
   Includes bibliographical references and index.
   ISBN 0-7817-2860-6
      1. Dental instruments and apparatus—Programmed instruction.   2. Dental
   hygiene—Programmed instruction.   I. Title: Periodontal instrumentation.   II. Title.
      [DNLM: 1. Dental Prophylaxis—instrumentation.   2. Dental Prophylaxis—methods. WU
   113 N6673f 2000]
   RK68I .N53 2000
   617.6'01—dc21
                                                                           00-042120

The publishers have made every effort to trace the copyright holders for borrowed material. If they have inadvertently overlooked any, they will be pleased to make the necessary arrangements at the first opportunity.

To purchase additional copies of this book, call our customer service department at **(800) 638-3030** or fax orders to **(301) 824-7390**. For other book services, including chapter reprints and large quantity sales, ask for the Special Sales department.

For all other calls originating outside of the United States, please call **(301) 714-2324**.

Visit Lippincott Williams & Wilkins on the Internet: **http://www.lww.com**. Lippincott Williams & Wilkins customer service representatives are available from 8:30 am to 6:00 pm, EST, Monday through Friday, for telephone access.

01 02 03 04
2 3 4 5 6 7 8 9 10

Preface

Fundamentals of Periodontal Instrumentation is designed to provide the learner with a detailed instructional guide to nonsurgical periodontal instrumentation. Over the years, many textbooks have addressed the cognitive "why" of periodontal instrumentation; this one, however, guides the learner step-by-step through the psychomotor "how" of instrumentation techique. The aim of *Fundamentals* has always been to make it easy for students to learn and faculty to teach instrumentation. To that end, the fourth edition has several new features designed to facilitate learning and teaching.

New Features

- Each module begins with a **module outline** that provides an overview of content and makes it easier to locate material within the module.

- Each module is subdivided into **Sections** to help the student recognize major content areas.

- **Key terms**, listed at the start of each module, call attention to important concepts in the module.

- **Terminology** pertinent to instrumentation and the periodontium is highlighted in bold type and clearly defined.

- Boxed **reference sheets, summary sheets** and **tables** emphasize important points and permit quick reference during technique practice and at-home review.

- **Flowcharts** help the student identify key steps in instrumentation technique.

- **Handle position landmarks** make it easier for students to learn to use instruments in the various treatment sextants.

- **Icons** indicating the treatment area, clock-position, patient head position, and handle position provide a quick reference for students in the technique practice sections of the book.

- **Rhyming Reminders** are poems that assist students in remembering basic instrumentation concepts in a whimsical manner.

- There are three new modules on the **mechanized instruments** that now play such an important role in nonsurgical periodontal instrumentation. Two chapters cover the theory behind and technique for ultrasonic instrumentation. A third module addresses the technique for using sonic instruments.

- **Redesigned skill evaluation checklists** are in a vertical, rather than horizontal, format and feature expanded criteria for skill attainment assessment.

Module Content and Sequencing

In the fourth edition, book content has been subdivided into more modules so that **each major topic area is addressed in a stand-alone module**. For example, there is a separate technique module for each design classification (anterior sickles, posterior sickles, universal curets, and area-specific curets). Each of these modules provides complete step-by-step instruction in the use of that instrument classification. For example, the module on universal curets provides complete instruction on the use of universal curets in posterior sextants (it does not rely on the student having a prior knowledge of the use of sickle scalers in posterior sextants.) This module structure means that it is not necessary to cover these modules in any particular order or even to include all instrument classifications. For example, if posterior sickle scalers are not part of the school's instrument kit, this module does not need to be included in the course outline.

New Module Content

Module 2, Principles of Positioning, includes additional information on **musculoskeletal disorders** and **neutral position** for the clinician. Also new **summary sheets** and **positioning references** for right- and left-handed clinicians are included.

Modules 4, 5, and 6 (Mirror and Finger Rests in Anterior Sextants, Mandibular Posterior, and Maxillary Posterior Sextants) introduce two new features in the fourth edition: (1) handle position landmarks and (2) quick reference icons. **Handle position landmarks** assist the student in learning where to position the handle in the grasp for anterior, mandibular posterior, and maxillary posterior sextants. **Quick reference icons** for clinician, patient, and handle position are used in the technique practice sections of these and other modules. All three Finger Rest modules feature summary tables for handle placement and right- and left-handed reference sheets for the treatment areas.

Module 18, Problem Identification: Difficulties in Instrumentation, has 10 new charts to aid students and faculty in **problem identification**.

Module 19, Instrument Sharpening, has two **Sharpening Guides** to assist students in achieving correct angulation of the sharpening stone to the instrument working-end.

Module 20, Instrumentation Strategies, has new content and learning activities on **instrument selection** and **treatment planning for calculus removal**.

Module 21, Basic Concepts of Ultrasonic Instrumentation, is a new module that covers the basic **theoretical concepts of ultrasonic instrumentation**. Module 21 represents an important addition to the book, given the significant role of ultrasonic instrumentation in the treatment of and supportive therapy for periodontal disease.

Module 24, Concepts in Periodontal Debridement, is a new module that summarizes research findings that are relevant to **periodontal debridement** and compares past concepts of scaling and root planing with the current concepts of debridement.

Features Retained from Previous Editions

- *Fundamentals* is still a **step-by-step, "how-to" guide** to periodontal instrumentation.
- Modules place **emphasis** on the **fundamental skills** of position, grasp, mirror use, and finger rests. These basic skills are introduced first to allow the learner to perfect them before tackling the use of instruments. Incorrect performance of one or more of these basic skills is the most common cause of poor skill attainment in instrumentation. These distinct instructional modules underscore for the learner the importance and universal application of these basic skills. A student who masters and consistently applies these skills will learn instrumentation with greater efficiency and ease.
- The Elements of Instrument Stroke section of the book introduces the learner to the **principles involved in stroke production** (adaptation, angulation, activation, pivot, handle roll, and instrumentation strokes). The three modules in this section guide the student through the steps involved in using any instrument to engage and remove calculus and provide technique practice independent of concerns about a particular instrument's design.
- Detailed instructions are provided for both **right-** and **left-handed** learners.
- Instrumentation technique is presented according to **instrument classifications** (e.g., universal curets) rather than by specific instruments (e.g., Columbia 13/14). It is unfortunate that many graduate practitioners, unable to recognize design characteristics, are reluctant to use any instruments other than those that they used while in school. Emphasis on instrument design characteristics provides students with concepts that they can apply to any instrument today or to new instrument designs in the future.
- **Step-by-step technique practice** is included for probes, explorers, sickle scalers, and curets in anterior and posterior treatment areas.
- **Skill Building Activities** are designed to allow the student to apply concepts presented in the book.
- Throughout the book, emphasis is placed on fostering the **autonomy and decision-making skills of the learner**. The step-by-step tutorial format allows the learner to work independently. This format provides the flexibility for the learner to spend more time on a skill that he or she finds difficult and to move on when a skill comes easily. The self-instructional format relieves the instructor from the task of endlessly repeating instructions and basic information, and frees him or her to demonstrate technique, observe student practice, and facilitate the process of skill acquisition.
- **Skill evaluation checklists** provide guidelines to student practice, promote student self-assessment skills, and provide benchmarks for faculty evaluation of student skill attainment. I encourage course instructors to require students to complete the self-evaluation portion of the checklists. The self-evaluation process helps students to develop the ability to assess their own level of competence rather than relying on instructor confirmation of skills.

I appreciate the enthusiastic comments and suggestions from educators and students about previous editions of *Fundamentals*, and welcome continued input. Being a dental healthcare provider is a special career and becoming one is a very challenging process. It is my sincere hope that this textbook will help the student to acquire the psychomotor skills that form a solid foundation for excellence in periodontal instrumentation.

Jill S. Nield-Gehrig

Acknowledgments

The author would like to acknowledge the contributions of these individuals whose help has been indispensable in bringing this book to completion.

Cynthia R. Biron, RDH, EMT, MA, Chairperson, Dental Hygiene Program, Tallahassee Community College, who made eminently helpful recommendations for the fourth edition, for her contributions to the module on advanced fulcrums, and, of course, for the Rhyming Reminders that appear in this edition. Also, to the **faculty and students of the Dental Hygiene Program at Tallahassee Community College** who use the *Fundamentals* text and contribute greatly to its improvement.

Rebecca Sroda, RDH, MS, and **Elizabeth Finnegan**, CDA, faculty at Asheville-Buncombe Technical Community College, Allied Dental Programs, for their support, patience, and contributions to the fourth edition. A special "thank you" to the **faculty and dental hygiene students at Asheville-Buncombe Technical Community College** for their support and suggestions.

I am grateful to the educators and reviewers who shared many helpful comments and suggestions with me. Most especially, dental hygiene educators, **Tina Daniels**, **Bea Hicks**, and **Leslie Delong** who took the time to provide me with detailed comments about what they would like to see in the fourth edition. I have tried to incorporate all the suggestions that I received.

Eros S. Chaves, DMD, MS, for his review of the Dental Implant module and contribution of clinical slides. **Nancy Snyder Whitten**, RDH, MEd, and **Christina S. Pellegrino**, CDA, RDH, MA, for their contributions to *Fundamentals*.

Charles D. Whitehead, the world's best medical illustrator, who created all the wonderful illustrations for the book. **Dee Robert Gehrig,** PE, Gehrig Photographic Studio, and **Al J. Julian**—the talented individuals who created the hundreds of photographs for this book.

The following individuals who were extremely generous with their time and knowledge—**Beth Beathard**, **Valerie Crane**, and **Annette Carswell** of EMS Electro Medical Systems; **Carol Hartman** of DENTSPLY Preventive Care; and **Susan Boyden** of Hu-Friedy Manufacturing. And **Craig Kilgore**, President, Kilgore International, Inc., for providing the dental typodonts for the book.

And finally, my editor, **Larry McGrew**, for his expertise and moral support.

Jill S. Nield-Gehrig

Registered Trademarks

The following are registered trademarks of:
American Eagle
    EagleLite Suregrip instrument handle
    Gracey +3 Access Curettes
    Gracey +3 Deep Pocket Curettes
DENTSPLY Preventive Care
    Cavitron ultrasonic scalers
    Cavitron SPS Ultrasonic Scaler with SPS Technology
    Dentsply BOBCAT ultrasonic scaler
    Steri-Mate sterilizable handpiece
    Midwest Quixonic sonic scaler
    Cavitron MED
    FSI Slimline (FSI-SLI) ultrasonic insert series
    Focused Spray (FSI) ultrasonic insert series
    Slimline (SLI) ultrasonic insert series
    Thru Flow (TFI) ultrasonic insert series
    DualSelect dispensing system
EMS (Electro Medical Systems)
    Piezon Master 400
Florida Probe
Hu-Friedy Manufacturing Company, Inc.
    After Five Gracey Curettes
    After Five 11/12 Explorer
    Mini Five
    Satin Steel instrument handle
    Vision Curvette instrument series
Impla-med Wiz-Stik implant instrument
Implant-Prophy+ implant instruments
Kilgore International, Inc.
    Dental hygiene and periodontal typodonts
Midwest
    Quixonic Sonic Scaler
Nobel Biocare Implant Instruments
Premier
    Periowise color-coded probe
    Premier implant scalers
SportsHealth Power Putty
Thompson Dental's Tactile Tone instrument handle

Contents

ELEMENTS OF INSTRUMENT STROKE

PATIENT ASSESSMENT

DEBRIDEMENT WITH HAND-ACTIVATED INSTRUMENTS

1
MODULE

Mathematical Principles and Anatomic Descriptors

This module contains a review of the mathematical principles and anatomic descriptors that you need to know when learning periodontal instrumentation. None of these concepts or terms is difficult, and you have probably studied them in the past. You should, however, review them now to be sure that you have a clear understanding of each principle or descriptor.

Required Equipment:

- red/blue pencil

1

Section 1: Mathematical Principles

Geometric Angles

The 90-degree angle and the 45-degree angle are commonly used reference points in instrumentation. For example, the cutting edge of an instrument meets the tooth surface at an angle that is less than 90-degrees but greater than 45-degrees. Review the every day examples of 90-degree and 45-degree angles shown below.

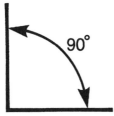

This is a 90-degree angle. It is also known as a "right-angle".

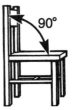

The seat of this chair is at a 90-degree angle to the chair back.

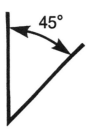

This is a 45-degree angle.

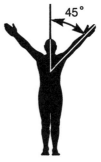

This man's arms are at a 45-degree angle to the midline of his body.

Parallel and Perpendicular

To correctly position an instrument, you will need to understand the terms parallel and perpendicular.

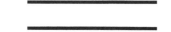

Parallel lines run in the same direction and will never meet.

Perpendicular lines meet at right angles.

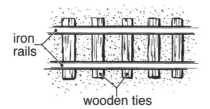

The iron rails and wooden ties of a railroad track can be used to explain the terms parallel and perpendicular. The iron rails are parallel. The wooden ties are perpendicular to the iron rails. The wooden ties also are parallel to each other.

Planes

To correctly move the instrument over the tooth, you will need to understand the terms vertical, oblique, and horizontal.

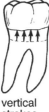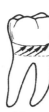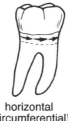

vertical strokes   oblique strokes   horizontal (circumferential) strokes

During instrumentation, instrument strokes are made across the tooth surface in vertical, oblique, and horizontal directions.

Cross Section

Cutting through an object, so that the incision is perpendicular to the object's long axis, will enable you to view the object in cross section.

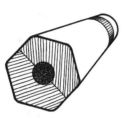

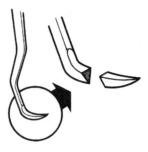

This lead pencil is hexagonal in cross section.

Certain instruments are triangular in cross section.

Millimeters

The anatomic features of the teeth are often measured in millimeters rather than in inches. The abbreviation for millimeters is "mm".

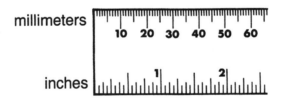

A probe is a periodontal instrument that is similar to a miniature ruler. The probe tip is marked in millimeter units and is used for making intraoral measurements.

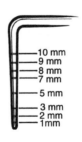

Section 2: Anatomic Descriptors

Long Axis of a Tooth

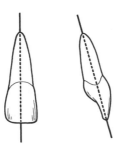

The long axis is an imaginary dividing line through the center of a tooth.

Apical and Coronal

If the working-end of an instrument moves in an **apical** direction, it is moved toward the tooth apex. If the working-end moves in a **coronal** direction, it is moved toward the tooth crown.

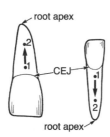

For both teeth shown here, moving from Point 1 to Point 2 is movement in an apical direction. It is also accurate to say that Point 1 is located apical to the cementoenamel junction (CEJ) on both illustrations.

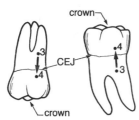

For both teeth shown here, moving from Point 3 to Point 4 is movement in a coronal direction. Also, Point 4 is *coronal* to the CEJ, Point 3 is *apical* to the CEJ, and Point 3 is *apical* to Point 4.

Midline

A structure can be divided into two equal halves at its midline.

A tooth may be divided into equal halves at the midline.

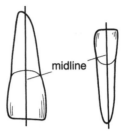

Quadrant

For purposes of identification, the dentition may be divided at the midline into four areas. Each area is referred to as a quadrant.

The four quadrants are:
- Maxillary right quadrant
- Maxillary left quadrant
- Mandibular left quadrant
- Mandibular right quadrant

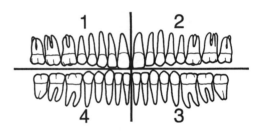

Sextant

For purposes of identification, the dentition may be divided into six areas. Each of the six areas is referred to as a sextant. There are two anterior sextants and four posterior sextants in the dental arch.

The six sextants of the dentition are:
- Maxillary right posterior sextant
- Maxillary anterior sextant
- Maxillary left posterior sextant
- Mandibular left posterior sextant
- Mandibular anterior sextant
- Mandibular right posterior sextant

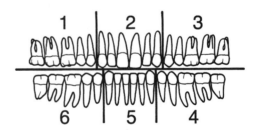

Line Angles

A line angle is an imaginary line formed where two tooth surfaces meet.

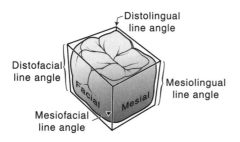

Each tooth has four line angles:
- Mesiofacial line angle
- Distofacial line angle
- Mesiolingual line angle
- Distolingual line angle

Facial and Lingual Aspects

A tooth, sextant, quadrant, or an arch may be divided into two aspects: (1) a facial aspect, and (2) a lingual aspect. When removing dental calculus from a sextant, the teeth are divided into aspects for instrumentation. For example, the calculus deposits may be removed first from the facial aspect of the teeth in the sextant. After all the calculus has been removed from the facial aspect, the lingual aspect of the teeth in the sextant will be instrumented.

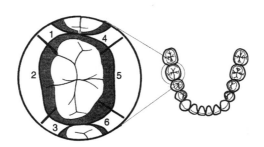

The **facial aspect** of a tooth is subdivided into three areas:
1—distofacial area
2—facial surface
3—mesiofacial area

The **lingual aspect** of a tooth is subdivided into three areas:
4—distolingual area
5—lingual surface
6—mesiolingual area

Section 3: Skill Building Activity

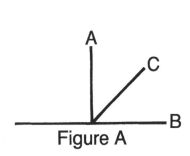

Figure A

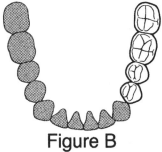

Figure B

Questions #1 to #5 refer to **Figure A**. Directions: circle the correct response.

1. Line A is: vertical   horizontal   oblique

2. Line C is: vertical   horizontal   oblique

3. Line(s) at 90-degree angle to Line A: B   C   both B & C

4. Line(s) at 45-degree angles to Line C: A   B   both A & B

5. Line(s) perpendicular to Line B: A   C   both A & C

6. Shape of a baseball in cross section: circular   triangular   rectangular

7. Shape of a pyramid in cross section: circular   triangular   rectangular

8. On **Figure B**, color the *facial aspect* of the mandibular left sextant in red. Color the *lingual aspect* in blue.

Principles of Positioning

In this module you will learn about positioning yourself and your patient. Correct positioning techniques help to prevent clinician discomfort and injury, permit a clear view of the tooth being worked on, allow easy access to the teeth, and facilitate efficient treatment of the patient.

This module contains information relating to the general principles for clinician and patient positioning; not all recommendations for positioning are suitable for everyone. If you experience any discomfort, consult a physician who specializes in the treatment of musculoskeletal disorders.

Required Equipment:

- a clinician stool
- a dental chair and unit, and
- a classmate or a dental typodont and manikin

Key Terms:

Ergonomics   Anterior surfaces toward the clinician
Musculoskeletal disorder   Anterior surfaces away from the clinician
Repetitive motion   Posterior aspect toward the clinician
Neutral position   Posterior aspect away from the clinician
Supine

Section 1: Musculoskeletal Disorders

The National Institute for Occupational Safety & Health (NIOSH), defines a **work-related musculoskeletal disorder (WMD)** as an injury affecting the musculoskeletal, peripheral nervous, and neurovascular systems that is caused or aggravated by occupational exposure to ergonomic hazards. Tools, equipment, and work tasks that are uncomfortable are **ergonomic hazards**. According to the U.S. Bureau of Labor Statistics, musculoskeletal disorders result in more than 60 percent of all newly reported occupational injuries.[1] Occupational injuries to the muscles, nerves, and tendon sheaths of the back, shoulders, neck, arms, elbows, wrists, and hands are common among dental healthcare workers.[2-8] Symptoms include loss of strength, tingling, numbness, and pain.

The human body was not designed to maintain the same body position or engage in repetitive movements for extended periods of time. B.A. Silverstein, in an article in the British Journal of Industrial Medicine, defined a **repetitive task** as one that performs the same fundamental element for more than 50% of the cycle.[9] A dental prophylaxis would certainly be categorized as a repetitive task under this definition. More than 50% of the time is spent performing very controlled, fast motions. The dental healthcare professional has a high risk of musculoskeletal injury when repetitive motions are combined with forceful movements, awkward postures, and insufficient recovery time.[9-12]

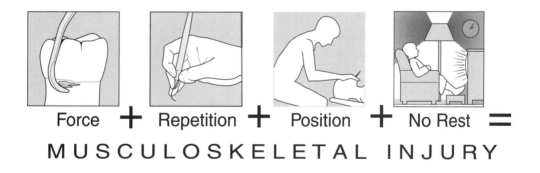

Force **+** Repetition **+** Position **+** No Rest **=**

M U S C U L O S K E L E T A L   I N J U R Y

WMDs Commonly Seen in Dental Healthcare Providers

Carpal tunnel syndrome is a painful disorder of the wrist and hand caused by compression of the median nerve within the carpal tunnel of the wrist. The nerve fibers that make up the median nerve originate in the spinal cord in the neck; therefore, poor posture can cause symptoms of CTS. Other ergonomic hazards for CTS include repeatedly bending the hand up, down, or from side-to-side at the wrist and continuously pinch-gripping an instrument without resting the muscles. Symptoms of CTS include numbness, pain, tingling in the thumb, index and middle fingers.

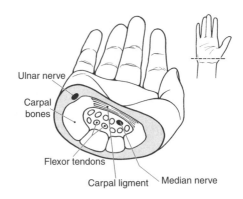

Ulnar nerve entrapment is a painful disorder of the lower arm and wrist caused by compression of the ulnar nerve of the arm as it passes through the wrist. Symptoms include numbness, tingling, and/or loss of strength in the lower arm or wrist. Ergonomic hazards include bending the hand up, down, or from side-to-side at the wrist and holding the little finger a full span away from the hand.

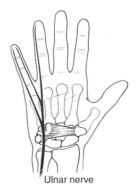

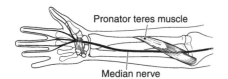

Pronator syndrome is a painful disorder of the wrist and hand caused by compression of the median nerve between the two heads of the pronator teres muscle. The symptoms are similar to those of carpal tunnel syndrome. An ergonomic hazard for this condition is holding the lower arm away from the body.

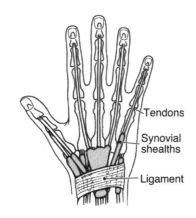

Tendinitis is a painful inflammation of the tendons of the wrist resulting from strain. Symptoms include pain in the wrist, especially on the outer edges of the hand, rather than through the center of the wrist. An ergonomic hazard for this condition is repeatedly extending the hand up or down at the wrist.

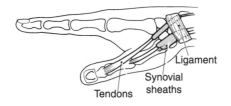

Tenosynovitis is a painful inflammation of the tendons on the side of the wrist and at the base of the thumb. Symptoms include pain on the side of the wrist and the base of the thumb; sometimes movement of the wrist yields a crackling noise. Ergonomic hazards include hand twisting, forceful gripping, bending the hand back or to the side.

Rotator cuff tendinitis is a painful inflammation of the muscle tendons in the shoulder region. Symptoms include severe pain and impaired function of the shoulder joint. Ergonomic hazards include holding the elbow above waist level and holding the upper arm away from the body.

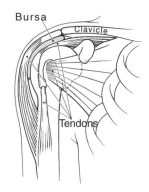

Extensor wad strain is a painful disorder of the fingers due to injury of the extensor muscles of the thumb and fingers. Symptoms include numbness, pain, and loss of strength in the fingers. An ergonomic hazard for this injury is extending the fingers independently of each other.

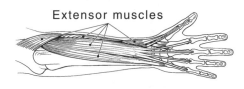

Thoracic outlet syndrome is a painful disorder of the fingers, hand, and/or wrist due to the compression of the brachial nerve plexus and vessels between the neck and shoulder. Symptoms include numbness, tingling, and/or pain in the fingers, hand, or wrist. Ergonomic hazards include tilting the head forward, hunching the shoulders forward, and continuously reaching overhead.

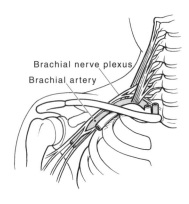

Section 2: Neutral Position for the Clinician

Research indicates that over 80 percent of dental hygienists complain of pain in the upper body and back.[2] This musculoskeletal pain often is the direct result of body positioning and movements made by dental healthcare professionals in their daily work. **Neutral position** is the ideal positioning of the body while performing work activities and is associated with decreased risk of musculoskeletal injury. It is generally believed that the more a joint deviates from the neutral position, the greater the risk of injury.

Neutral Seated Position

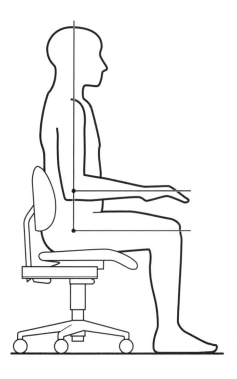

- Forearms parallel to the floor.

- Weight evenly balanced.

- Thighs parallel to the floor.

- Hip angle of 90°.

- Seat height positioned low enough so that you are able to rest the heels of your feet on the floor.

- When working from clock positions 9-12:00 (or 12-3:00), spread feet apart so that your legs and the chair base form a tripod, somewhat like the legs of a three-legged stool. This tripod formation creates a very stable position from which to work.

- **AVOID** positioning your legs under the back of the patient chair. In this position the patient chair will be too high and you will need to raise your upper arms to reach the patient's mouth.

Neutral Neck Position

- Head tilt of 0° to 15°
- The line from your eyes to the treatment area should be as near to vertical as possible

AVOID:

- Head tipped too far forward
- Head tilted to one side

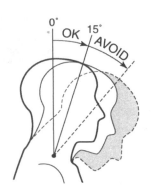

Neutral Shoulder Position

- Shoulders in horizontal line
- Weight evenly balanced when seated

AVOID:

- Shoulders lifted up toward ears
- Shoulders hunched forward
- Sitting with weight on one hip

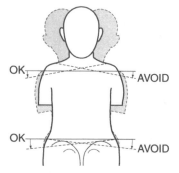

Neutral Back Position

- Leaning forward slightly from the waist or hips
- Trunk flexion of 0° to 20°

AVOID:

- Over flexion of the spine (curved back)

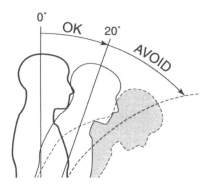

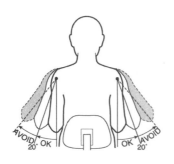

Neutral Upper Arm Position
- Upper arms hang in a vertical line parallel to long axis of torso
- Elbows at waist level held slightly away from body

AVOID:
- Greater than 20° of abduction of elbows away from the body
- Elbows held above waist level

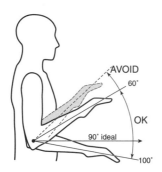

Neutral Forearm Position
- Held parallel to the floor
- Raised or lowered, if necessary, by pivoting at the elbow joint

AVOID:
- Angle between forearm and upper arm of less than 60°

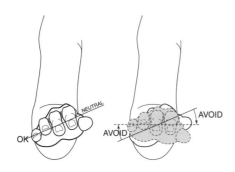

Neutral Hand Position
- Little finger-side of palm is slightly lower than thumb-side of palm
- Wrist aligned with forearm

AVOID:
- Thumb-side of palm rotated down so that palm is parallel to floor
- Hand and wrist bent up or down

Section 3: Patient Position

Supine Patient Position

Supine position—the position of the patient during dental treatment, with the patient lying on his or her back in a horizontal position and the chair back nearly parallel to the floor.

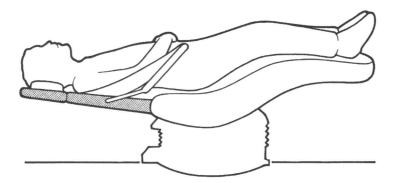

The Supine Patient Position	
Recommended Position	
Body	The patient's heels should be slightly higher than the tip of his or her nose. This position maintains good blood flow to the head. An apprehensive patient is more likely to faint if positioned with the head **higher** than the heels. The chair back should be nearly parallel to the floor for maxillary treatment areas. The chair back may be raised slightly for mandibular treatment areas.
Head	The top of the patient's head should be even with the upper edge of the headrest. If necessary, ask the patient to slide up in the chair to assume this position.
Headrest	If the headrest is adjustable, raise or lower it so that the patient's neck and head are aligned with the torso.

Patient Head Positions

The patient's head position is an important factor in determining whether the clinician can see and access the teeth in a treatment area. Unfortunately, many clinicians ignore this important aspect of patient positioning. A clinician may contort his or her body into an uncomfortable position instead of asking the patient to change head positions. Working in this manner not only causes stress on the clinician's musculoskeletal system, but also makes it difficult to see the treatment area. Remember that the patient is only in the chair for a limited period of time while the clinician spends hours at chairside day after day.

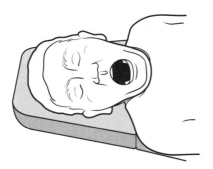

The patient should be asked to adjust his head position to provide the clinician with the best view of the treatment area.

Basic Patient Head Positioning	
Recommended Position	
Position on headrest	For you to be able to see and reach the patient's mouth comfortably, the top of the patient's head must be even with the end of the headrest.
Mandibular areas	Ask your patient to open the mouth and tilt the head downward. The term for this patient head position is the *chin-down* position.
Maxillary areas	Ask your patient to open the mouth and position the head in a neutral position. The term for this patient head position is the *chin-up* position.

Section 4: Clinician Stool and Patient Chair

The Adjustable Clinician Chair

Ergonomics is the science of adjusting the design of tools, equipment, tasks, and environments for safe, comfortable and effective human use. Manufacturers of dental equipment are constantly working to design seating for clinicians that is more ergonomic in design. Blood circulation to your legs, thighs, and feet is maintained by adjusting the stool to a proper height. Minimize stress on your spine by moving the chair back closer or farther away from the seat so that your upper arms and torso are aligned with the long axis of your body. Each individual who uses the chair should readjust it to fit his or her own body. A chair that is adjusted correctly for another person may be uncomfortable for you. Just as each driver of the family car must change the position of the driver's seat and mirrors, you should adjust the stool height and seat back to conform to your own body proportions and height.

The chair should have the following design characteristics [13]:
1. Legs—five legs for stability; casters for easy movement

2. Height
   - Should allow clinician to sit with thighs parallel to the floor. A seat height range of 14 to 20 inches will accommodate both tall and short clinicians.
   - Should be easily adjustable from a seated position.

3. Seat
   - Fabric that breathes (ex: cloth rather than vinyl).
   - Front edge of seat should have a waterfall shape (rounded front edge).
   - Should not be too heavily padded; thick padding requires constant minor readjustments in order to maintain balance.
   - When seated with the back against the backrest, the seat length should not impinge on the back of the clinician's knees. A seat length of 15 to 16 inches will fit most clinicians.

4. Backrest
   - Should be adjustable in both vertical and horizontal directions so that it can be positioned to touch the lumbar region of the back when comfortably seated.
   - Angle between the seat and the chair back should be between 85- and 100-degrees.

Patient Position Relative to the Clinician

Once comfortably seated, several other factors influence the clinician's ability to maintain correct neutral positioning. While working, the clinician must be able to gain access to the patient's mouth and the dental unit without bending, stretching, or holding his or her elbows above waist level. To maintain neutral position, the patient and the dental unit must be positioned correctly in relation to the clinician.

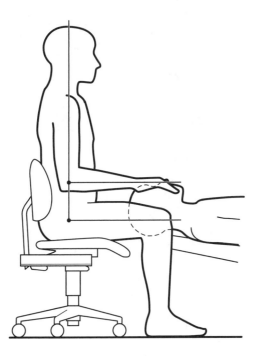

Establishing neutral position:

1. First, adjust the height of the clinician chair to establish a hip angle of 90°.
2. Next, lower the patient chair until the tip of the patient's nose is below waist level. Your elbow angle should be at 90° when your fingers are touching the teeth in the treatment area.

An Easy Technique for Establishing Neutral Position in Relation to the Patient

The most common ergonomic hazard during instrumentation is positioning the patient too high in relation to the clinician.

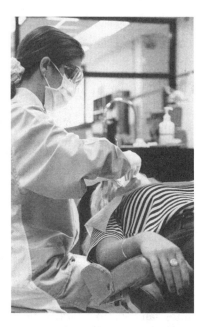

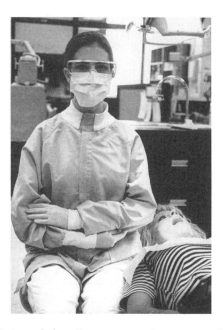

Incorrect positioning—patient too high.

Note how the clinician must hold her elbows up in a stressful position in order to reach the patient's mouth.

This error is often due to a misconception that the clinician can see better if the patient is closer. Actually, the reverse is true; the clinician has improved vision of the mouth when the patient is in a lower position.

Determining the proper placement of the patient.

Sit alongside of the patient with your arms against your sides and crossed at your waist. The patient's open mouth should be *below* the point of your elbow.

With the patient in this position, the clinician will be able to reach the mouth without placing stress on the muscles of her shoulders or arms.

Summary Sheet: Relationship to Patient and Dental Unit	
	Description
Clinician chair	Your thighs should be parallel to the floor and you should be able to rest your heels on the floor.
	When working from clock positions 9-12:00 (or 12-3:00), your legs and the stool base should form a tripod, somewhat like the legs of a three-legged stool. This tripod formation creates a very stable position from which to work.
Height of patient chair	TEST FOR PROPER NEUTRAL POSITION: Fold your arms across your waist. The tip of the patient's noise should be lower than your elbows.
Clinician's body position	You should not have to raise your elbows above waist level when working in the patient's mouth.
	Your *lower arms* should be in a horizontal position or raised slightly so that the angle formed between your lower and upper arms is slightly less than 90 degrees. In this position, your muscles are well positioned to control fine wrist and finger movements.
	Your shoulders should be level and should not be hunched up toward your ears.
Bracket table	Position it slightly above the patient's body. The lower the tray level, the easier it will be for you to see the periodontal instruments resting on it.
Dental light	Position the light as far away from the patient's face as possible while still keeping it within easy reach.

Dental Light Position

Mandibular Treatment Areas

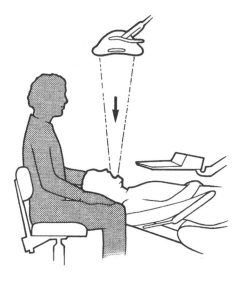

For the mandibular treatment areas, position the dental light directly above the patient's head, so that the light beam shines directly down into the patient's mouth. Remember to keep the light at arm's length.

Maxillary Treatment Areas

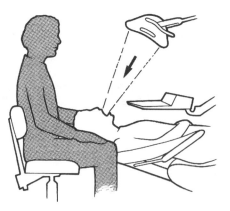

Position the dental light above the patient's chest area for maxillary treatment areas. Tilt the dental light so the light beam shines into the patient's mouth at an angle. Remember to keep the light at arm's length.

Positioning Terminology

- **Anterior surfaces toward the clinician**—the surfaces of the anterior teeth that are closest to the clinician.
- **Anterior surfaces away from the clinician**—the surfaces of the anterior teeth that are farthest from the clinician.

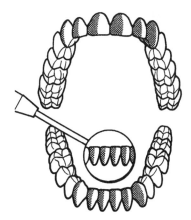

RIGHT-Handed clinicians: The **shaded** anterior surfaces in this illustration are the anterior surfaces toward the right-handed clinician.

LEFT-Handed clinicians: The **unshaded** (white) anterior surfaces in this illustration are the anterior surfaces toward the left-handed clinician.

- **Posterior aspects toward the clinician**—the aspects of the posterior sextants that are closest to the clinician.
- **Posterior aspects away from the clinician**—the aspects of the posterior sextants that are farthest from the clinician.

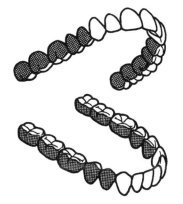

RIGHT-Handed clinician: The **shaded** surfaces in this illustration are the posterior aspects toward a right-handed clinician.

LEFT-Handed clinicians—The **shaded** surfaces in this illustration are the posterior aspects away from a left-handed clinician.

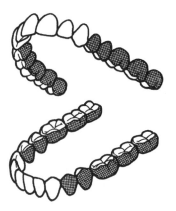

RIGHT-Handed clinicians—The **shaded** surfaces in this illustration are the posterior aspects away from a right-handed clinician.

LEFT-Handed clinician: The **shaded** surfaces in this illustration are the posterior aspects toward a left-handed clinician.

Directions for Sections 5 and 6 of this Module:

1. The next two sections of this Module contain instructions for positioning yourself to obtain the best possible access to each of the treatment areas. For some treatment areas, there is a range of clock positions in which you can sit.
2. For this module, you should concentrate on mastering your positioning for each treatment area. Work without dental instruments and just concentrate on learning positioning.
3. You will not be able to obtain a clear view of all the teeth as you practice your positioning in this module. In Modules 4, 5, and 6 you will learn to use a dental mouth mirror to view these "hidden" tooth surfaces.
4. When practicing on a classmate, you should use infection control techniques including the use of protective attire and barrier techniques, handwashing, sterilization or disinfection and cleaning of instruments, equipment, and environmental surfaces.

RIGHT-Handed clinicians: Turn to Section 5 on page 27. When you are finished with this section, turn to page 43.

LEFT-Handed clinicians: Turn to Section 6 on page 35. When you are finished with this section, turn to page 43.

Section 5: Position for RIGHT-Handed Clinician

Clock Positions

Instrumentation of the various treatment areas may be accomplished from one of four basic clinician positions. The four basic clinician positions are usually identified in relation to a 12-hour clock face:

1. the 8 o'clock position, to the front of the patient's head,
2. the 9 o'clock position, to the side of the patient's head,
3. the 10 to 11 o'clock position, to the back of the patient's head, or
4. the 12 o'clock position, directly behind the patient's head.

The four clock positions are described in detail on pages 28 and 29.

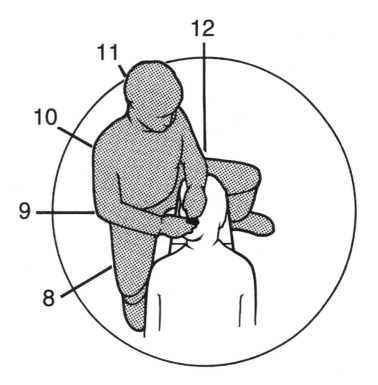

The 8 o'clock Position (Front Position)

- Sit facing the patient with your hips in line with the patient's elbows.

- To reach the patient's mouth, hold your arms slightly away from your sides. Hold your lower right arm over the patient's chest. The side of your left hand rests in the area of the patient's right cheekbone and upper lip. NOTE: Do not rest your arm on the patient's head or chest.

- Your line of vision is straight ahead, into the patient's mouth.

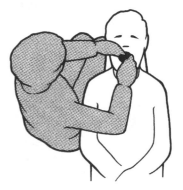

The 9 o'clock Position (Side Position)

- Sit facing the side of the patient's head. The midline of your torso is even with the patient's mouth.

- To reach the patient's mouth, hold the lower half of your right arm in approximate alignment with the patient's shoulder. Hold your left hand and wrist over the region of patient's right eye.

- Your line of vision is straight down into the mouth.

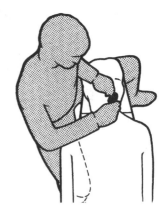

The 10 to 11 o'clock Position (Back Position)

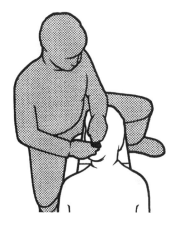

- Sit at the top right corner of the headrest; the midline of your torso is even with the temple region of the patient's head.

- To reach the patient's mouth, hold your right hand directly across the corner of the patient's mouth. Hold your left hand and wrist above the patient's nose and forehead.

- Your line of vision is straight down into the mouth.

The 12 o'clock Position (Directly Behind Patient)

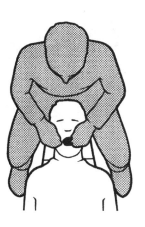

- Sit directly behind the patient's head.

- To reach the patient's mouth, hold your wrists and hands above the region of the patient's ears and cheeks.

- Your line of vision is straight down into the patient's mouth.

Positioning for the Anterior Sextants

Anterior Surfaces Toward the Clinician

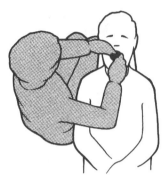

8 to 9 o'clock position

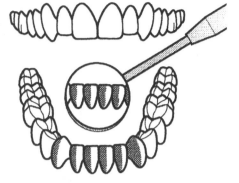

1. Head turned slightly toward the clinician
2. Chin-down position

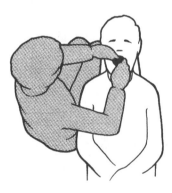

8 to 9 o'clock position

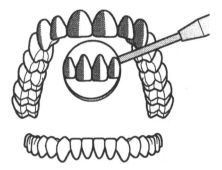

1. Head turned slightly toward the clinician
2. Chin-up position

Anterior Surfaces Away From the Clinician

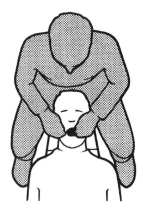

12 o'clock position

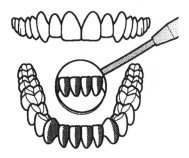

1. Head turned slightly toward the clinician
2. Chin-down position

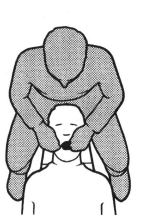

12 o'clock position

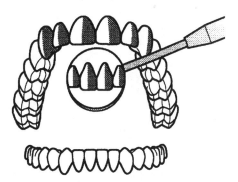

1. Head turned slightly toward the clinician
2. Chin-up position

Positioning for the Posterior Sextants

Posterior Aspects Toward the Clinician

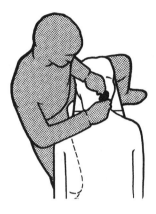

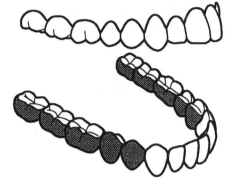

9 o'clock position

1. Head turned slightly away from the clinician
2. Chin-down position

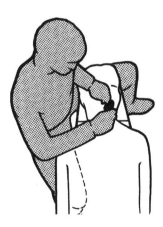

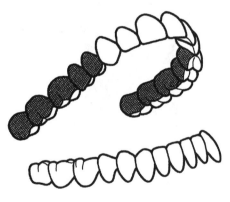

9 to 10 o'clock position

1. Head turned slightly away from the clinician
2. Chin-up position

Posterior Aspects Away From the Clinician

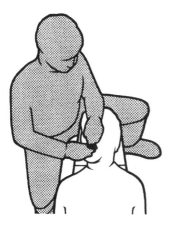

10 to 11 o'clock position

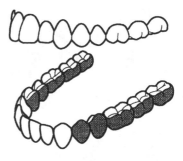

1. Head turned toward the clinician
2. Chin-down position

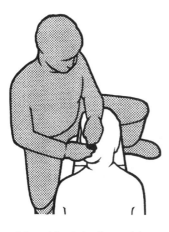

10 to 11 o'clock position

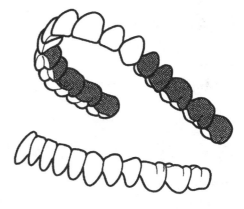

1. Head turned toward the clinician
2. Chin-up position

Reference Sheet: Positioning for the RIGHT-Handed Clinician

Photocopy this page and use it for quick reference as you practice your positioning skills. Place the photocopied reference sheet in a plastic page protector for longer use.

Positioning Summary		
Treatment Area	**Clock Position**	**Patient Head Position**
Anterior surfaces, toward Mandibular arch	8 – 9:00	Slightly toward Chin-down
Anterior surfaces, toward Maxillary arch	8 – 9:00	Slightly toward Chin-up
Anterior surfaces, away Mandibular arch	12:00	Slightly toward Chin-down
Anterior surfaces, away Maxillary arch	12:00	Slightly toward Chin-up
Posterior aspects, toward Mandibular arch (right facial and left lingual)	9:00	Slightly away Chin-down
Posterior aspects, toward Maxillary arch (right facial and left lingual)	9:00	Slightly away Chin-up
Posterior aspects, away Mandibular arch (right lingual and left facial)	10 – 11:00	Toward Chin-down
Posterior aspects, away Maxillary arch (right lingual and left facial)	10 – 11:00	Toward Chin-up

Note: This ends the section for RIGHT-Handed Clinician. Turn to **page 43** for the Activity, References, and Evaluations section.

Section 6: Position for LEFT-Handed Clinician

Clock Positions

Instrumentation of the various treatment areas may be accomplished from one of four basic clinician positions. The four basic clinician positions are usually identified in relation to a 12-hour clock face:

1. the 4 o'clock position, to the front of the patient's head,
2. the 3 o'clock position, to the side of the patient's head,
3. the 2 to 1 o'clock position, to the back of the patient's head, or
4. the 12 o'clock position, directly behind the patient's head.

The four clock positions are described in detail on pages 36 and 37.

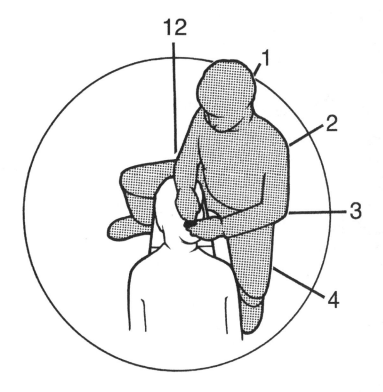

The 4 o'clock Position (Front Position)

- Sit facing the patient with your hips in line with the patient's elbows.

- To reach the patient's mouth, hold your arms slightly away from your sides. Hold your lower left arm over the patient's chest. The side of your right hand rests in the area of the patient's left cheekbone and upper lip. NOTE: Do not rest your arm on the patient's head or chest.

- Your line of vision is straight ahead, into the patient's mouth.

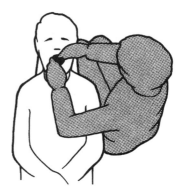

The 3 o'clock Position (Side Position)

- Sit facing the side of the patient's head. The midline of your torso is even with the patient's mouth.

- To reach the patient's mouth hold the lower half of your left arm in approximate alignment with the patient's shoulder. Hold your right hand and wrist over the region of patient's left eye.

- Your line of vision is straight down into the mouth.

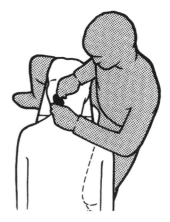

The 2 to 1 o'clock Position (Back Position)

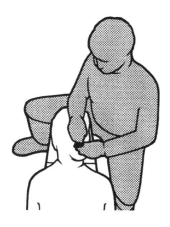

- Sit at the top left corner of the headrest; the midline of your torso is even with the temple region of the patient's head.

- To reach the patient's mouth hold your left hand directly across the corner of the patient's mouth. Hold your right hand and wrist above the patient's nose and forehead.

- Your line of vision is straight down into the mouth.

The 12 o'clock Position (Directly Behind Patient)

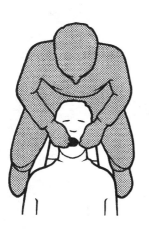

- Sit directly behind the patient's head.

- To reach the patient's mouth, hold your wrists and hands above the region of the patient's ears and cheeks.

- Your line of vision is straight down into the patient's mouth.

Positioning for the Anterior Sextants

Anterior Surfaces Toward the Clinician

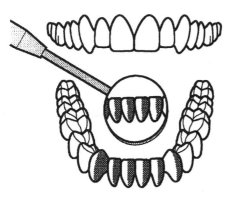

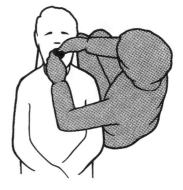

1. Head turned slightly toward the clinician
2. Chin-down position

4 to 3 o'clock position

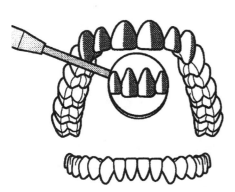

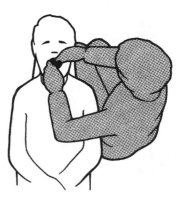

1. Head turned slightly toward the clinician
2. Chin-up position

4 to 3 o'clock position

Anterior Surfaces Away From the Clinician

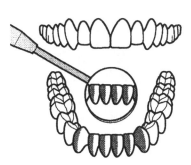

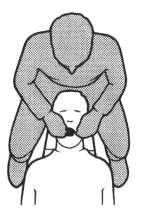

1. Head turned slightly toward the clinician
2. Chin-down position

12 o'clock position

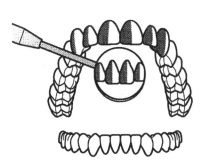

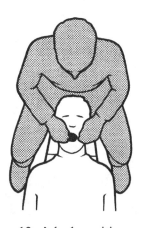

1. Head turned slightly toward the clinician
2. Chin-up position

12 o'clock position

Positioning for the Posterior Sextants

Posterior Aspects Toward the Clinician

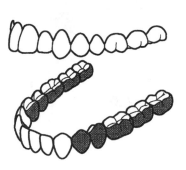

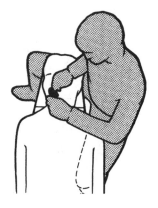

1. Head turned slightly away from the clinician
2. Chin-down position

3 o'clock position

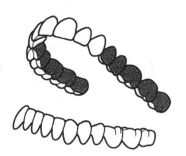

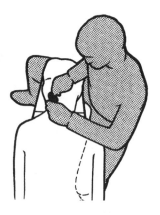

1. Head turned slightly away from the clinician
2. Chin-up position

3 o'clock position

Posterior Aspects Away From the Clinician

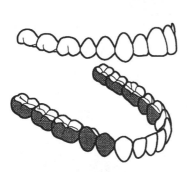

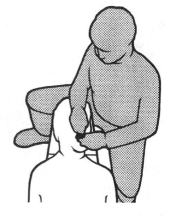

1. Head turned toward the clinician
2. Chin-down position

2 to 1 o'clock position

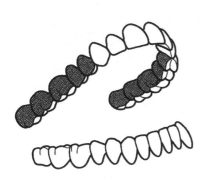

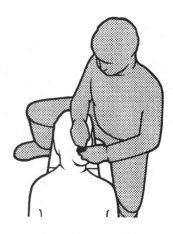

1. Head turned toward the clinician
2. Chin-up position

2 to 1 o'clock position

Reference Sheet: Positioning for the LEFT-Handed Clinician

Photocopy this page and use it for quick reference as you practice your positioning skills. Place the photocopied reference sheet in a plastic page protector for longer use.

Positioning Summary		
Treatment Area	**Clock Position**	**Patient Head Position**
Anterior surfaces, toward Mandibular arch	4 – 3:00	Slightly toward Chin-down
Anterior surfaces, toward Maxillary arch	4 – 3:00	Slightly toward Chin-up
Anterior surfaces, away Mandibular arch	12:00	Slightly toward Chin-down
Anterior surfaces, away Maxillary arch	12:00	Slightly toward Chin-up
Posterior aspects, toward Mandibular arch (left facial and right lingual)	3:00	Slightly away Chin-down
Posterior aspects, toward Maxillary arch (left facial and right lingual)	3:00	Slightly away Chin-up
Posterior aspects, away Mandibular arch (left lingual and right facial)	2 – 1:00	Toward Chin-down
Posterior aspects, away Maxillary arch (left lingual and right facial)	2 – 1:00	Toward Chin-up

Section 7: Activity, References, and Evaluations

Rhyming Reminder

Rhyming Reminders are poems written to help you remember important concepts in an interesting manner. You will find Rhyming Reminders in several modules of the book. Originally, these poems were written for the dental hygiene students at Tallahassee Community College by their program director, Cynthia Biron.

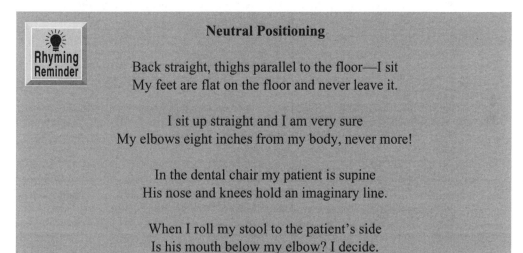

Neutral Positioning

Back straight, thighs parallel to the floor—I sit
My feet are flat on the floor and never leave it.

I sit up straight and I am very sure
My elbows eight inches from my body, never more!

In the dental chair my patient is supine
His nose and knees hold an imaginary line.

When I roll my stool to the patient's side
Is his mouth below my elbow? I decide.

Skill Building Activity

Position your patient so that the tip of his or her nose is level with the mid-region of your chest. Try reaching each of the 12 treatment areas with your patient positioned in this manner. What kind of muscle strain do you think that you would experience if you were to work for several hours with the patient positioned in this manner?

References

1. Silverstein, B.A., et al., *Work-related musculoskeletal disorders: comparison of data sources for surveillance.* Am J Ind Med, 1997. **31**(5): p. 600-8.

2. Jacobsen, N., and A. Hensten-Pettersen, *Occupational health problems among dental hygienists.* Community Dent Oral Epidemiol, 1995. **23**(3): p. 177-81.

3. Jacobsen, N., T. Derand, and A. Hensten-Pettersen, *Profile of work-related health complaints among Swedish dental laboratory technicians.* Community Dent Oral Epidemiol, 1996. **24**(2): p. 138-44.

4. Moen, B.E., and K. Bjorvatn, *Musculoskeletal symptoms among dentists in a dental school.* Occup Med (Lond), 1996. **46**(1): p. 65-8.

5. Reitemeier, B., *Psychophysiological and epidemiological investigations on the dentist.* Rev Environ Health, 1996. **11**(1-2): p. 57-63.

6. Rundcrantz, B.L., B. Johnsson, and U. Moritz, *Cervical pain and discomfort among dentists. Epidemiological, clinical and therapeutic aspects. Part 1. A survey of pain and discomfort.* Swed Dent J, 1990. **14**(2): p. 71-80.

7. Rundcrantz, B.L., B. Johnsson, and U. Moritz, *Pain and discomfort in the musculoskeletal system among dentists. A prospective study.* Swed Dent J, 1991. **15**(5): p. 219-28.

8. Rundcrantz, B.L., *Pain and discomfort in the musculoskeletal system among dentists.* Swed Dent J Suppl, 1991. **76**: p. 1-102.

9. Silverstein, B.A., L.J. Fine, and T.J. Armstrong, *Hand wrist cumulative trauma disorders in industry.* Br J Ind Med, 1986. **43**(11): p. 779-84.

10. Latko, W.A., et al., *Development and evaluation of an observational method for assessing repetition in hand tasks.* Am Ind Hyg Assoc J, 1997. **58**(4): p. 278-85.

11. Kilbom, S., et al., *Musculoskeletal Disorders: Work-related risk factors and prevention.* Int J Occup Environ Health, 1996. **2**(3): p. 239-246.

12. Silverstein, B.A., L.J. Fine, and T.J. Armstrong, *Occupational factors and carpal tunnel syndrome.* Am J Ind Med, 1987. **11**(3): p. 343-58.

13. Occhipinti, E., et al., *Criteria for the ergonomic evaluation of work chairs.* Med Lav, 1993. **84**(4): p. 274-85.

Skill Evaluation #1: Position, Mandibular Sextants

Student: _____   Area 1 = anterior sextant, facial aspect

Evaluator: _____   Area 2 = anterior sextant, lingual aspect

Date: _____   Area 3 = right posterior sextant, facial aspect

Area 4 = right posterior sextant, lingual aspect

Area 5 = left posterior sextant, facial aspect

Area 6 = left posterior sextant, lingual aspect

DIRECTIONS: For each area, use **Column S** for student self-evaluation and **Column I** for instructor evaluation. For each skill evaluated, indicate the skill level as: **S** (satisfactory), **I** (improvement needed), or **U** (unsatisfactory).

CRITERIA:	Area 1		Area 2		Area 3		Area 4		Area 5		Area 6	
	S	I	S	I	S	I	S	I	S	I	S	I
Adjusts clinician chair correctly												
Positions patient chair correctly												
Assures that patient's head is even with top of headrest												
Positions bracket table within easy reach												
Positions unit light at arm's length												
Assumes recommended clock position												
Asks patient to adjust head position												
Adjusts patient chair so that clinician's elbows are at waist level when fingers touch teeth in treatment area												
Maintains neutral position												
Directs unit light to illuminate tx. area												

Skill Evaluation #1: Position, Mandibular Sextants

Student: _____

Evaluator Comments:

_____

_____

_____

_____

_____

_____

_____

_____

_____

_____

_____

_____

_____

_____

_____

_____

_____

Box for sketches pertaining to written comments.

Skill Evaluation #2: Position, Maxillary Sextants

Student: _____

Evaluator: _____

Date: _____

Area 1 = anterior sextant, facial aspect

Area 2 = anterior sextant, lingual aspect

Area 3 = right posterior sextant, facial aspect

Area 4 = right posterior sextant, lingual aspect

Area 5 = left posterior sextant, facial aspect

Area 6 = left posterior sextant, lingual aspect

DIRECTIONS: For each area, use **Column S** for student self-evaluation and **Column I** for instructor evaluation. For each skill evaluated, indicate the skill level as: **S** (satisfactory), **I** (improvement needed), or **U** (unsatisfactory).

CRITERIA:	Area 1		Area 2		Area 3		Area 4		Area 5		Area 6	
	S	I	S	I	S	I	S	I	S	I	S	I
Adjusts clinician chair correctly												
Positions patient chair correctly												
Assures that patient's head is even with top of headrest												
Positions bracket table within easy reach												
Positions unit light at arm's length												
Assumes recommended clock position												
Asks patient to adjust head position												
Adjusts patient chair so that clinician's elbows are at waist level when fingers touch teeth in treatment area												
Maintains neutral position												
Directs unit light to illuminate tx. area												

Skill Evaluations—Note to Course Instructor

The Skill Evaluation pages for all modules are designed so that these forms may be torn from the book without loss of text content. If you like, the forms may be used for evaluation and then removed for your records at completion of each module or upon completion of the course.

Skill Evaluation #2: Position, Maxillary Sextants

Student: _____

Evaluator Comments:

_____

_____

_____

_____

_____

_____

_____

_____

_____

_____

_____

_____

_____

_____

_____

_____

_____

_____

_____

Box for sketches pertaining to written comments.

3
MODULE

Instrument Grasp

In this module you will learn about the parts of a periodontal instrument and the correct grasp for holding a periodontal instrument.

Required Equipment:

You will need a dental mirror and a variety of periodontal instruments to use while learning to identify the parts of the instruments. Ask your instructor to help you find a sickle scaler, curet, periodontal explorer and probe from your instrument kit. Don't be concerned about the names of the instruments at this time; you will learn this information in another module.

Key Terms:

Handle   Working-end
Shank   Modified pen grasp

Section 1: Parts of the Periodontal Instrument

A correct instrument grasp requires precise finger placement on the instrument. In order to follow the instructions for the grasp, you must be able to identify the parts of a periodontal instrument.

Handle—the part of a periodontal instrument used for holding the instrument.

Shank—a rod-shaped length of metal located between the handle and the working-end of a dental instrument. The shank is an extension device that increases the length of the instrument so that the working-end can be positioned on the tooth root. Look closely at the instrument handle; usually you will be able to see a line or edge where the handle joins the shank. The shank is usually much smaller in diameter than the handle. The shank may be straight or it may be bent in one or more places.

Working-End—the part of a dental instrument that does the work of the instrument. The working end begins where the instrument shank ends. While the shank is circular and smooth, the working-end is shaped or flattened on some of its surfaces. The working-end may terminate in sharp point or a rounded surface. It may be thin and wire-like or look somewhat like a tiny measuring stick. In some cases, the working-end is a small mirror. An instrument may have one working-end or two working-ends.

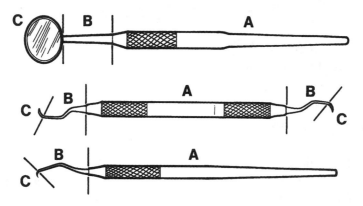

A. Handle, **B.** Shank, **C.** Working-end

Section 2: Modified Pen Grasp

Introduction to the Modified Pen Grasp

The **modified pen grasp** is the recommended grasp for holding a periodontal instrument. This grasp allows precise control of the working-end, permits a wide range of movement and facilitates good tactile conduction. **Tactile sensitivity** is the ability to detect tooth irregularities by feeling vibrations transferred from the working-end of an instrument to the shank and handle. As the working-end moves across rough tooth surfaces or deposits, it vibrates. These vibrations of the working-end cannot be seen but can be felt. The placement of the fingers in the modified pen grasp permits the clinician to feel vibrations transmitted from the working end through the instrument shank. Placing the middle finger on the instrument shank provides the most tactile information to the clinician's fingers.

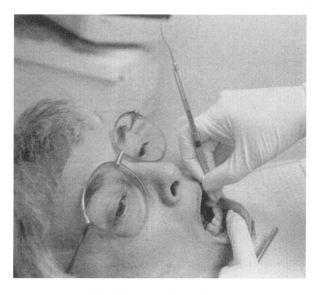

The Modified Pen Grasp

Finger Identification for the Grasp

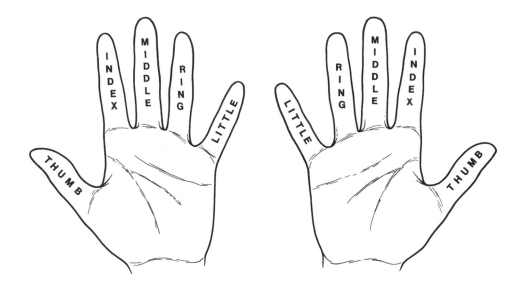

Finger Placement and Function		
Digit(s)	**Placement**	**Function**
Index and Thumb	On the instrument handle	Hold the instrument
Middle Finger	Rests lightly on the shank	Helps to guide the working-end
		Feels vibrations transmitted from the working-end to the shank
Ring Finger	On oral structure; often a tooth surface	Stabilizes the hand for control and strength
Little Finger	Near ring finger, held in a natural, relaxed manner	Has no function in the grasp

RIGHT-Handed Clinician: Modified Pen Grasp

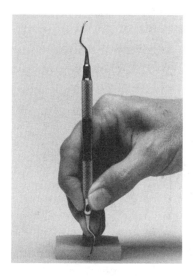

Right-handed clinician: side view

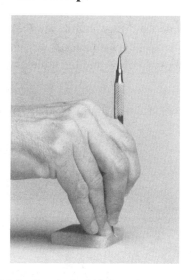

Right-handed clinician: front view

LEFT-Handed Clinician: Modified Pen Grasp

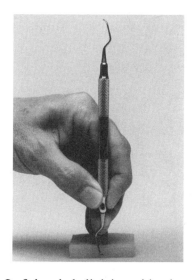

Left-handed clinician: side view

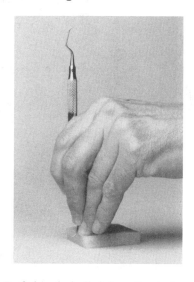

Left-handed clinician: front view

Fine-Tuning Your Grasp

Successful instrumentation technique depends to a great degree on the precise placement of each finger of your dominant hand in the modified pen grasp. Use the illustrations below and the table on page 55 to fine-tune your grasp.

Right-Handed Clinician

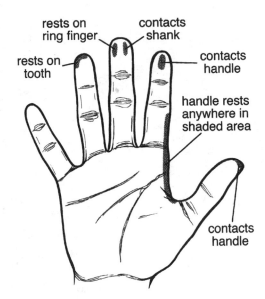

Left-Handed Clinician

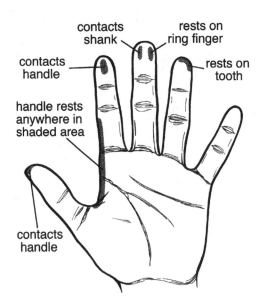

Reference Sheet: Modified Pen Grasp

Correct Finger Placement	
Digit	**Recommended Position**
Middle	One side of the finger **pad** rests *lightly* on the instrument shank (see illustration on page 54). The other side of the finger **pad** rests against (or *slightly* overlaps) the ring finger. Not used to hold the instrument. You should be able to lift your finger off of the shank without dropping the instrument. If you drop the instrument, then you are incorrectly using the middle finger to help hold the instrument.
Index and Thumb	The finger **pads** rest opposite each other at or near the junction of the handle and the shank. The fingers do not overlap; there is a tiny space between them. These fingers should hold the handle in a relaxed manner. If your fingers are blanched, you are holding too tightly. The index finger and thumb curve outward from the handle in a C-shape; this position places the finger pads on the handle in the best position for instrumentation. These fingers should not bend inward toward the handle in a U-shape. This U-shape causes the pads to lift off of the handle making it difficult to roll the instrument during instrumentation.
Ring	Fingertip, not the pad, balances *firmly* on the tooth to support the weight of the hand and instrument. When grasping the dental mirror, the rest may be on a tooth or against the patient's lip or cheek area. The finger is held straight and upright to act as a strong support beam for the hand. The finger should not feel tense, but it should not be held limply on the tooth.
Little	This finger should be held in a relaxed manner.

Section 3: Glove Use

Proper Fit

Proper glove fit is important in avoiding muscle strain during instrumentation. In fact, **surgical glove-induced injury** is a type of musculoskeletal disorder that is caused by improperly fitting gloves. Symptoms include numbness, tingling or pain in the wrist, hand, and/or fingers. This disorder is caused by wearing gloves that are too tight or by wearing ambidextrous gloves. It is best to wear right- and left-fitted gloves.

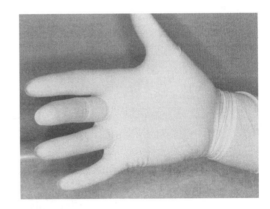

AVOID: Gloves that are tight fitting across the palm and/or wrist area of your hand can cause muscle strain during instrumentation.

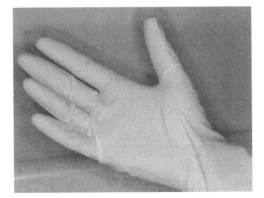

The index finger of your opposite hand should slip easily under the wrist area of the gloved hand.

Effective Glove Use Fact Sheet	
	Recommendations
Type	• Latex—the most durable; good flexibility; some individuals are allergic to latex • Nitrile—provides good dexterity and is tougher than latex • Neoprene or Polymer—much less durable than latex • Vinyl—least durable; not flexible, breaks rather than gives
Hand Care	• Maintain short fingernails to prevent punctures • During non-work hours, apply hand lotion to maintain skin integrity
Lotions	Avoid using lotions under gloves that can compromise the integrity of the glove material. Avoid petroleum-based lotions or those containing lanolin, cocoa butter, mineral oil, jojoba oil.
Jewelry	• Remove jewelry prior to donning gloves; it presents a puncture hazard • Jewelry interferes with thorough washing and rinsing of hands and increases the risk of skin irritation
Size	• Select right- and left-hand fitted gloves that come in a full range of sizes (i.e.: 5 1/2, 6, 6 1/2, etc. rather than S, M, L) • Gloves should never be tight across the palm or at the wrist
Use	• Change gloves every hour; the probability of punctures increases over time • Gloves have been on too long if hands are sweaty or skin is wrinkled • Wash and rinse hands thoroughly in-between glove changes

Section 4: Improving Muscle Strength

Well-conditioned muscles have improved control and endurance; allow for freer wrist movement; and reduce the likelihood of injury. The hand exercises shown here will help you to develop and maintain muscle strength for instrumentation.

Directions: The exercises shown here use Power Putty, a silicone rubber material that resists both squeezing and stretching forces. For each exercise illustrated, squeeze or stretch the Power Putty for the suggested number of repetitions. The exercise set, for both hands doing all 9 exercises, should take no more than 10 to 20 minutes. When exercising, maintain your hands at waist level.

> **Caution**: Not all exercise programs are suitable for everyone, discontinue any exercise that causes you discomfort and consult a medical expert. If you have or suspect that you may have a musculoskeletal injury, do not attempt these exercises without the permission of a physician. Any user assumes the risk of injury resulting from performing the exercises. The creators and authors disclaim any liabilities in connection with the exercises and advice herein.

   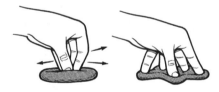

1. Full Grip (flexor muscles).
Squeeze putty with your fingers against the palm of your hand. Roll it over and around in your hand and repeat as rapidly and with as much strength as possible.
Suggested Repetitions: 10

2. All Finger Spread (extensor and abductor muscles).
Form putty into a thick pancake shape and place on a tabletop. Bunch fingertips together and place in putty. Spread fingers out as fast as possible.
Suggested Repetitions: 3

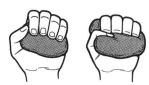

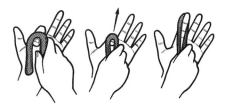

3. Fingers Dig (flexor muscles).

Place putty in the palm of your hand and dig fingertips deep into the putty. Release the fingers, roll putty over and repeat.
Suggested Repetitions: 10

4. Finger Extension (extensor muscles).

Close one finger into palm of hand. Wrap putty over tip of finger and hold loose ends with the other hand. As quickly as possible, extend finger to a fully opened position. Regulate difficulty by increasing or decreasing thickness of putty wrapped over the fingertip. Repeat with each finger.
Suggested Repetitions: 3

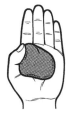

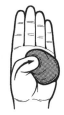

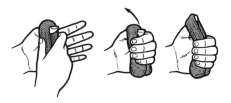

5. Thumb Press (flexor muscles).

Form putty into a barrel shape and place in the palm of your hand. Press your thumb into the putty with as much force as you can. Reform putty and repeat.
Suggested Repetitions: 5

6. Thumb Extension (extensor muscles).

Bend your thumb toward the palm of the hand; wrap putty over the thumb tip. Hold the loose ends down and extend the thumb open as quickly as possible. Regulate difficulty by increasing or decreasing the thickness of putty wrapped over tip of thumb.
Suggested Repetitions: 3

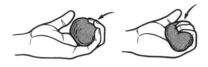

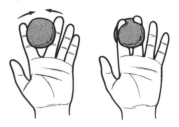

7. Fingers Only (flexor muscles).
Lay putty across fingers and squeeze with fingertips only. Keep the palm of your hand flat and open. Rotate putty with thumb and repeat.
Suggested Repetitions: 10

8. Finger Scissors (adductor muscles).
Form putty into the shape of a ball and place between any two fingers. Squeeze fingers together in scissors-like motion. Repeat with each pair of fingers.
Suggested Repetitions: 3

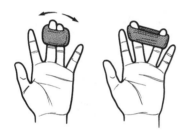

9. Finger Splits (abductor muscles).
Mold putty around any two fingers while they are closed together. Spread fingers apart as quickly as possible. Repeat exercise with each pair of fingers.
Suggested Repetitions: 3

Hand exercises are reprinted with permission of *SportsHealth*. Power Putty™ is available in four levels of rigidity: soft, soft/medium, medium/firm, and hard. Power Putty can be purchased in sport stores or directly from: *SportsHealth,* 527 West Windsor Road, Glendale, California 91204 USA, (818) 240-7170.

Skill Evaluation: Instrument Grasp

Student: _____   1 = Grasp with mirror hand

Evaluator: _____   2 = Grasp with instrument hand

Date: _____

DIRECTIONS: For each grasp, use **Column S** for student self-evaluation and **Column I** for instructor evaluation. For each grasp evaluated, indicate the skill level as: **S** (satisfactory), **I** (improvement needed), or **U** (unsatisfactory).

CRITERIA:	Grasp 1		Grasp 2	
	S	I	S	I
Identifies handle, shank, and working end(s) of mirror or instrument				
Describes the function each finger serves in the grasp				
Describes criteria for proper glove fit				
Holds handle with pad tips of index finger and thumb				
Thumb and index finger positioned opposite one another on handle				
Thumb and index finger do not touch or overlap				
Pad of middle finger rests lightly on shank				
Pad of middle finger touches the ring finger				
Thumb, index, and middle fingers are bent and relaxed (form "C" shape)				
Ring finger is straight and supports weight of hand				
Instrument handle rests against hand				
Grasp is relaxed (no blanching of fingers)				

Skill Evaluation: Instrument Grasp

Student: _____

Evaluator Comments:

_____

_____

_____

_____

_____

_____

_____

_____

_____

_____

_____

_____

_____

_____

_____

_____

Box for sketches pertaining to written comments.

4
MODULE

Mirror and Finger Rests in Anterior Sextants

This module will guide you through the use of a dental mirror and establishing finger rests in the anterior treatment areas. It begins by discussing the dental mirror and its uses. Covered next is information on recommended wrist position and hand placement during instrumentation. The third section of the module presents information on fulcrums and finger rests. The final section is a technique practice for using a mirror and finger rests in the anterior treatment sextants. When using the mirror and finger rests, you will need to apply the skills of correct positioning and instrument grasp that you practiced in previous modules.

Required Equipment:

- a dental mirror and a dental mirror handle or a periodontal probe
- a manikin and typodont and/or a fellow student
- protective attire for clinician and patient safety glasses, if applicable

Key Terms:

Indirect vision   Finger rest
Retraction   Extraoral fulcrum
Indirect illumination   Intraoral fulcrum
Transillumination   Dominant hand
Fulcrum   Non-dominant hand

Section 1: The Dental Mirror

Types of Dental Mirrors

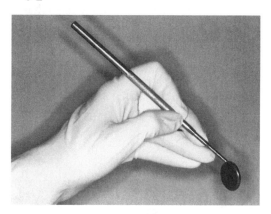

The dental mirror, or mouth mirror, is a hand instrument. The working-end has a reflecting mirrored surface used to view tooth surfaces that cannot be seen directly.

Types of Mirror Surfaces	
Type	**Characteristics**
Front Surface	Reflecting surface is on the front surface of the glass Produces a clear mirror image with no distortion Most commonly used type because of good image quality Reflecting surface of mirror is easily scratched
Concave	Reflecting surface is on the front surface of the mirror lens Produces a magnified image (image is enlarged) Not recommended because the magnification distorts the image
Plane (Flat Surface)	Reflecting surface is on the back surface of the mirror lens Produces a double image (ghost image) Not recommended because double image is distracting

Uses of the Dental Mirror

The dental mirror has the following functions during instrumentation:

1. **Indirect vision** is the use of a dental mirror to view a tooth surface or intraoral structure that cannot be seen directly.
2. **Retraction** is use of the mirror head to hold the patient's cheek or tongue so that the clinician can view tooth surfaces or other structures that are otherwise hidden from view by the cheeks or tongue. The clinician's fingers also are used for retraction, especially to retract the patient's lips.
3. **Indirect illumination** is the use of the mirror surface to reflect light onto a tooth surface in a dark area of the mouth.
4. **Transillumination** is the use of the mirror surface to reflect light through the anterior teeth [*trans* = through + *illumination* = lighting up].

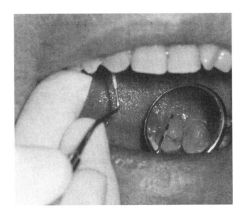

Indirect Vision. Use of a dental mirror to view the lingual surfaces of the maxillary right first premolar. Note that you can see the periodontal probe in the mirror.

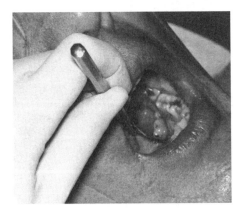

Retraction. Use of the dental mirror to retract the tongue away from the lingual surfaces of the mandibular premolars.

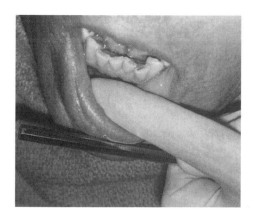

Retraction. The index finger or thumb is used to retract the lip away from the facial aspect of anterior teeth. The patient will be more comfortable if you use your finger, rather than the mirror, for retraction in anterior sextants.

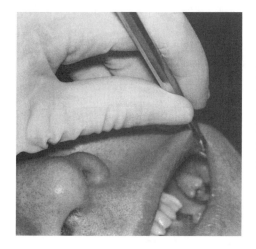

Retraction. Use of a dental mirror to retract the buccal mucosa away from the facial surfaces of the maxillary left posterior teeth. In this instance, the mirror is used both for retraction and to view the tooth surfaces indirectly.

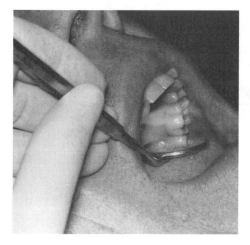

Indirect Illumination. The mirror is being used to direct additional light on the lingual surfaces of the maxillary left molars. The reflecting surface of the mirror is used to redirect light to a dark area of the mouth.

Transillumination

When transilluminating a tooth, the mirror is used to reflect light through the tooth surface. As light is reflected off the mirror surface, the light beams pass through the tooth. The transilluminated tooth almost will appear to glow. A carious lesion, hidden beneath the intact outer enamel surface, appears as a shadow when an anterior tooth is transilluminated. Transillumination is effective only with anterior teeth because they are thin enough to allow light to pass through.

The procedure for transillumination is as follows:
1. Position yourself in the 12:00 position.
2. Using a modified pen grasp, hold the mirror in your non-dominant (mirror) hand. Bring your arm up and over the patient's face. Gently rest your ring finger on the side of the patient's lip or cheek.
3. Hold the dental mirror behind the central incisors so that the reflecting surface is parallel to the lingual surfaces. Position the unit light so that the light beams shine on the dental mirror at a 90-degree angle to the mirror's reflecting surface.
4. If you have correctly positioned the light and the mirror, the central incisors will appear to "glow". Remember, in this case, you are looking directly at the teeth (the mirror is not used for indirect vision, only to reflect light back through the teeth). You probably will not see any shadows in your classmate's teeth since he or she, most likely, does not have untreated interproximal decay.

Lingual surfaces of the maxillary anterior teeth, viewed without transillumination. (From Langlais, R.P., and C.S. Miller, *Color Atlas of Common Oral Diseases*, 2nd. ed., Lippincott Williams & Wilkins, 1998, page 39.)

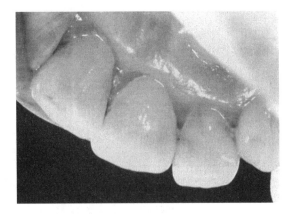

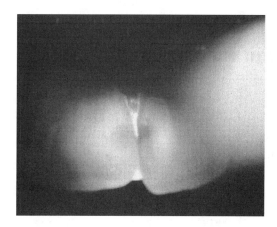

Transillumination. On the same patient, transillumination reveals interproximal decay between the central and lateral incisors. (From Langlais, R.P. and Miller, C.S.: Color Atlas of Common Oral Diseases, 2nd. ed., Lippincott Williams & Wilkins, 1998, page 39.)

Techniques With a Dental Mirror

Use direct vision whenever possible. In many instances, however, you will need to use a combination of direct and indirect vision.

Use one of the following techniques to stop fogging of the reflecting surface:
- Warm the reflecting surface against the patient's buccal mucosa,
- Ask patient to breathe through the nose,
- Wipe the reflecting surface with a commercial defogging solution.

Avoid using the mirror with the reflecting surface against the buccal mucosa. Instead, keep the reflecting surface exposed so that it is ready for use when needed for indirect vision.

Avoid hitting the mirror head against the patient's teeth or resting the outer rim of the mirror head against the patient's gingival tissues.

Section 2: Wrist Position for Instrumentation

Neutral Wrist Position

Proper wrist position during instrumentation is an important component in avoiding muscle discomfort and painful musculoskeletal injuries.

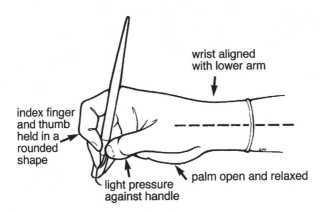

Neutral position of the wrist and fingers:
- Wrist aligned with the long axis of the lower arm.
- Little finger-side of the palm rotated slightly downward.
- Fingers held in a rounded shape, light finger pressure against handle.
- Palm open and relaxed.

OK:
Wrist aligned with the long axis of the forearm

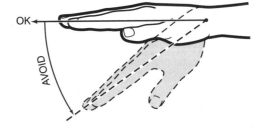

AVOID:
Bending the wrist and hand down towards the palm (flexion)

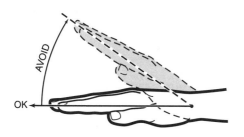

OK:
Wrist in alignment with the forearm

AVOID:
Bending the wrist and hand up and back
(extension)

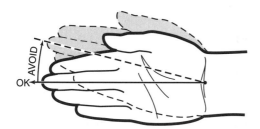

OK:
Wrist aligned with long axis of forearm

AVOID:
Bending the wrist toward the thumb
(radial deviation)

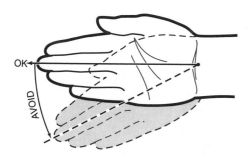

OK:
Wrist in alignment with the long axis of
the forearm

AVOID:
Bending the wrist toward the little finger
(ulnar deviation)

Section 3: The Fulcrum

The **fulcrum** stabilizes the clinician's hand during instrumentation. In periodontal instrumentation, the ring finger serves as the fulcrum finger acting as a "support beam" for the weight of the hand during instrumentation. The fulcrum, also, enables the hand and instrument to move as a unit as instrumentation strokes are made against the tooth. Without a fulcrum, the clinician would not be able to control the movement of the working-end. The fulcrum allows the clinician to make precise instrumentation strokes in an exacting manner against the tooth surface. There are two basic types of fulcrums: extraoral fulcrums and intraoral fulcrums.

An **intraoral fulcrum** is a stabilizing point inside the patient's mouth against a tooth surface. The basic intraoral fulcrum uses a finger rest on a tooth surface. A **finger rest** is the place where fulcrum finger rests and pushes against during instrumentation. Intraoral fulcrums also are used with advanced instrumentation techniques. The basic intraoral fulcrum has the following characteristics:

- It is positioned on the same arch as the tooth being instrumented (worked on)
- It rests on the (1) incisal or occlusal surface or (2) the occlusofacial or occlusolingual line angle of a stable tooth near the tooth being instrumented

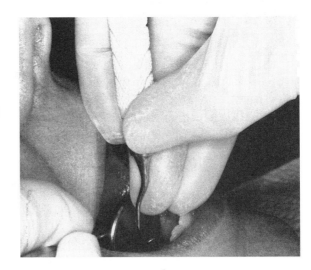

Intraoral Fulcrum. This clinician is using an intraoral fulcrum to stabilize the periodontal instrument in the mouth.

Summary Sheet: Basic Intraoral Fulcrum	
	Technique
Grasp	Hold the instrument in a modified pen grasp.
Fulcrum	Keep ring finger straight, with the tip of the finger supporting the weight of the hand.
Finger rest	Place the finger rest on the same arch as the tooth being instrumented.
Location	Position the finger rest near the tooth being instrumented. Depending on the tooth being instrumented and the size of your hand, the finger rest may be 1 to 4 teeth away from the tooth on which you are working.
Surface	Rest the fingertip of the fulcrum finger on an incisal (or occlusal) surface or on the occlusofacial or occlusolingual line angle of a tooth. The teeth are saliva-covered, so you will be more likely to slip if you establish a finger rest on the facial or lingual surface. Avoid resting on a mobile tooth or one with a large carious lesion.

An **extraoral fulcrum** is a stabilizing point outside the patient's mouth (for example, against the patient's chin or cheek). An extraoral fulcrum may be used to stabilize the dental mirror in the patient's mouth.

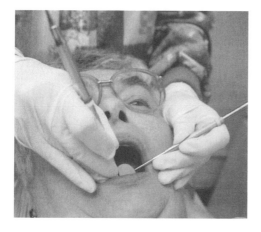

Extraoral Fulcrum. The clinician is using an extraoral fulcrum on the patient's cheek to stabilize the dental mirror in the mouth.

Fulcrum Characteristics
• Provides stable support for the hand. • Enables the hand and instrument to move as a unit. • Facilitates precise stroke pressure against the tooth surface. • Decreases the likelihood of injury to the patient or clinician if the patient moves unexpectedly during instrumentation.

Directions for Technique Practice (Sections 4 and 5)

1. The photographs in Section 4 and 5 depict the use of a dental mirror and finger rests in the anterior treatment areas.
   - Some photographs were taken on a patient.
   - Others were taken using a manikin and without gloves so that you can easily see the finger placement in the grasp.
2. The focus of your attention should be on mastering mirror use, wrist position, and the finger rests for anterior sextants. Do not use an instrument with a cutting edge because the sharp working end will distract your attention from these skills. Use the following instruments in this module:
   For your non-dominant (mirror) hand—Use a dental mirror.
   For your dominant (instrument) hand—(a) Remove the mirror head from one of your dental mirrors and use the mirror handle as if it were a periodontal instrument or (b) use a periodontal probe to represent the periodontal instrument in this module.
3. If possible divide your practice time between working on a dental manikin and with a classmate. These two forms of practice both offer certain advantages.
   Manikin practice: Without gloves you can monitor the pressure of your grasp; if your fingers blanch, you are grasping the instrument too tightly.
   Classmate practice: Provides practice in establishing finger rests on slippery tooth surfaces.
4. The photographs will provide a *general guideline* for the intraoral finger rests, however, the location of your own finger rest depends on the size and length of your fingers. You may need to fulcrum closer to or farther from the tooth being treated than is shown in the photograph.

Step-by-Step Approach to Technique Practice Sessions

Your practice will progress better if you do each task in a step-by-step manner:
1. Establish your clock position.
2. Establish the patient head position.
3. Grasp the mirror in your non-dominant hand.
4. Establish a finger rest with your mirror hand.
5. Grasp the instrument in your dominant hand.
6. Establish a finger rest with your instrument hand.

Icon Symbol Key

Icons will appear throughout the book to assist you with identifying the treatment area and in positioning yourself, the patient, and the instrument handle. The four types of icon symbols are sextant icons, clock position icons, patient head position icons, and handle placement icons.

Technique Icons	
Sextant Icon	Clock Position Icon
Patient Head Position Icon	Handle Placement Icon

Key: Patient Head Position Icons		
RIGHT-Handed Icons	**Description**	**LEFT-Handed Icons**
	Chin down, turned toward clinician	
	Chin down, head slightly toward clinician	
	Chin down, slightly away from clinician	
	Chin up, turned toward clinician	
	Chin up, head slightly toward clinician	
	Chin up, slightly away from clinician	

Sections 4 and 5 of this Module are divided into **RIGHT-Handed clinician** and **LEFT-Handed clinician** sections. The RIGHT-Handed section begins on the next page. LEFT-Handed clinicians should turn to **page 96**.

Section 4: Skills for RIGHT-Handed Clinician

Handle Position for Mandibular Anteriors

For instrumentation of the mandibular arch, the hand is held in a palm down position and the handle extends upward.

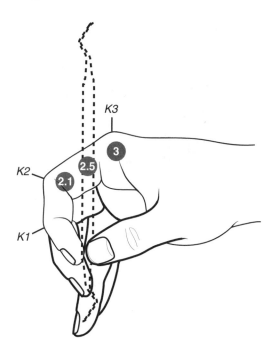

The anatomic landmarks for handle placement when working on the mandibular anteriors are the:

- first knuckle (K1)
- second knuckle (K2)
- third knuckle (K3)

Summary Table: Handle Placement for Mandibular Anteriors
2.1 (area on index finger just past knuckle 2)
2.5 (area halfway between knuckle 2 and 3)

Technique Practice: Mandibular Anterior Teeth

Mandibular Anterior Sextant, Facial Aspect: Surfaces Toward

Position Overview

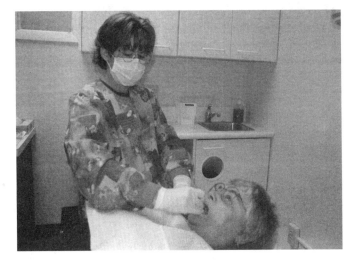

Retraction

Retract the lip with your
finger or thumb.

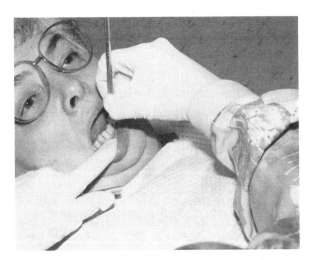

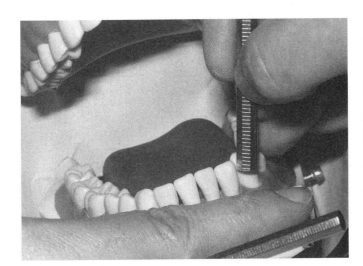

Task 1—mesial surface of the left canine

Finger rest on an occlusofacial line angle.

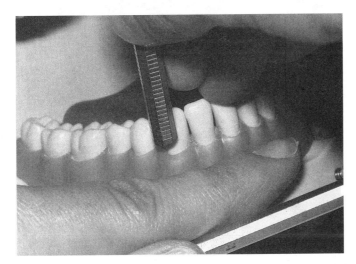

Task 2—distal surface of right canine

Finger rest on an incisal edge.

Mandibular Anterior Sextant, Lingual Aspect: Surfaces Toward

Position Overview

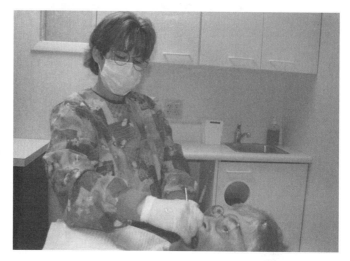

Mirror

Use the mirror head to push the tongue away gently so the lingual surfaces of the anterior teeth can be seen.

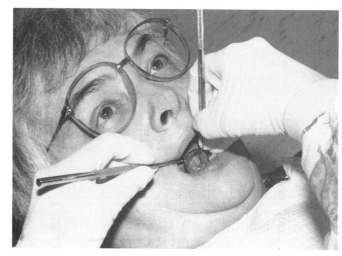

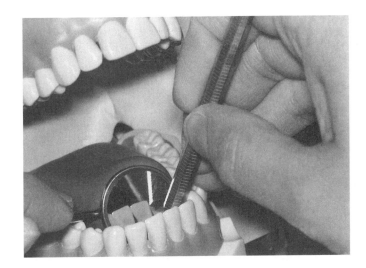

Task 1—mesial surface of the left canine

Finger rest on an occlusofacial line angle.

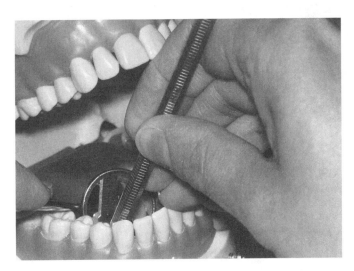

Task 2—distal surface of right canine

Finger rest on an incisal edge.

Mandibular Anterior Sextant, Facial Aspect: Surfaces Away

Position Overview

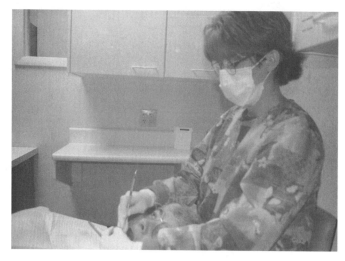

Retraction

Retract the lip with your finger or thumb.

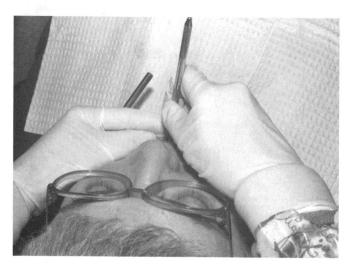

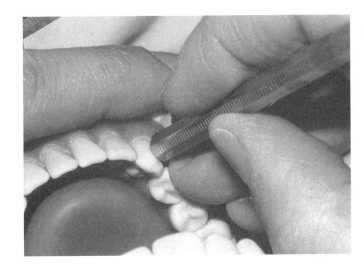

Task 1—mesial surface of the right canine

Finger rest on an occlusofacial line angle.

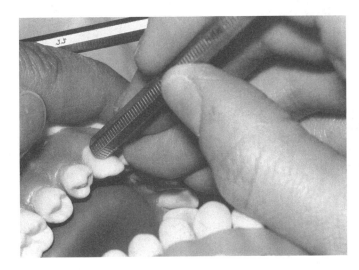

Task 2—distal surface of the left canine

Finger rest on an incisal edge.

Mandibular Anterior Sextant, Lingual Aspect: Surfaces Away

Position Overview

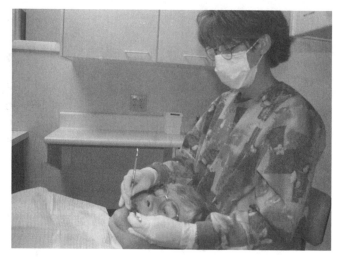

Mirror

Use the mirror head to push the tongue back gently so that the lingual surfaces of the teeth can be seen.

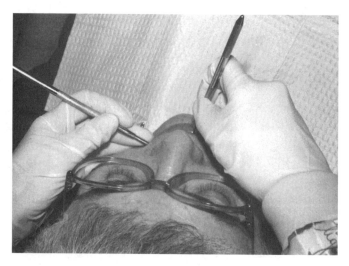

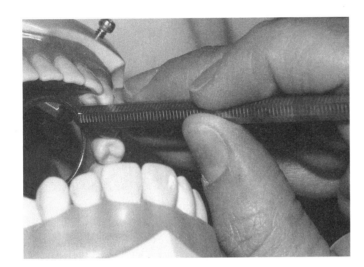

Task 1—mesial surface of the right canine

Finger rest on an occlusofacial line angle.

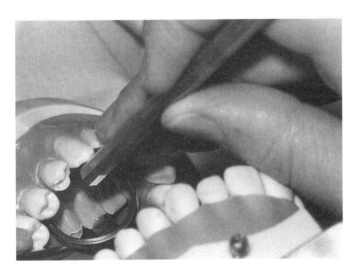

Task 2—distal surface of the left canine

Finger rest on an incisal edge.

Handle Position for Maxillary Anteriors

For instrumentation of the maxillary arch, the hand is held in a palm-up position and the handle extends down.

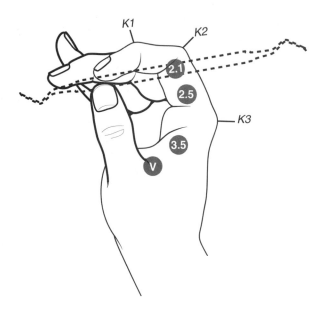

The anatomic landmarks for handle placement when working on the maxillary anteriors are the:

- first knuckle (K1)
- second knuckle (K2)
- third knuckle (K3)
- "V" of the hand (V)

Summary Table: Handle Placement for Maxillary Anteriors
2.1 (area on index finger just past knuckle 2)
2.5 (area halfway between knuckle 2 and 3)
V (area between the base of the index finger and the thumb)

Technique Practice: Maxillary Anterior Teeth

Maxillary Anterior Sextant, Facial Aspect: Surfaces Toward

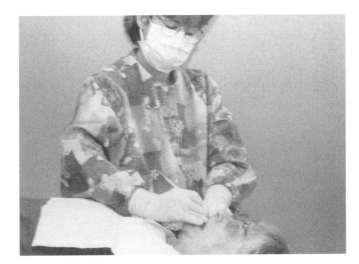

Position Overview

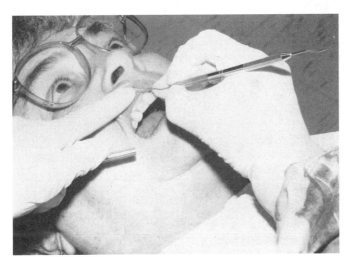

Retraction

Retract the lip with your finger or thumb.

Task 1—mesial surface of the left canine

Finger rest on an occlusofacial line angle.

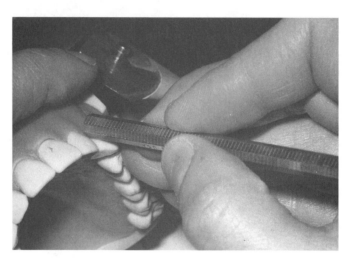

Task 2—distal surface of right canine

Finger rest on an incisal edge.

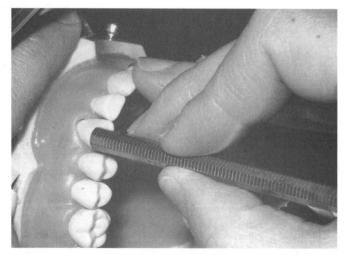

Maxillary Anterior Sextant, Lingual Aspect: Surfaces Toward

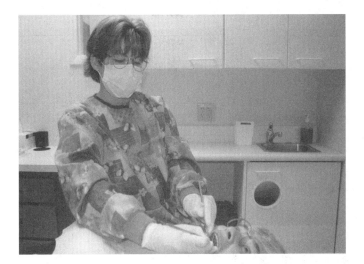

Position Overview

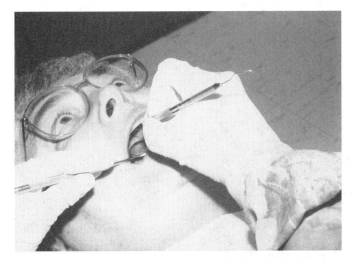

Mirror

Position the mirror so that the lingual surfaces of the anterior teeth can be seen.

Task 1—mesial surface of the left canine

Finger rest on an occlusofacial line angle.

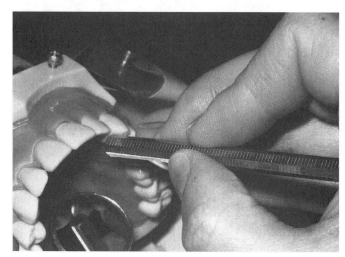

Task 2—distal surface of right canine

Finger rest on an incisal edge.

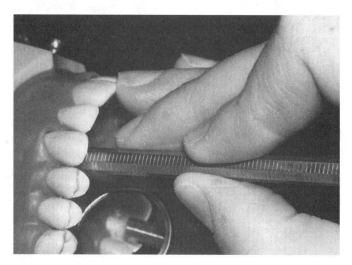

Maxillary Anterior Sextant, Facial Aspect: Surfaces Away

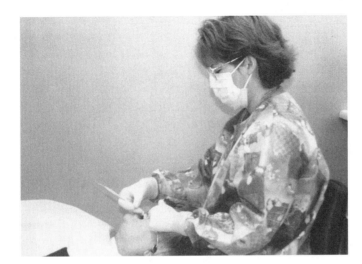

Position Overview

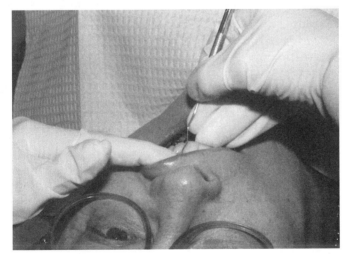

Retraction

Retract the lip with your finger or thumb.

**Task 1—mesial surface
of the right canine**

Finger rest on an occlusal
surface.

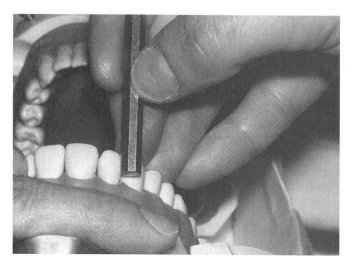

**Task 2—distal surface
of left canine**

Finger rest on an incisal
edge.

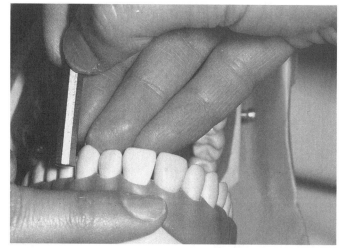

Maxillary Anterior Sextant, Lingual Aspect: Surfaces Away

Position Overview

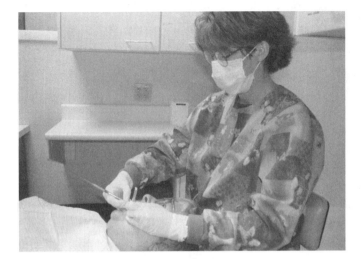

Mirror

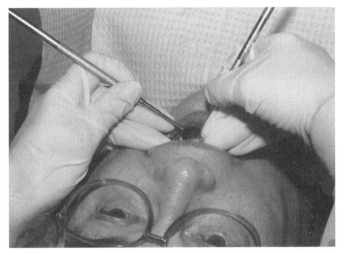

Position the mirror so that the lingual surfaces of the anterior teeth can be seen.

Task 1—mesial surface of the right canine

Finger rest on an occlusal line angle.

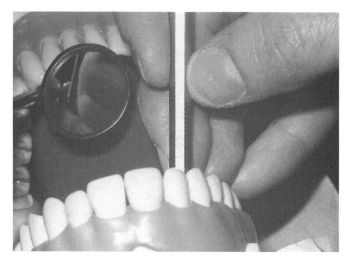

Task 2—distal surface of the left canine

Finger rest on an incisal edge.

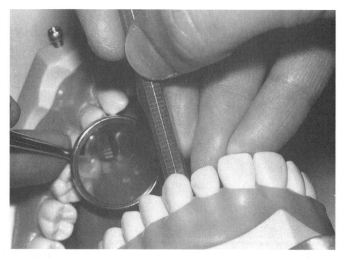

Reference Sheet: Anterior Sextants (RIGHT-Handed Clinician)

Photocopy this page and use it for quick reference as you practice your skills. Place the photocopied reference sheet in a plastic page protector for longer use.

Mandibular Anterior Treatment Areas			
Sextant	Clock Position	Patient's Head	Handle
Facial surfaces toward	8—9:00	Slightly toward chin-down	2.5
Lingual surfaces toward	8—9:00	Slightly toward chin-down	2.5
Facial surfaces away	12:00	Slightly toward chin-down	2.1
Lingual surfaces away	12:00	Slightly toward chin-down	2.1
Maxillary Anterior Treatment Areas			
Sextant	Clock Position	Patient's Head	Handle
Facial surfaces toward	8—9:00	Slightly toward chin-up	V
Lingual surfaces toward	8—9:00	Slightly toward chin-up	V
Facial surfaces away	12:00	Slightly toward chin-up	2.1
Lingual surfaces away	12:00	Slightly toward chin-up	2.1

Note: This ends the section for RIGHT-Handed Clinicians. Turn to **page 115** for the Skill Evaluation.

Section 5: Skills for LEFT-Handed Clinician

Handle Position for Mandibular Anteriors

For instrumentation of the mandibular arch, the hand is held in a palm down position and the handle extends upward.

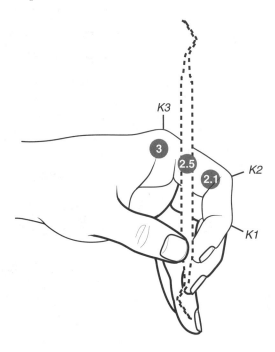

The anatomic landmarks for handle placement when working on the mandibular anteriors are the:
- first knuckle (K1)
- second knuckle (K2)
- third knuckle (K3)

Summary Table: Handle Placement for Mandibular Anteriors
2.1 (area on index finger just past knuckle 2)
2.5 (area halfway between knuckle 2 and 3)

Technique Practice: Mandibular Anterior Teeth

Mandibular Anterior Sextant, Facial Aspect: Surfaces Toward

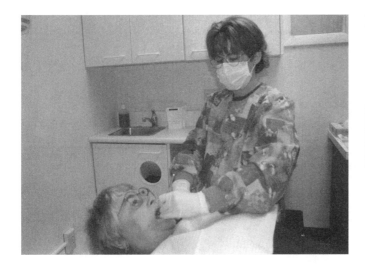

Position Overview

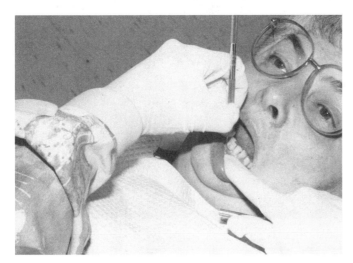

Retraction

Retract the lip with your finger or thumb.

Task 1—mesial surface of the right canine

Finger rest on an occlusofacial line angle.

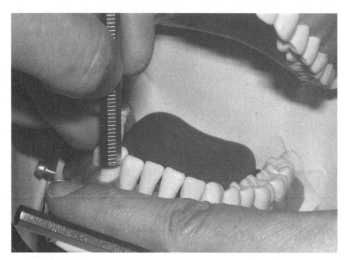

Task 2—distal surface of left canine

Finger rest on an incisal edge.

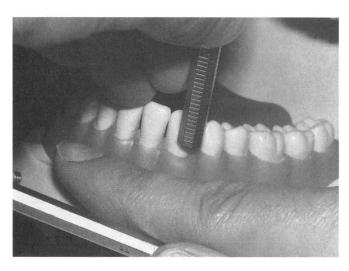

Mandibular Anterior Sextant, Lingual Aspect: Surfaces Toward

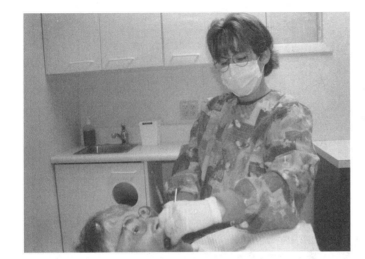

Position Overview

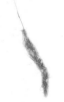

Mirror

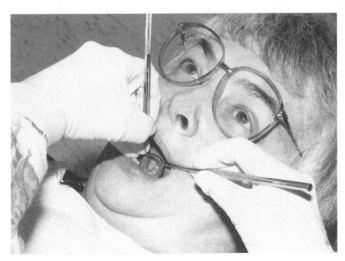

Use the mirror head to push the tongue away gently so the lingual surfaces of the anterior teeth can be seen.

Task 1—mesial surface of the right canine

Finger rest on an occlusofacial line angle.

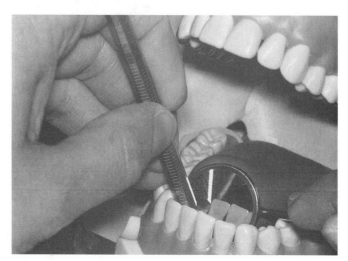

Task 2—distal surface of left canine

Finger rest on an incisal edge.

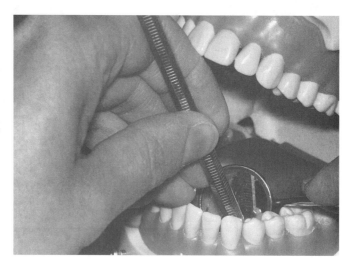

Mandibular Anterior Sextant, Facial Aspect: Surfaces Away

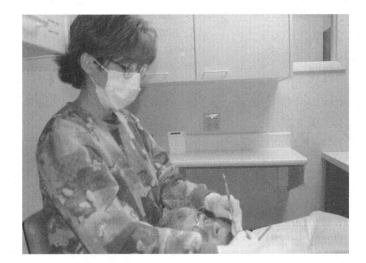

Position Overview

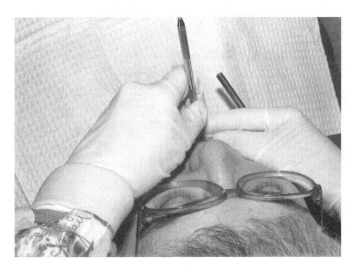

Retraction

Retract the lip with your finger or thumb.

Task 1—mesial surface of the left canine

Finger rest on an occlusofacial line angle.

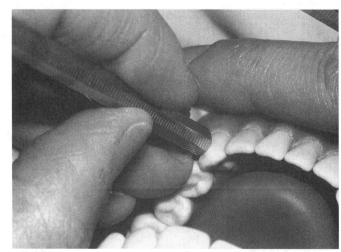

Task 2—distal surface of the right canine

Finger rest on an incisal edge.

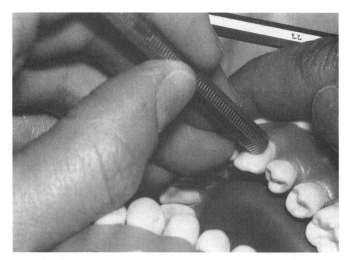

Mandibular Anterior Sextant, Lingual Aspect: Surfaces Away

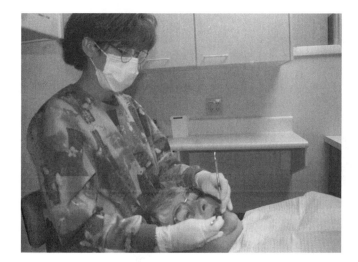

Position Overview

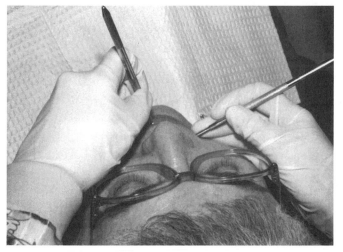

Mirror

Use the mirror head to push the tongue back gently so that the lingual surfaces of the teeth can be seen.

Task 1—mesial surface of the left canine

Finger rest on an occlusofacial line angle.

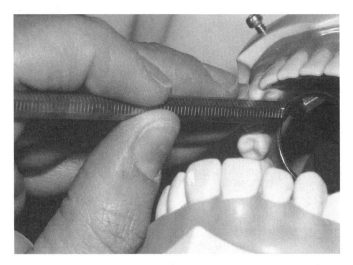

Task 2—distal surface of the right canine

Finger rest on an incisal edge.

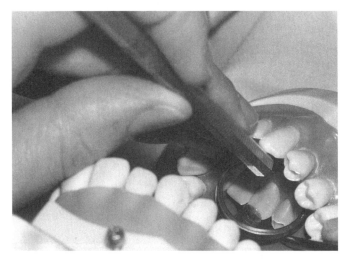

Handle Position for Maxillary Anteriors

For instrumentation of the maxillary arch, the hand is held in a palm-up position and the handle extends down.

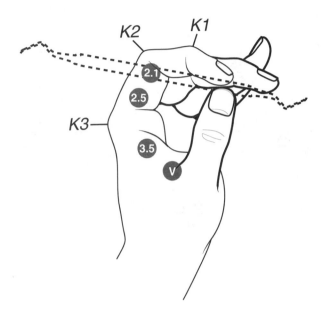

The anatomic landmarks for handle placement when working on the maxillary anteriors are the:
- first knuckle (K1)
- second knuckle (K2)
- third knuckle (K3)
- "V" of the hand (V)

Summary Table: Handle Placement for Maxillary Anteriors
2.1 (area on index finger just past knuckle 2)
2.5 (area halfway between knuckle 2 and 3)
V (area between the base of the index finger and the thumb)

Technique Practice: Maxillary Anterior Teeth

Maxillary Anterior Sextant, Facial Aspect: Surfaces Toward

Position Overview

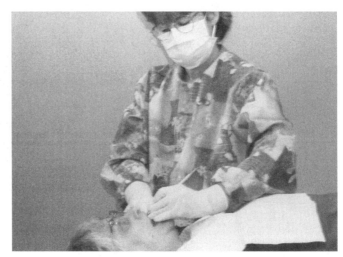

Retraction

Retract the lip with your finger or thumb.

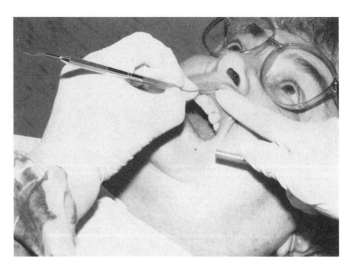

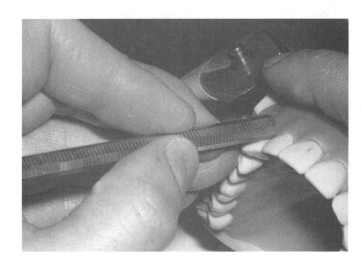

Task 1—mesial surface of the right canine

Finger rest on an occlusofacial line angle.

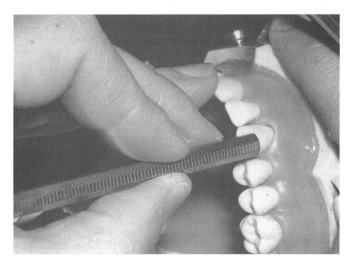

Task 2—distal surface of left canine

Finger rest on an incisal edge.

Maxillary Anterior Sextant, Lingual Aspect: Surfaces Toward

Position Overview

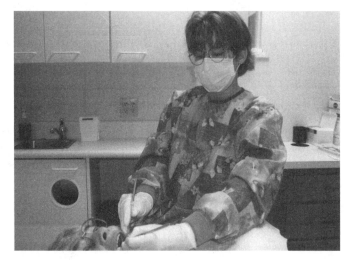

Mirror

Position the mirror so that the lingual surfaces of the anterior teeth can be seen.

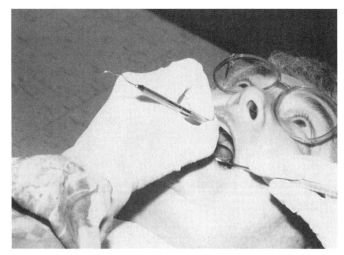

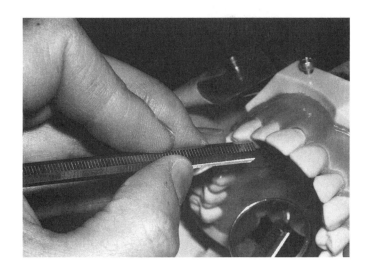

Task 1—mesial surface of the right canine

Finger rest on an occlusofacial line angle.

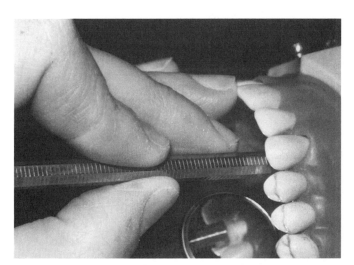

Task 2—distal surface of left canine

Finger rest on an incisal edge.

Maxillary Anterior Sextant, Facial Aspect: Surfaces Away

Position Overview

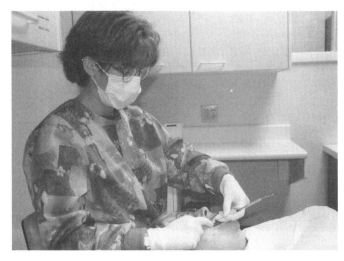

Retraction

Retract the lip with your finger or thumb.

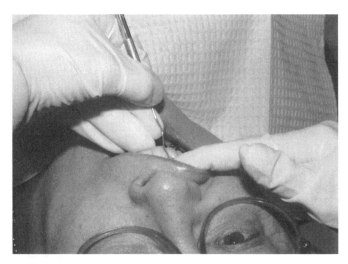

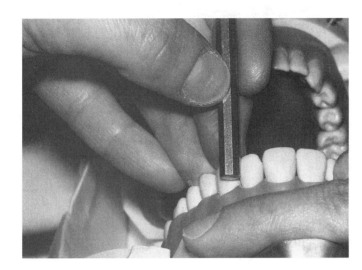

Task 1—mesial surface of the left canine

Finger rest on an occlusal surface.

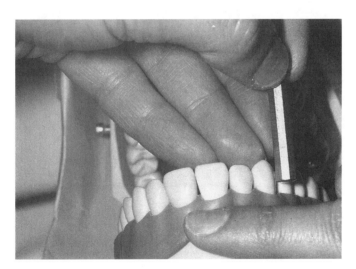

Task 2—distal surface of the right canine

Finger rest on an incisal edge.

Maxillary Anterior Sextant, Lingual Aspect: Surfaces Away

Position Overview

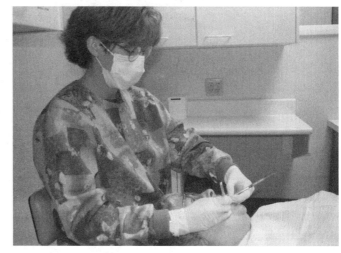

Mirror

Position the mirror so that the lingual surfaces of the anterior teeth can be seen.

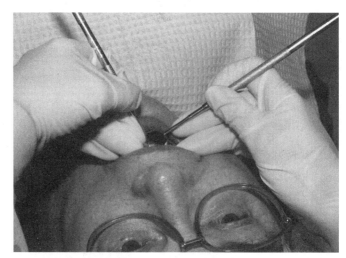

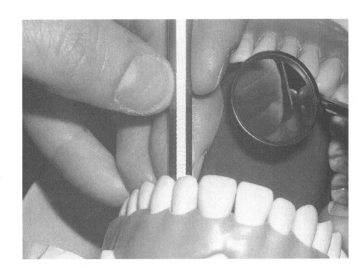

Task 1—mesial surface of the left canine

Finger rest on an occlusal line angle.

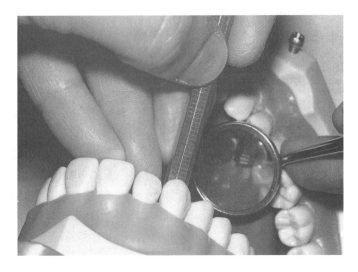

Task 2—distal surface of the right canine

Finger rest on an incisal edge.

Reference Sheet: Anterior Sextants (LEFT-Handed Clinician)

Photocopy this page and use it for quick reference as you practice your skills. Place the photocopied reference sheet in a plastic page protector for longer use.

Mandibular Anterior Treatment Areas			
Sextant	**Clock Position**	**Patient's Head**	**Handle**
Facial surfaces toward	4:00—3:00	Slightly toward chin-down	2.5
Lingual surfaces toward	4:00—3:00	Slightly toward chin-down	2.5
Facial surfaces away	12:00	Slightly toward chin-down	2.1
Lingual surfaces away	12:00	Slightly toward chin-down	2.1
Maxillary Anterior Treatment Areas			
Sextant	**Clock Position**	**Patient's Head**	**Handle**
Facial surfaces toward	4:00—3:00	Slightly toward chin-up	V
Lingual surfaces toward	4:00—3:00	Slightly toward chin-up	V
Facial surfaces away	12:00	Slightly toward chin-up	2.1
Lingual surfaces away	12:00	Slightly toward chin-up	2.1

Note to Course Instructor

One excellent source of periodontal typodonts is Kilgore International, Inc. (800) 892-9999. They have a dental hygiene typodont with flexible gingiva and synthetic calculus, as well, as a variety of other periodontal typodonts with flexible gingiva.

Skill Evaluation: Mirror and Finger Rests in Anterior Sextants

Student: _____ Area 1 = mandibular anteriors, facial aspect

Evaluator: _____ Area 2 = mandibular anteriors, lingual aspect

Date: _____ Area 3 = maxillary anteriors, facial aspect

Area 4 = maxillary anteriors, lingual aspect

DIRECTIONS: For each area, use **Column S** for student self-evaluation and **Column I** for instructor evaluation. For each skill evaluated, indicate the skill level as: **S** (satisfactory), **I** (improvement needed), or **U** (unsatisfactory).

CRITERIA:	Area 1 S	Area 1 I	Area 2 S	Area 2 I	Area 3 S	Area 3 I	Area 4 S	Area 4 I
Position: Positioned correctly on clinician stool								
Positioned correctly in relation to patient, dental equipment, and treatment area								
Uses correct patient head position								
Dental Mirror: States four uses of the dental mirror								
Uses correct grasp with mirror								
Establishes secure rest with mirror								
Assures patient comfort by not hitting teeth or resting the rim of mirror head against gingiva								
Demonstrates use of mirror for indirect vision, indirect illumination, and retraction								
Instrument Grasp: Uses all criteria for correct grasp								
Basic Intraoral Fulcrum: Balances hand on tip of ring finger								
Holds ring finger straight to act as a "support beam" for hand								
Fulcrums on same arch, near tooth being instrumented								

Skill Evaluation: Mirror and Finger Rests in Anterior Sextants

Student: _____

Evaluator Comments:

_____

_____

_____

_____

_____

_____

_____

_____

_____

_____

_____

_____

_____

_____

_____

_____

_____

Box for sketches pertaining to written comments.

Mirror and Finger Rests in Mandibular Posterior Sextants

This module will guide you through the use of a dental mirror and establishing finger rests in the mandibular posterior sextants.

Required Equipment:

- a dental mirror and a dental mirror handle or a periodontal probe
- a manikin and typodont and/or a classmate
- protective attire for clinician and patient safety glasses, if applicable

Section 1: Technique Practice with Mirror

Directions: Retracting the buccal mucosa away from the facial surfaces of the posterior teeth can be a challenging task, especially if your patient tenses his or her cheek muscles. It is a good idea to practice this technique first before attempting the technique practice section for posterior finger rests. Follow the steps listed below to practice this important technique.

Technique Practice: Retracting the Cheek

Practice viewing the facial aspect of mandibular posterior teeth.

1. *RIGHT-Handed clinicians*: View mandibular left posteriors, facial aspect. Sit in the 11:00 position.
   LEFT-Handed clinicians: View mandibular right posteriors, facial aspect. Sit in the 1:00 position.

2. Grasp the dental mirror in your non-dominant hand.

3. Place the mirror head between the dental arches with the reflecting surface parallel to the occlusal surfaces of the maxillary teeth ("Frisbee position").

4. Slide the mirror back until it is in line with the second molar.

5. Roll the mirror handle between your fingers until the mirror head is parallel to the buccal mucosa (back of mirror head is against the buccal mucosa).

6. Gently retract the buccal mucosa down and out from the teeth.

7. Establish a finger rest on the side of the patient's cheek.

8. Use your arm muscles for retraction. Trying to pull with only your finger muscles is a difficult and tiring way to retract the cheek.

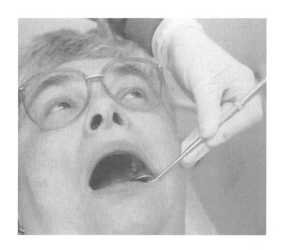

Insert mirror with the reflecting surface parallel to the maxillary occlusal surfaces ("Frisbee-style"). The photographs show a RIGHT-Handed clinician.

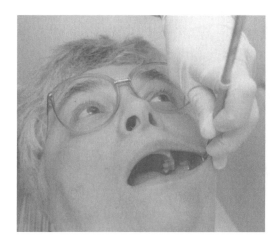

Position mirror for retraction by turning the mirror handle until the mirror head is parallel to the buccal mucosa.

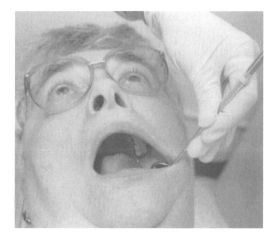

Do NOT use the instrument shank for retraction. Retracting in this manner will be uncomfortable for your patient.

When practicing finger rests, it is extremely helpful to do each task in a step-by-step manner.

Reference Sheet: Sequence for Establishing a Fulcrum

Establish the clock position

↓

Establish patient head position

↓

Grasp mirror and establish finger rest

↓

Grasp instrument
Pause and do self-check of finger placement in grasp

↓

Establish a finger rest near the tooth being instrumented

↓

Pause and do self-check of your finger rest
- Is the tip of the ring finger on a secure tooth surface?
- Is ring finger straight, acting as a support beam for hand?
- Is each finger still in the recommended position for grasp?

↓

Position the instrument handle so that it is as vertical as possible.
(It will NOT be possible to hold the handle in a true
vertical position because of the maxillary arch.)

Section 2: Skills for RIGHT-Handed Clinician

Handle Placement in Grasp: Mandibular Posteriors

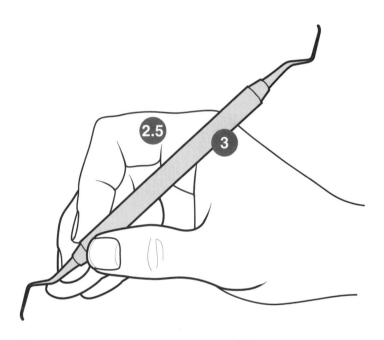

Summary Table: Handle Placement for Mandibular Posterior Teeth	
Area:	**Handle Position:**
Left posteriors, lingual aspect	at or close to 3
Right posteriors, facial aspect	at or close to 3
Left posteriors, facial aspect	at or close to 3
Right posteriors, lingual aspect	at or close to 3

Technique Practice: Mandibular Posterior Sextants

Mandibular Right Posterior Sextant, Facial
Aspect: Posterior Aspect, Toward

Position Overview

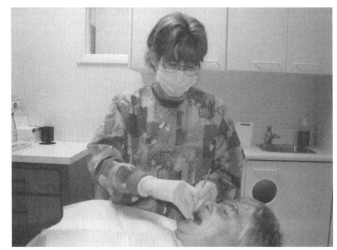

Retraction

Retract the buccal mucosa with the mirror. Use the mirror for indirect vision, particularly to view the distal surfaces in this aspect.

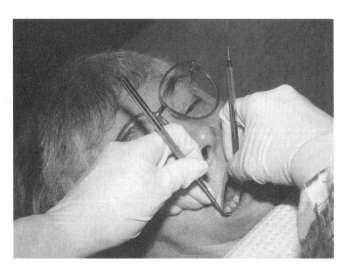

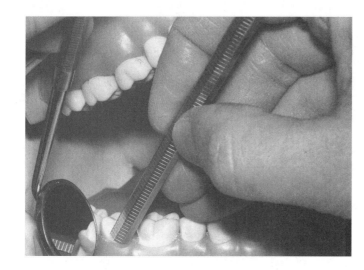

Task 1—second molar, facial aspect

Finger rest on an occlusal surface.

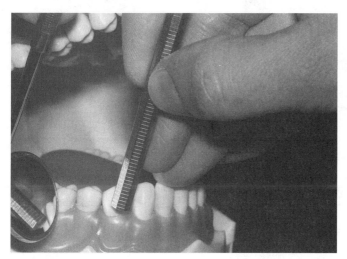

Task 2—first premolar, facial aspect

Finger rest on an incisal surface of one of the mandibular anteriors.

Mandibular Left Posterior Sextant, Lingual Aspect: Posterior Aspect, Toward

Position Overview

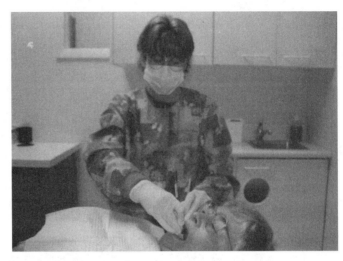

Mirror

Use mirror to gently pull the tongue away from the teeth, toward the midline of the mouth.

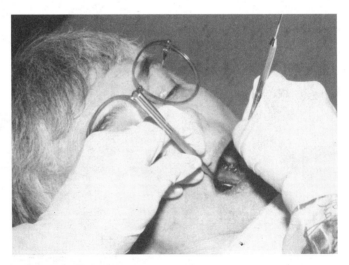

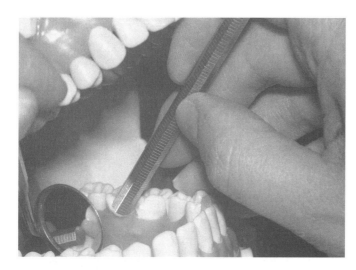

Task 1—second molar, lingual aspect

Finger rest on an occlusofacial line angle.

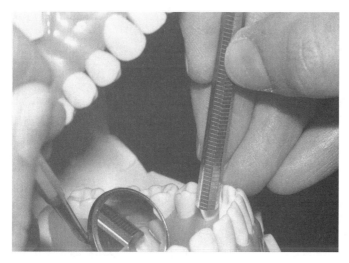

Task 2—first premolar, lingual aspect

Finger rest on an incisal edge of one of the mandibular anterior teeth.

Mandibular Left Posterior Sextant, Facial Aspect: Posterior Aspect, Away

Position Overview

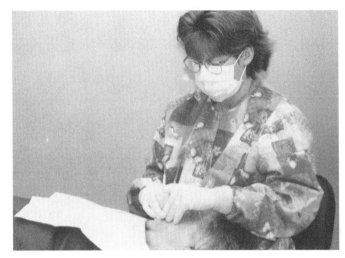

Retraction

Use the mirror to retract the buccal mucosa down and away from the teeth.

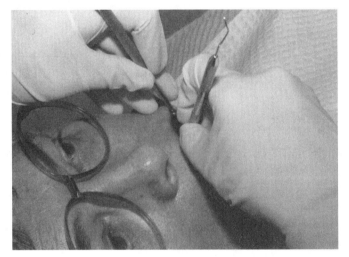

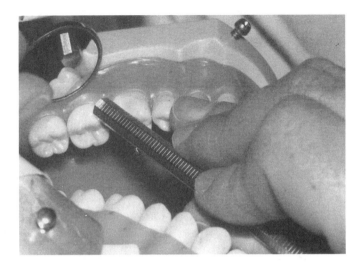

Task 1—second molar, facial aspect

Finger rest on an occlusofacial line angle.

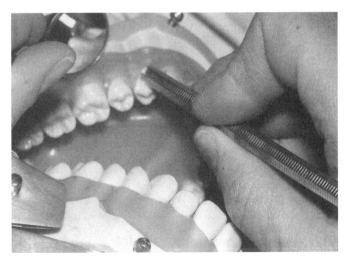

Task 2—first premolar, facial aspect

Finger rest on an incisal edge of an anterior tooth.

Mandibular Right Posterior Sextant, Lingual Aspect: Posterior Aspect, Away

Position Overview

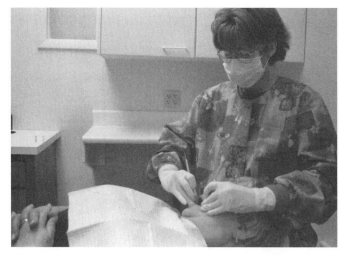

Mirror

Use the mirror head to push the tongue back gently so that the lingual surfaces of the teeth can be seen.

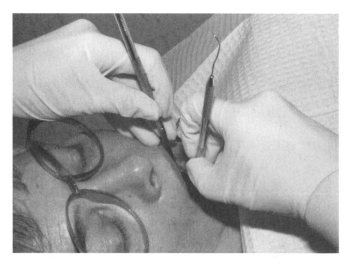

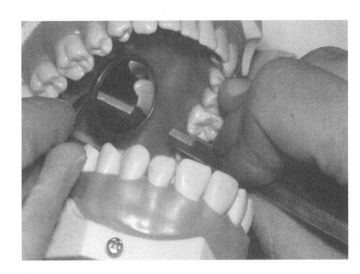

Task 1—second molar, lingual aspect

Finger rest on an occlusal surface.

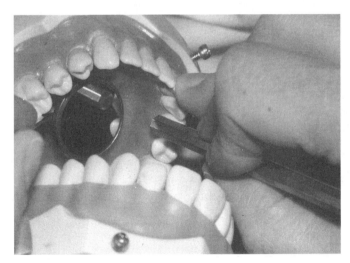

Task 2—first premolar, lingual aspect

Finger rest on an incisal edge of an anterior tooth.

Reference Sheet: RIGHT-Handed Clinician

Photocopy this page and use it for quick reference as you practice your skills. Place the photocopied reference sheet in a plastic page protector for longer use.

Mandibular Posterior Treatment Areas			
Sextant	**Clock Position**	**Patient's Head**	**Handle**
Right posterior, facial aspect (aspect toward)	9:00	Straight or slightly away chin-down	at or close to 3
Left posterior, lingual aspect (aspect toward)	9:00	Slightly away chin-down	at or close to 3
Right posterior, lingual aspect (aspect away)	10 – 11:00	Toward chin-down	at or close to 3
Left posterior, facial aspect (aspect away)	10 – 11:00	Toward chin-down	at or close to 3

Note: This ends the Section for RIGHT-Handed Clinicians. Turn to **page 141** for the Skill Evaluation.

Section 3: Skills for LEFT-Handed Clinician

Handle Placement in Grasp: Mandibular Posteriors

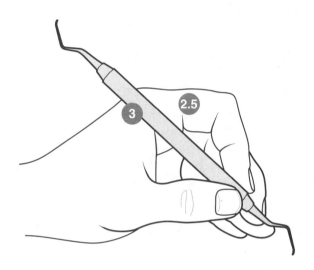

Summary Table: Handle Placement for Mandibular Posterior Teeth	
Area:	**Handle Position:**
Left posteriors, facial aspect	at or close to 3
Right posteriors, lingual aspect	at or close to 3
Left posteriors, lingual aspect	at or close to 3
Right posteriors, facial aspect	at or close to 3

Technique Practice: Mandibular Posterior Sextants

Mandibular Left Posterior Sextant, Facial Aspect: Posterior Aspect, Toward

Position Overview

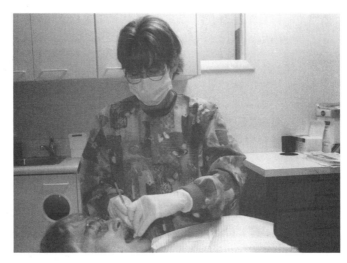

Retraction

Retract the buccal mucosa with the mirror. Use the mirror for indirect vision, particularly to view the distal surfaces in this aspect.

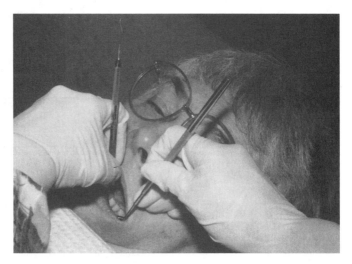

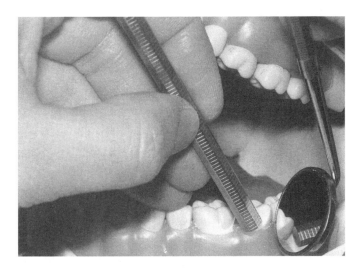

Task 1—second molar, facial aspect

Finger rest on an occlusal surface.

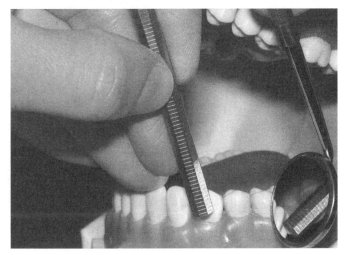

Task 2—first premolar, facial aspect

Finger rest on an incisal surface of one of the mandibular anteriors.

Mandibular Right Posterior Sextant, Lingual Aspect: Posterior Aspect, Toward

Position Overview

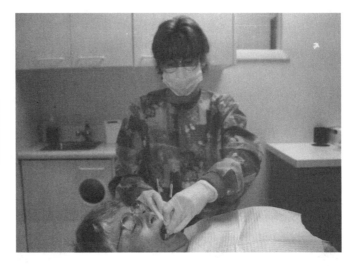

Mirror

Use mirror to gently pull the tongue away from the teeth, toward the midline of the mouth.

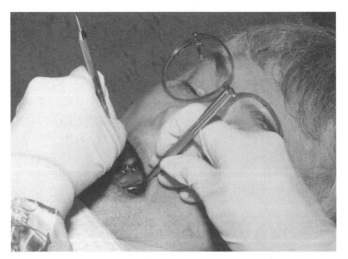

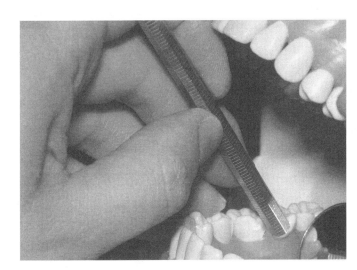

Task 1—second molar, lingual aspect

Finger rest on an occlusofacial line angle.

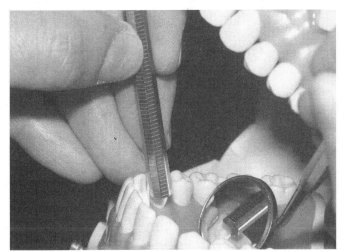

Task 2—first premolar, lingual aspect

Finger rest on an incisal edge of one of the mandibular anterior teeth.

Mandibular Right Posterior Sextant, Facial Aspect: Posterior Aspect, Away

Position Overview

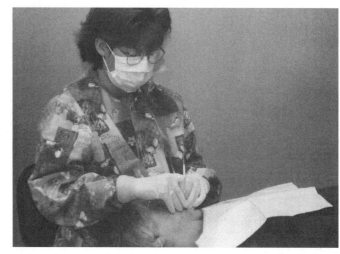

Retraction

Use the mirror to retract the buccal mucosa down and away from the teeth.

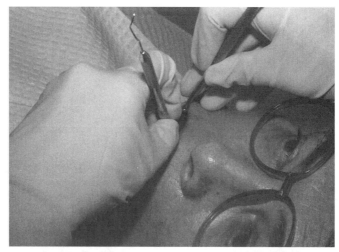

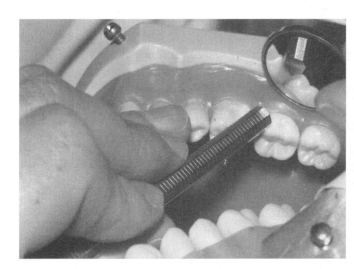

Task 1—second molar, facial aspect

Finger rest on an occlusofacial line angle.

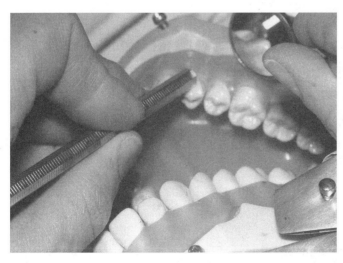

Task 2—first premolar, facial aspect

Finger rest on an incisal edge of an anterior tooth.

Mandibular Left Posterior Sextant, Lingual Aspect: Posterior Aspect, Away

Position Overview

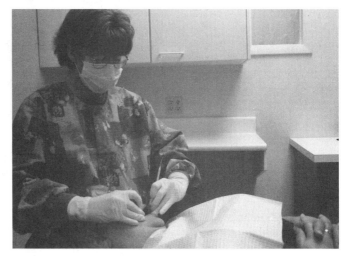

Mirror

Use the mirror head to push the tongue back gently so that the lingual surfaces of the teeth can be seen.

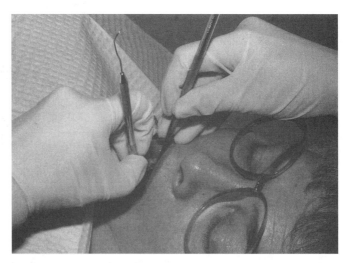

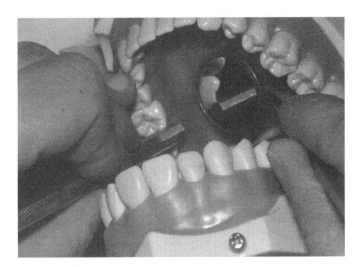

Task 1—second molar, lingual aspect

Finger rest on an occlusal surface.

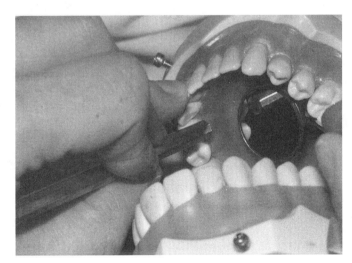

Task 2—first premolar, lingual aspect

Finger rest on an incisal edge of an anterior tooth.

Reference Sheet: LEFT-Handed Clinician

Photocopy this page and use it for quick reference as you practice your skills. Place the photocopied reference sheet in a plastic page protector for longer use.

Mandibular Posterior Treatment Areas			
Sextant	**Clock Position**	**Patient's Head**	**Handle**
Left posterior, facial aspect (aspect toward)	3:00	Straight or slightly away chin-down	at or close to 3
Right posterior, lingual aspect (aspect toward)	3:00	Slightly away chin-down	at or close to 3
Right posterior, facial aspect (aspect away)	2 – 1:00	Toward chin-down	at or close to 3
Left posterior, lingual aspect (aspect away)	2 – 1:00	Toward chin-down	at or close to 3

Skill Evaluation: Mirror and Rests in Mandibular Posterior Sextants

Student: _____

Area 1 = right posterior, facial aspect

Evaluator: _____

Area 2 = right posterior, lingual aspect

Date: _____

Area 3 = left posterior, facial aspect

Area 4 = left posterior, lingual aspect

DIRECTIONS: For each area, use **Column S** for student self-evaluation and **Column I** for instructor evaluation. For each skill evaluated, indicate the skill level as: **S** (satisfactory), **I** (improvement needed), or **U** (unsatisfactory).

CRITERIA:	Area 1		Area 2		Area 3		Area 4	
	S	I	S	I	S	I	S	I
Position: Positioned correctly on clinician stool.								
Positioned correctly in relation to patient, dental equipment, and treatment area.								
Uses correct patient head position.								
Dental Mirror Uses correct grasp with mirror.								
Establishes secure rest with mirror.								
Assures patient comfort by not hitting teeth, resting the rim against gingiva, or pulling on corner of mouth.								
Uses mirror for indirect vision and illumination, and retraction, as appropriate.								
Instrument Grasp: Uses all criteria for correct grasp.								
Basic Intraoral Fulcrum: Balances hand on tip of ring finger.								
Holds ring finger straight to act as a "support beam" for hand.								
Fulcrums on same arch, near tooth being instrumented.								

Skill Evaluation: Mirror and Rests in Mandibular Posterior Sextants

Student: _____

Evaluator Comments:

_____

_____

_____

_____

_____

_____

_____

_____

_____

_____

_____

_____

_____

_____

_____

_____

_____

Box for sketches pertaining to written comments.

Mirror and Finger Rests in Maxillary Posterior Sextants

This module will guide you through the use of a dental mirror and establishing finger rests in the maxillary posterior sextants.

Required Equipment:

- a dental mirror and a dental mirror handle or a periodontal probe
- a manikin and typodont and/or a classmate
- protective attire for clinician and patient safety glasses, if applicable

Section 1: Wrist Position for Maxillary Posteriors

The most common error in instrumenting the maxillary posterior treatment areas is failing to maintain a neutral wrist position. Incorrect wrist position results when the clinician bends the wrist rather than adjusting the handle placement in the grasp.

The clinician pictured here has incorrectly placed the handle in the 2.1 position while working on the maxillary posterior sextants. With the handle in this position, the clinician must bend the wrist in order to place the working-end on the tooth surface.

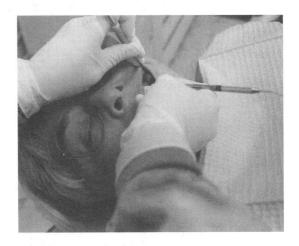

Here the clinician is working with the wrist in a neutral position. The wrist position is corrected by placing the handle in the "V" of the hand.

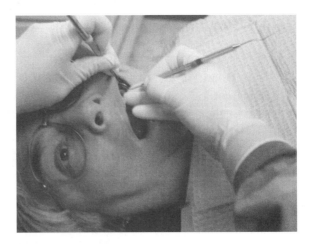

Section 2: Skills for RIGHT-Handed Clinician

Handle Placement in Grasp: Maxillary Posteriors

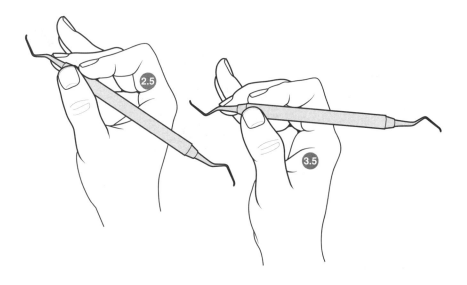

Summary Table: Handle Placement for Maxillary Posterior Teeth		
Area:	**Handle Position With Probe:**	**Handle Position Other Instruments:**
Right posteriors, facial aspect	2.5	3.5 to V
Left posteriors, lingual aspect	2.5	3.5 to V
Right posteriors, lingual aspect	2.5	3.5 to V
Left posteriors, facial aspect	2.5	3.5 to V

Technique Practice: Maxillary Posterior Teeth

Maxillary Right Posterior Sextant, Facial
Aspect: Posterior Aspect, Toward

Position Overview

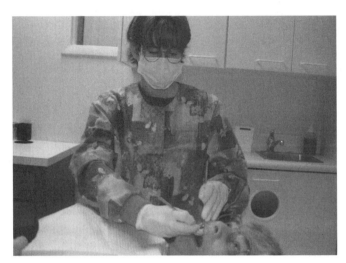

Retraction

Retract the buccal mucosa
with the mirror. Use the
mirror for indirect vision,
particularly to view the
distal surfaces in this aspect.

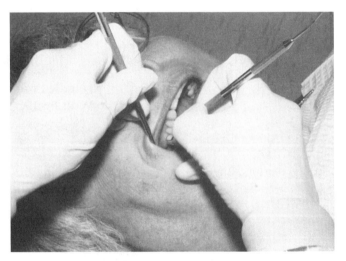

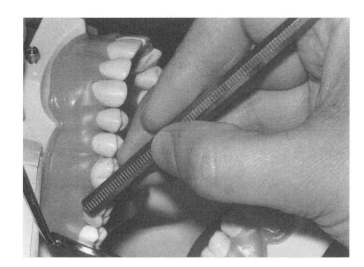

Task 1—second molar, facial aspect

Finger rest on an occlusal surface.

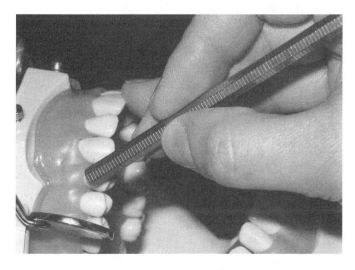

Task 2—first premolar, facial aspect

Finger rest on an incisal surface of one of the maxillary anteriors.

Maxillary Left Posterior Sextant, Lingual Aspect: Posterior Aspect, Toward

Position Overview

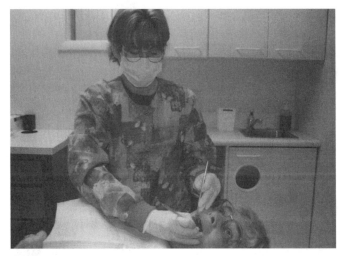

Mirror

Use mirror to view the distal surfaces of the teeth in this aspect.

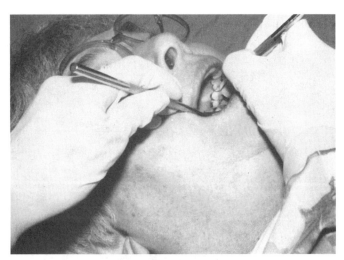

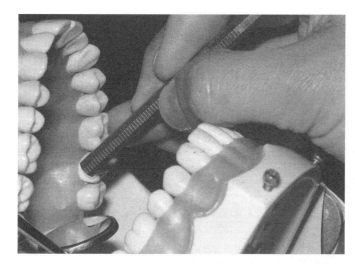

Task 1—second molar, lingual aspect

Finger rest on an occlusofacial line angle.

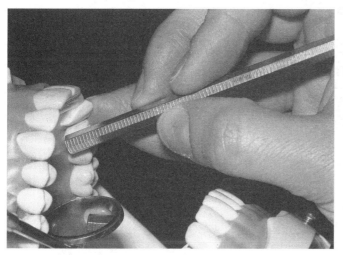

Task 2—first premolar, lingual aspect

Finger rest on the occlusofacial line angle or an incisal edge.

Maxillary Left Posterior Sextant, Facial Aspect: Posterior Aspect, Away

Position Overview

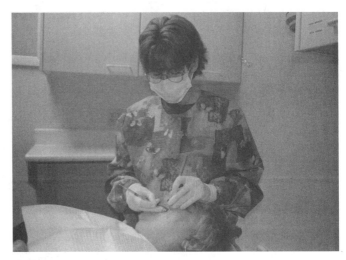

Retraction

Use the mirror to retract the buccal mucosa up and away from the teeth.

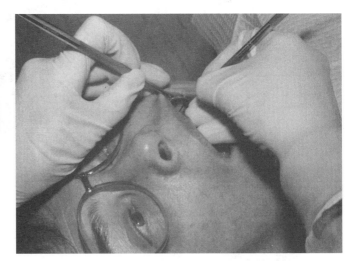

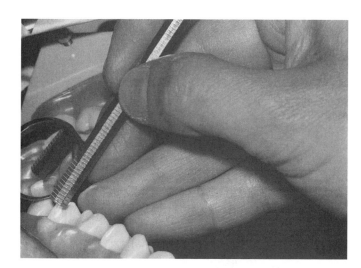

Task 1—second molar, facial aspect

Finger rest on an occlusal surface.

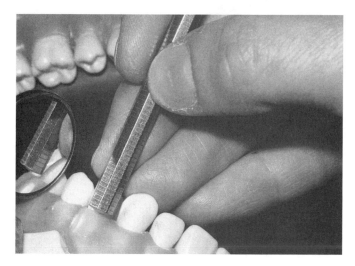

Task 2—first premolar, facial aspect

Finger rest on an incisal edge of an anterior tooth.

Maxillary Right Posterior Sextant, Lingual Aspect: Posterior Aspect, Away

Position Overview

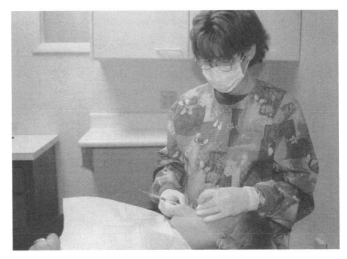

Mirror

Use the mirror head for indirect vision.

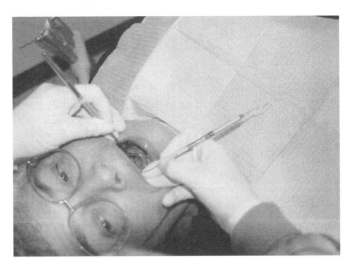

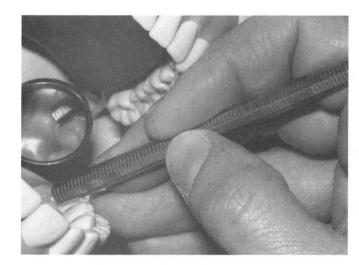

Task 1—second molar, lingual aspect

Finger rest on an occlusal surface.

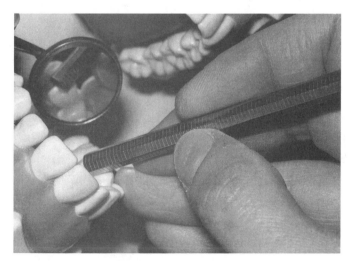

Task 2—first premolar, lingual aspect

Finger rest on the occlusal surface or an incisal edge.

Reference Sheet: RIGHT-Handed Clinician

Photocopy this page and use it for quick reference as you practice your skills. Place the photocopied reference sheet in a plastic page protector for longer use.

Maxillary Posterior Treatment Areas			
Sextant	**Clock Position**	**Patient's Head**	**Handle**
Right posterior, facial aspect (aspect toward)	9:00	Straight or slightly away chin-up	2.5 to 3.5
Left posterior, lingual aspect (aspect toward)	9:00	Slightly away chin-up	2.5 to 3.5
Right posterior, lingual aspect (aspect away)	10 – 11:00	Toward chin-up	2.5 to 3.5
Left posterior, facial aspect (aspect away)	10 – 11:00	Toward chin-up	2.5 to 3.5

Note: This ends the Section for RIGHT-Handed Clinicians. Turn to **page 165** for the the Checklist, Activities, and Evaluation section.

Section 3: Skills for LEFT-Handed Clinician

Handle Placement in Grasp: Maxillary Posteriors

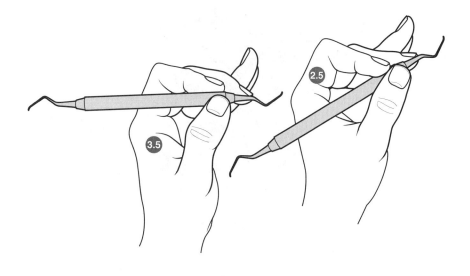

Summary Table: Handle Placement for Maxillary Posterior Teeth		
Area:	**Handle Position With Probe:**	**Handle Position, Other Instruments:**
Right posteriors, facial aspect	2.5	3.5 to V
Left posteriors, lingual aspect	2.5	3.5 to V
Right posteriors, lingual aspect	2.5	3.5 to V
Left posteriors, facial aspect	2.5	3.5 to V

Technique Practice: Maxillary Posterior Teeth

Maxillary Left Posterior Sextant, Facial Aspect: Posterior Aspect, Toward

Position Overview

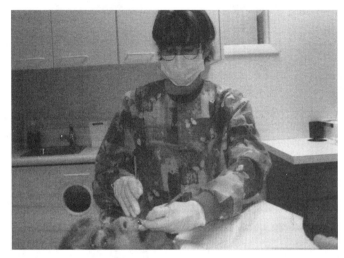

Retraction

Retract the buccal mucosa with the mirror. Use the mirror for indirect vision, particularly to view the distal surfaces in this aspect.

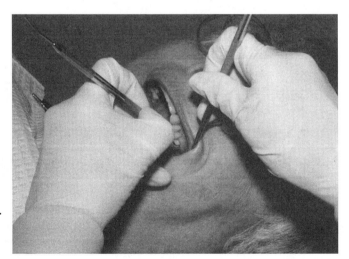

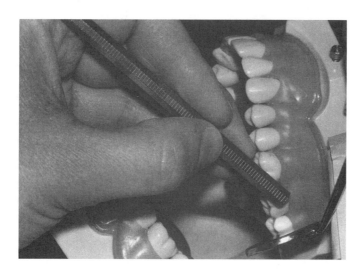

Task 1—second molar, facial aspect

Finger rest on an occlusal surface.

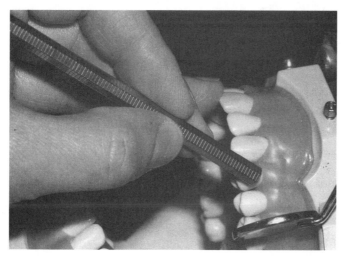

Task 2—first premolar, facial aspect

Finger rest on an incisal surface of one of the maxillary anteriors.

Maxillary Right Posterior Sextant, Lingual Aspect: Posterior Aspect, Toward

Position Overview

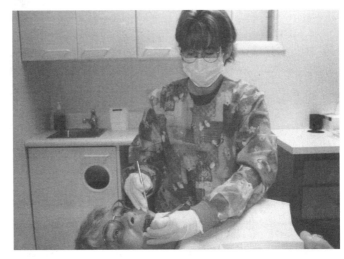

Mirror

Use mirror to view the distal surfaces of the teeth in this aspect.

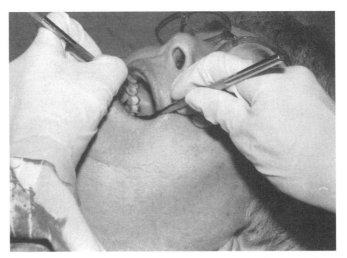

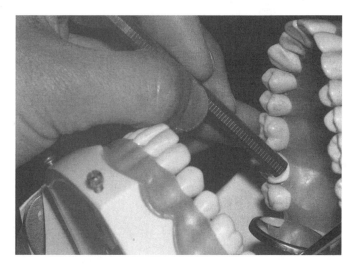

Task 1—second molar, lingual aspect

Finger rest on an occlusofacial line angle.

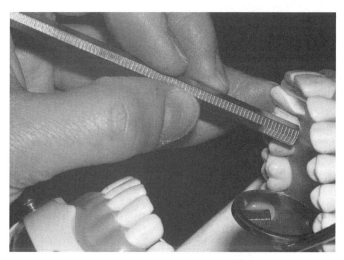

Task 2—first premolar, lingual aspect

Finger rest on the occlusofacial line angle or an incisal edge.

Maxillary Right Posterior Sextant, Facial Aspect: Posterior Aspect, Away

Position Overview

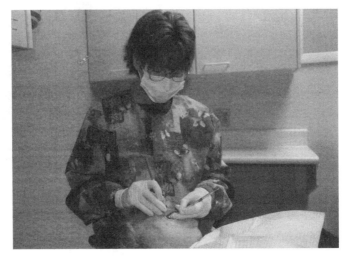

Retraction

Use the mirror to retract the buccal mucosa up and away from the teeth.

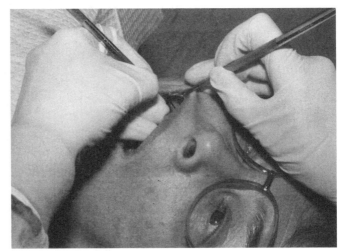

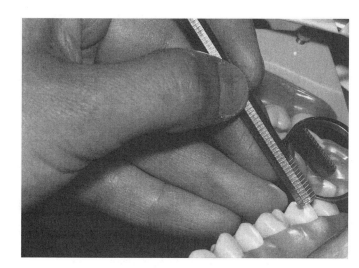

Task 1—second molar, facial aspect

Finger rest on an occlusal surface.

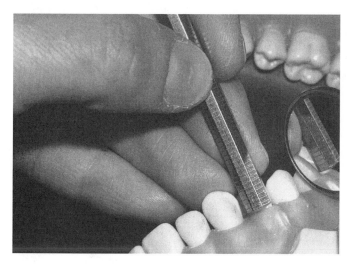

Task 2—first premolar, facial aspect

Finger rest on an incisal edge of an anterior tooth.

Maxillary Left Posterior Sextant, Lingual Aspect: Posterior Aspect, Away

Position Overview

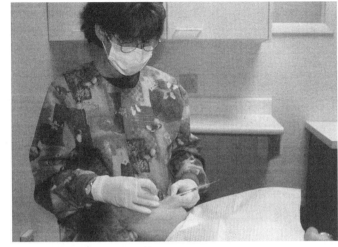

Mirror

Use the mirror for indirect vision.

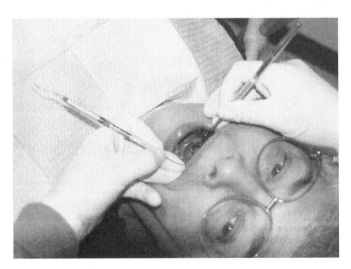

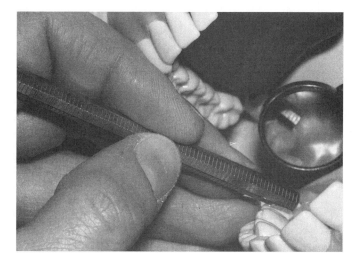

Task 1—second molar, lingual aspect

Finger rest on an occlusal surface.

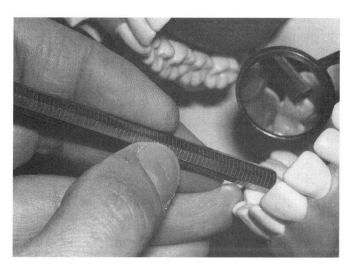

Task 2—first premolar, lingual aspect

Finger rest on the occlusal surface or an incisal edge.

Reference Sheet: LEFT-Handed Clinician

Photocopy this page and use it for quick reference as you practice your skills. Place the photocopied reference sheet in a plastic page protector for longer use.

Maxillary Posterior Treatment Areas			
Sextant	**Clock Position**	**Patient's Head**	**Handle**
Left posterior, facial aspect (aspect toward)	3:00	Straight or slightly away chin-up	2.5 to 3.5
Right posterior, lingual aspect (aspect toward)	3:00	Slightly away chin-up	2.5 to 3.5
Left posterior, lingual aspect (aspect away)	2 – 1:00	Toward chin-up	2.5 to 3.5
Right posterior, facial aspect (aspect away)	2 – 1:00	Toward chin-up	2.5 to 3.5

Section 4: Checklist, Activities, and Evaluation

Do you sometimes forget about neutral body position as you concentrate on the finger rests? Use this checklist to assess your habits. *A "YES" answer means that changes are indicated.*

Body Breakers Risk Assessment Questionnaire			
Structure	**Incorrect Body Mechanics**	**YES**	**NO**
Head	Tilted to one side?	☐	☐
	Tipped too far forward?	☐	☐
Shoulders	Lifted up toward ears?	☐	☐
	Tense?	☐	☐
	Hunched forward?	☐	☐
Upper Arms	Held more than 20-degrees away from body?	☐	☐
Elbows	Raised above waist level?	☐	☐
Wrists	Hand bent up? down?	☐	☐
	Hand angled toward thumb? toward little finger?	☐	☐
	Thumb-side of palm tipped down?	☐	☐
Hands	Gloves too tight?	☐	☐
	Fingers blanched in grasp?	☐	☐
	Fingers tense?	☐	☐
Back	Rounded back?	☐	☐
Hips	Perched forward on seat?	☐	☐
	All weight on one hip?	☐	☐
Legs	Under back of patient's chair?	☐	☐
	Thighs "cut" by edge of chair seat?	☐	☐
	Legs crossed?	☐	☐
Feet	Dangling?	☐	☐
	Ankles crossed?	☐	☐

Skill Building Activities

Activity #1: Indirect Vision

Materials and Equipment: a box of straight pins, a dental mirror, and cotton pliers or tweezers.

1. Pile approximately 10 to 15 pins in a haphazard heap.
2. Grasp the pliers in your dominant hand and the dental mirror with your non-dominant hand. Position the mirror behind the pile of pins.
3. Looking in the mirror (not directly at the pins), pick up the pins one-by-one by the pinhead and put them aside.
4. Repeat the activity, this time picking up the pins by grasping the center portion of each pin.
5. Repeat the activity, grasping the pins near the point ends.

Activity #2: Precise Instrument Control

This activity simulates the skills you will need to use when placing the instrument's working end on the various tooth surfaces while using indirect vision. It was designed by Margaret Starr, R.D.H. when she was a student learning instrumentation. Can you name several tooth surfaces that can best be seen with indirect vision?

Materials and Equipment: Printed page from a textbook or magazine, a dental mirror, and a sharpened pencil.

1. Lay the printed page flat on a desk or tabletop. Hold a dental mirror in your non-dominant hand and position it on the page. Angle the mirror head so that you are able to see several letters reflected in the mirror. How do the letters appear?
2. Still looking in the mirror, locate a letter "e" in one of the words. Grasp the pencil in a modified pen grasp and touch the pencil point to the "e" *on the paper*.
3. Move the mirror to a different location on the paper. Looking in the mirror, select a letter and touch it with the pencil point.

Skill Evaluation: Mirror and Rests in Maxillary Posterior Sextants

Student: _____

Evaluator: _____

Date: _____

Area 1 = right posterior, facial aspect

Area 2 = right posterior, lingual aspect

Area 3 = left posterior, facial aspect

Area 4 = left posterior, lingual aspect

DIRECTIONS: For each area, use **Column S** for student self-evaluation and **Column I** for instructor evaluation. For each skill evaluated, indicate the skill level as: **S** (satisfactory), **I** (improvement needed), or **U** (unsatisfactory).

CRITERIA:	Area 1 S	Area 1 I	Area 2 S	Area 2 I	Area 3 S	Area 3 I	Area 4 S	Area 4 I
Position: Positioned correctly on clinician stool.								
Positioned correctly in relation to patient, dental equipment, and treatment area.								
Uses correct patient head position.								
Dental Mirror Uses correct grasp with mirror.								
Establishes secure rest with mirror.								
Assures patient comfort by not hitting teeth, resting the rim against gingiva, or pulling on corner of mouth.								
Uses mirror for indirect vision and illumination, and retraction, as appropriate.								
Instrument Grasp: Uses all criteria for correct grasp.								
Basic Intraoral Fulcrum: Balances hand on tip of ring finger.								
Holds ring finger straight to act as a "support beam" for hand.								
Fulcrums on same arch, near tooth being instrumented.								

Skill Evaluation: Mirror and Rests in Maxillary Posterior Sextants

Student: _____

Evaluator Comments:

_____

_____

_____

_____

_____

_____

_____

_____

_____

_____

_____

_____

_____

_____

_____

_____

_____

_____

Box for sketches pertaining to written comments.

7

MODULE

Design of
Hand-Activated Instruments

This module will introduce you to the various design characteristics of periodontal instruments. Instrument handles, shanks, and working-ends all have design features that you will need to understand when selecting an instrument.

Required Equipment:

For this module, ask your instructor to help you find at least one example of a probe, explorer, sickle scaler, universal and area-specific curet.

Key Terms:

Functional shank	Working-end	Lateral surface
Lower shank	Face	Cutting edge
Complex shank design	Back	Cross section

Section 1: The Periodontal Instrument

Instrument Identification

Periodontal instruments are available in single-ended and double-ended configurations. Single-ended instruments are less efficient to use since the clinician must stop more often to lay down one instrument and pick up another. Double-ended instruments allow the clinician to simply flip the instrument in order to use the other working-end. Most double-ended instruments are paired, having working-ends that are exact mirror images of each other. Some double-ended instruments have unpaired (different) working-ends. An example of a double-ended instrument with unpaired working-ends is an explorer and a probe combination.

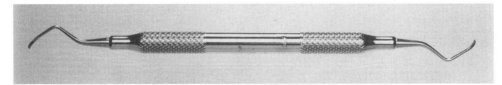

Paired working-ends are exact mirror images of each other.

A unique design name and number identify each periodontal instrument. The **design name** is marked on the instrument handle and usually identifies a group or "family" of instruments. Instruments often are named after the designer or an academic institution. A well-known example is the design name "Gracey". In the late 1930s, Dr. Clayton H. Gracey designed the 14 original single-ended instruments in this series that bears his name. The **design number** is marked on the instrument handle and when combined with the design name, provides an exact identification of the instrument's working-ends. Using the Gracey series as an example, the "Gracey 5" is the design name and number that identifies a specific instrument in this instrument series.

A double-ended instrument will have two design numbers, one to identify each working-end of the instrument. For example, the original Gracey series of instruments includes 7 double-ended instruments, such as, the Gracey 3/4, Gracey 5/6, Gracey 11/12, and Gracey 13/14.

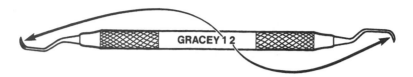

The design name and number may be marked horizontally along the length of the instrument handle. In this case, each working-end is identified by the number closest to it.

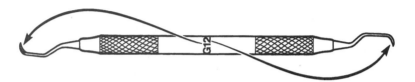

The design name and number may be marked across the instrument handle. In this case, the first number (on the left) identifies the working-end at the top and the second number identifies the working-end at the lower end of the handle.

Instrument Handles

Instrument handles are available in a variety of diameters and textures. Handle design is an important component in the prevention of musculoskeletal injury during instrumentation. In selecting an instrument handle, there are three characteristics to consider: (1) weight, (2) diameter, and (3) texture. Select an instrument handle that is lightweight with bumpy texturing. Avoid small diameter handles that are more difficult to grasp and tend to cause muscle cramping. Select large diameter handles that can be held more easily in a pinch-grip. It may be helpful to select handles in a range of larger diameters; thus, providing some variety for the muscles of your fingers.

Handle Selection Criteria	
Recommended:	**Avoid:**
Large diameter (3/8-inch)	Small diameter (3/17-inch)
Lightweight, hollow handle	Heavy, solid metal handle
Bumpy texturing	Smooth or flat texturing

Handle Selection. The handle at the top of the photograph, with a small diameter and limited texturing, is not recommended. The handle pictured at the bottom of the photograph is an example of a recommended handle design with a large diameter and bumpy texturing.

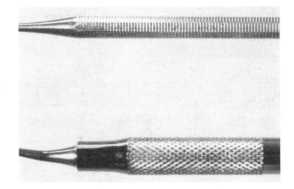

The Hu-Friedy Satin Steel instrument handle has texturing that extends onto the tapered portion of the handle. This feature reduces muscle strain for short-fingered clinicians who must grip the tapered portion of the handle.

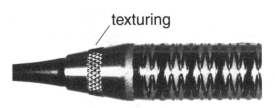

texturing

Instrument Balance

An instrument is **balanced** if the centers of the working-ends are aligned with the center axis of the handle. Balance insures that finger pressure applied against the handle and shank is transferred to the working-end resulting in pressure against the tooth. An instrument that is not balanced is more difficult to use and stresses the muscles of the hand and arm. An easy way to determine if an instrument is balanced is to place it on a line of a lined writing tablet. Align the midline of the handle with a line on the paper; the instrument is balanced if the working-ends are centered on the line.

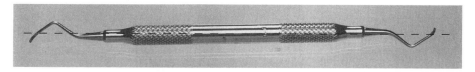

An instrument is balanced if the working-ends are centered on an imaginary line running through the long axis of the handle.

Instrument Shanks

The part of the shank that allows the working-end to be adapted to the tooth surface is called the **functional shank**. The functional shank extends from the first bend in the shank (nearest the handle) up to the working-end. Instruments with short functional shanks are used on the coronal surfaces of the teeth. Instruments with long functional shanks may be used on both the crown and roots of the teeth or when using advanced fulcruming techniques.

The **lower shank** is the bent section of the shank nearest to the working-end. Another name for the lower shank is the **terminal shank**. The ability to identify the lower shank is important during instrumentation. The working-end of a Gracey instrument is positioned correctly on the tooth when the lower shank is parallel to the surface to be instrumented. For this reason, the lower shank is a visual clue that will help you during instrumentation.

The **functional shank** extends from the first bend in the shank (nearest the handle) up to the working-end.

The **lower shank** is the bent section of the shank nearest to the working-end.

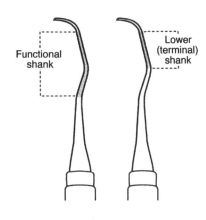

Some instruments have **extended lower shanks** that are ideal for working in deep periodontal pockets or when using advanced fulcruming techniques. The lower shanks on these instruments are 3 mm longer than a standard shank.

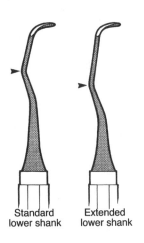

Simple and Complex Shank Design

The shanks of most periodontal instruments have bends in one or more places. Without shank bends, the working-end could not be applied effectively to the tooth surfaces. A shank that is bent in *one plane* (front-to-back) has a **simple shank** design. Instruments with simple shanks are used primarily on anterior teeth.

A shank that is bent in two planes (front-to-back and side-to-side) has a **complex shank** design. Complex shank designs were developed to allow instrumentation of posterior teeth. The crowns of posterior teeth are rounded and overhang their roots. An instrument with a complex shank is needed to reach around the crown and onto the root surface.

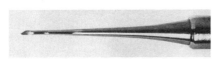

Simple Shank. Instruments with simple shank design have no shank bends in a side-to-side direction. An anterior sickle scaler is an example of an instrument with simple shank design.

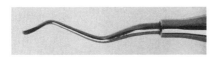

Complex Shank. Instruments with complex shank design have shank bends in a front-to-back and a side-to-side direction. Gracey curets are examples of instruments with complex shank design.

Simple Shank. The crowns of anterior teeth are wedge-shaped. A simple shank design is adequate to reach along the crown and onto the root surface.

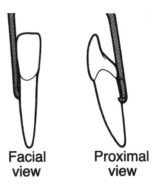

Facial view   Proximal view

Complex Shank. The illustration shows a left mandibular molar when viewed from the mesial aspect. The front-to-back shank bends allow the clinician to reach the lingual and facial surfaces of the root.

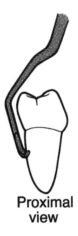

Proximal view

Complex Shank. The illustration shows a mandibular left molar when viewed from the facial aspect. The side-to-side bends allow the clinician to reach the mesial and distal surfaces of the tooth.

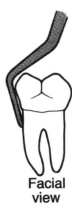

Facial view

Shank Flexibility

An important characteristic of an instrument shank is how strong it is. The type and diameter of metal used in a shank will determine its strength. Instrument shanks are classified as either rigid or flexible in design. During instrumentation, the clinician applies pressure against the handle and shank to press the working-end against the tooth surface. A calculus deposit can be removed more quickly and with less effort if the instrument has a rigid shank. As the working-end encounters a piece of calculus, a rigid shank will withstand the force applied against the deposit; a flexible shank will bend or flex as pressure is applied against the deposit. For this reason, a rigid shank design is desirable for instruments that are used for calculus removal.

Visual information is of limited use during subgingival instrumentation. Instead, the clinician relies on his or her sense of touch to locate calculus deposits hidden beneath the gingival margin. Vibrations are created when the working-end quivers slightly as it moves over irregularities on the surface of the tooth. These vibrations are transmitted from the working-end, through the shank, and into the handle. **Tactile sensitivity** is the ability to detect tooth irregularities by feeling vibrations transferred from the working-end to the handle. The clinician feels the vibrations with his or her fingers as they rest on the shank and handle.

Flexible shanks enhance the amount of tactile information transferred to the clinician's fingers. For this reason, a flexible shank design is desirable for instruments (explorers) that are used to locate calculus deposits.

Shank Flexibility		
	Flexible Shank Design	Rigid Shank Design
Strength	Shank flexes when force is applied during instrumentation	Shank will withstand strong forces during instrumentation
Use	Best for detection of calculus deposits	Best for removing calculus deposits

Section 2: Working-Ends

An instrument's use is determined, primarily, by the design of its working-end. The characteristics of the working-end of a particular instrument may vary slightly from manufacturer to manufacturer. If you examine three Gracey 13/14 instruments from three manufacturers, you will probably notice differences in the working-ends. The working-end from one manufacturer may be larger or more curved than that of another manufacturer. The important consideration in choosing a manufacturer is which instrument works best in your hand. The best instrument for one clinician may not be the best for another. With experience, you will learn which instruments are most effective for you.

Some manufacturers produce instruments with standard and miniature working-ends. Miniature working-ends are thinner and shorter than standard working-ends and are used in narrow deep pockets, root concavities, and furcation areas. Examples of instruments with miniature working-ends are the "Mini Five Gracey Curettes"; these instruments have working-ends that are thinner and shortened to half the length of the standard Gracey working-ends.

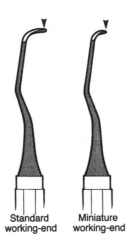

Standard
working-end

Miniature
working-end

Parts of the Working-End

To determine an instrument's use you must recognize the design characteristics of the face, back, lateral surfaces, and cutting edges of the working-end.

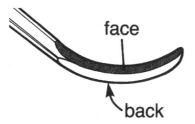

The shaded surface on this illustration is the instrument **face**.

The surface opposite the face is the instrument **back**.

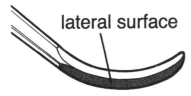

The shaded surfaces on either side of the face are called the **lateral surfaces** of the instrument.

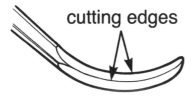

The line formed where the face and a lateral surface meet is the **cutting edge** of the instrument. Hand-activated periodontal instruments have one or more sharp cutting edges.

The Working-End in Cross Section

An important characteristic of an instrument's working-end is its shape in cross section. An instrument's cross section determines whether the instrument can be used subgingivally.

A **cross section** is the shape of an object when a horizontal cutting is made through the object perpendicular to its long axis. At first, understanding cross sections may seem difficult, but looking at an everyday object should help you to understand this concept.

Imagine that you are sawing a lead pencil into two parts by cutting it in the middle perpendicular to the long axis of the pencil.

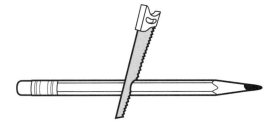

When the pencil has been cut, you can view its shape in cross section.

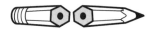

In cross section, the pencil is hexagonal in shape. (A hexagon is a six-sided figure.)

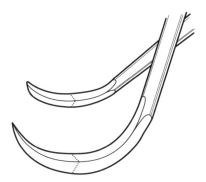

In a similar manner, imagine that you are going to cut the working-ends of these instruments in half.

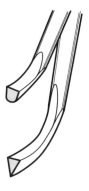

After the cut is made, you can view the cross sections of the working-ends of these two instruments.

The top instrument is semi-circular in cross section. The bottom instrument is triangular in cross section.

Section 3: Skill Building Activity

This activity is designed to help you learn to identify parts of the working-end and the functional and lower shanks on various instruments.

Equipment: Ask your instructor to help you assemble the following instruments—a sickle scaler, universal curet, and an area-specific curet.

Materials: Several bottles of brightly colored nail polish, and nail polish remover or orange solvent (to remove nail polish from your instruments at the completion of this activity).

1. Paint the **lateral surfaces** of each working-end with one color of nail polish.

2. Use a contrasting color of polish to paint the **face** of each instrument.

3. Paint the **functional shank** on each instrument. How does the functional shank differ from the overall shank length? Compare the functional shank lengths on the various instruments.

4. Use a contrasting color of polish to paint the **lower shank** on each instrument.

5. Ask an instructor to check your work.

Skill Evaluation:
The Skill Evaluation for this module and Module 8 are combined. The evaluation can be found at the end of Module 8. Students should complete Module 8 before attempting the skill evaluation.

8

MODULE

Instrument Classification

Periodontal instruments are divided into types, or classifications, based upon the specific design features of the working-end. In selecting an instrument for a specific task, one of the most important considerations is the classification of the working-end.

Required Equipment:

For this module, you should assemble an assortment of periodontal instruments for identification and study. Try to examine at least one example of each instrument classification (probe, explorer, sickle scaler, periodontal file, universal curet, and area-specific curet.)

Section 1: Terminology

This section contains an overview of terminology used in this and following modules that may be new to you.

Assessment is the evaluation of a tooth to determine tooth anatomy and for the detection of irregularities, carious lesions, and plaque-retentive factors, such as calculus deposits or restorations with over hanging margins.

Periodontal debridement is the removal or disruption of bacterial plaque, its byproducts, and plaque-retentive calculus deposits from crown and root surfaces, and within the sulcus or pocket space, as indicated, for periodontal healing and repair. Instrumentation is limited to that needed to return the adjacent soft tissues to a healthy state.

Deplaquing is the disruption or removal of *subgingival* bacterial plaque and its byproducts from cemental surfaces and the pocket space following the completion of subgingival instrumentation.

Instrumenting is using periodontal instruments on the tooth surface.

Free gingiva is the unattached portion of the gingiva that encircles the tooth to form the gingival sulcus. It extends from the gingival margin to the attached gingiva.

Attached gingiva is the portion of the gingiva extending from the free gingiva to the mucogingival junction. It is firmly attached to the cementum of the tooth and alveolar bone.

The **sulcus** is the shallow space between the inner aspect of the free gingiva and the tooth. Healthy sulci range in depth from 0.5 to 3 mm.

The **junctional epithelium** is a thin layer of epithelium that forms the base of the sulcus and provides the epithelial attachment to the tooth surface.

A **periodontal pocket** is a diseased sulcus that has been deepened by the apical migration of the junctional epithelium along the root surface and destruction of the periodontal ligament and alveolar bone.

The **clinical attachment level** is the distance from the cementoenamel junction (CEJ) to the junctional epithelium as measured with a calibrated periodontal probe.

Supragingival—located *coronal* to the gingival margin. For example, supragingival calculus is a deposit that is located on the tooth coronal to the gingival margin. This calculus is visible to the eye when dried with compressed air.

Subgingival—located *apical* to the gingival margin within the sulcus or pocket. For example, subgingival calculus is a deposit that is located on the tooth apical to the gingival margin. This calculus is hidden beneath the gingival margin and must be detected with an explorer.

The **furcation area** is the area between the roots of a multirooted tooth. In health, the furcation area is filled with alveolar bone.

Bacterial plaque (microbial dental plaque) is a mass of densely packed complex colonies of microorganisms in an intermicrobial matrix. Bacterial plaque grows on and tenaciously attaches to the teeth and other oral structures and forms as loosely attached plaque between the tooth and the soft tissue wall of the sulcus or pocket. It causes dental caries and infections of the gingival tissues.

Bacterial byproducts are substances produced by bacteria that irritate and produce changes in the periodontal tissues. These substances are cytotoxic to the tissues and must be removed for healing to occur. Bacterial byproducts include toxins, enzymes, bacterial antigens, bacterial waste products, and invasion factors.

Calculus is calcified plaque. It is commonly known as tartar. Calculus deposits are **plaque-retentive**, meaning that the outer surface of a calculus deposit is covered with dental plaque.

Residual calculus deposits are minute remnants of calculus located on the outer layers of the root surface.

A **carious lesion** is a decayed area on the tooth crown or root.

Section 2: Working-End Utilization

To select an appropriate instrument for a task, you will need to recognize each instrument's classification, design characteristics, application, and function.

Classification and Design Characteristics

The **classification** of an instrument is determined by the design characteristics of the working-end(s). Non-surgical, hand-activated periodontal instruments are classified as periodontal probes, explorers, sickle scalers, periodontal files, universal curets, area-specific curets, hoes, or chisels. (Hoes and chisels are rarely used; mechanized instruments have largely replaced their function.) Instrument **design characteristics** include the (1) design of the cutting edges, back, lateral surfaces, and shank; (2) working-end cross section; and (3) relationship of the face to the lower shank.

Application

The instrument's **application** refers to the tooth surfaces or areas of the mouth on which the instrument can be used. Each instrument is limited to one of the following applications:

1. Anterior use—one single-ended instrument can be used to instrument all tooth surfaces (facial, lingual, mesial, and distal) in the mandibular and maxillary anterior sextants.
2. Posterior use—one double-ended instrument can be used to instrument all tooth surfaces of the four posterior sextants.
3. Universal use—one double-ended instrument can be used to instrument all tooth surfaces in the dentition (anterior and posterior teeth).
4. Area-specific use—an instrument can be applied only to specific surfaces and areas of the mouth. A set comprised of several area-specific instruments is needed to instrument the entire dentition.

Function

In general, non-surgical periodontal instruments have one or more of the following functions:

1. Assessment of teeth and/or soft tissues
2. Debridement of tooth surfaces (the removal or disruption of calculus deposits, bacterial plaque and its byproducts)

Section 3: Assessment Instruments

Periodontal Probes

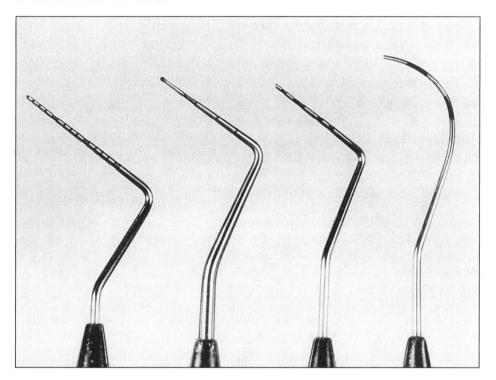

The **periodontal probe** is a slender assessment instrument used to evaluate the periodontal health of the tissues. Probes have blunt, rod-shaped working-ends that are circular or rectangular in cross section.

There are two basic types: **calibrated** and **furcation** probes. Calibrated probes are marked in millimeter increments and are used like miniature rulers for making intraoral measurements. Furcation probes are used to evaluate bone support in the furcation areas of bifurcated and trifurcated teeth. Findings from an examination with a calibrated probe are an important part of a comprehensive periodontal assessment.

The calibrated periodontal probe is used to measure sulcus and pocket depths, measure clinical attachment levels, determine the width of attached gingiva, assess for the presence of bleeding, and/or purulent exudate (pus), and measure the size of oral lesions.

Millimeter Markings

Calibrated probes are used like miniature intraoral rulers. The working-end of the probe is marked at millimeter intervals. Each millimeter may be indicated on the probe or only certain millimeter increments may be marked. Color-coded probes are marked in bands (often black in color) with each band being several millimeters in width. If you are uncertain how a probe is calibrated, you can use a millimeter ruler to determine the millimeter markings.

Examples of Probe Markings		
Type	**Marking Pattern**	**mm Increments**
UNC15	All mm from 1-15 marked	1 to 15
Glickman 26G	No mark at 6 mm	1-2-3-5-7-8-9-10
Goldman Fox	No mark at 6 mm	1-2-3-5-7-8-9-10
Merritt	No mark at 6 mm	1-2-3-5-7-8-9-10
Williams	No mark at 6 mm	1-2-3-5-7-8-9-10
Maryland Moffitt	No mark at 6 mm; ball-end	1-2-3-5-7-8-9-10
Michigan "O"	Marks at 3, 6, and 8 mm	3-6-8
PSR Screening	Colored band from 3.5-5.5; marks at 8.5 and 11.5 mm; ball-end	3.5-5.5-8.5-11.5
CP-18	Colored bands from 3-5 and 8-10	3-5-8-10
CP-11	Colored bands from 3-6 and 8-11	3-6-8-11
CP-12	Colored bands from 3-6 and 9-12	3-6-9-12
Hu-Friedy Novatech	Right-angled probe; available in a wide variety of designs.	

The UNC 15 probe has millimeter markings at 1, 2, 3, 4, 5, 6, 7, 8, 9, 10, 11, 12, 13, 14, and 15 millimeters.

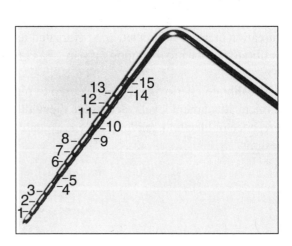

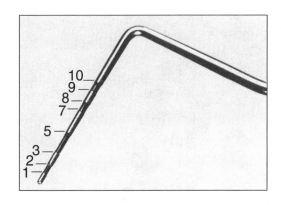

This probe has millimeter markings at 1-2-3-5-7-8-9-10 and a black band from 3-5 mm.

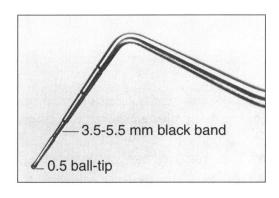

This probe has a 0.5 ball-tip and a black band from 3.5-5.5 mm. Read more about this probe in Module 12.

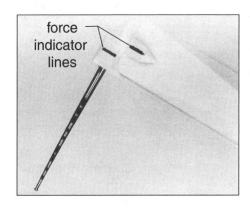

This TPS Probe from Vivadent uses force indicator lines to aid the clinician in applying a consistent probing force. This TPS probe has marks at 1.5, 2.5 mm and a black band from 3.5 to 5.5 mm; marks at 6.5, 7.5 mm and a black band from 8.5 to 11.5 mm.

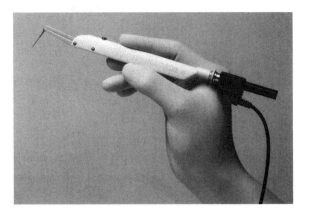

This is a computer-assisted probe. The probe is connected to a computer unit that will store information on recession, pocket depth, furcation involvement, and mobility. (Photograph courtesy of Florida Probe Corporation.)

Furcation Probes

Furcation probes are curved, blunt-tipped assessment instruments used to detect bone loss in the furcation areas. Examples of furcation probes are the Nabers 1N and 2N.

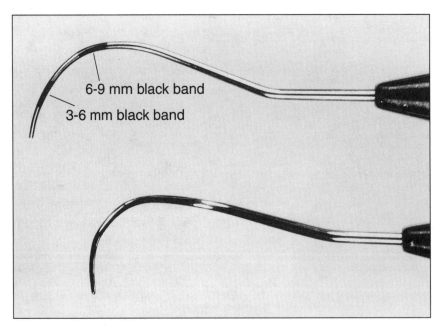

6-9 mm black band

3-6 mm black band

Furcation Probes. The probe on the top has black bands from 3-6 mm and 6-9 mm. Most furcation probes, like the one at the bottom of the photograph, do not have millimeter markings.

Explorers

An **explorer** is an assessment instrument with a fine, wire-like working-end. It is made of flexible metal and is circular in cross section. Explorers provide the best tactile information to the clinician's fingers and are used to locate calculus deposits, tooth surface irregularities, defective margins on restorations, decalcified areas, and carious lesions.

The working-end of an explorer is 1 to 2 mm in length and is referred to as its tip. The actual point of the explorer is not used to detect dental calculus; rather the side of explorer tip is applied to the tooth surface. Explorers are available in a variety of design types. All design types are not well suited to subgingival use; therefore, the clinician must be knowledgeable about the recommended use of each design type.

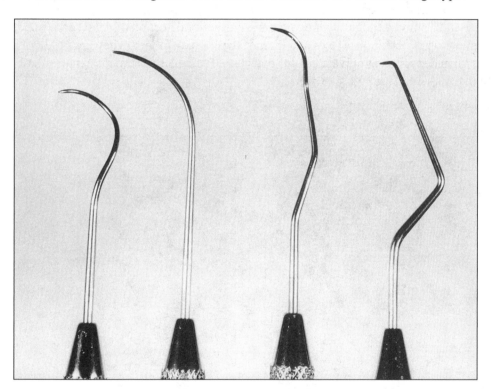

Shepherd Hook and Straight Explorer Designs

The *Shepherd Hook* is an unpaired explorer; one working-end can be used throughout the dentition. This explorer has two design limitations. The short lower shank restricts it to use on the crown of the tooth. The second design limitation is the sharp, pointed tip. When used subgingivally, the sharp point of the explorer is directed toward the junctional epithelium. Subgingival use of a Shepherd Hook explorer could result in trauma to the base of the sulcus. Therefore, these explorers are NOT recommended for calculus detection. Shepherd Hook explorers are used for detection of dental caries and examination of occlusal surfaces and restorations. Examples of Shepherd Hook explorers include the 23 and 54 explorers.

The *straight explorer* is an unpaired explorer; one working-end can be used throughout the dentition. This explorer type has the design limitations of a short lower shank and a pointed tip. Straight explorers are used for detection of dental caries and examination of occlusal surfaces and the surfaces of restorations. They are NOT recommended for subgingival calculus detection. Examples of straight explorers are the 6, 6A, 6L, and the 6XL explorers.

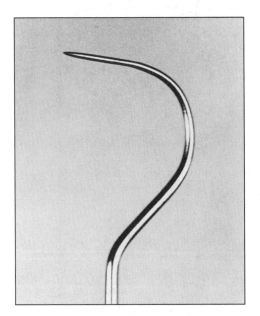

Shepherd Hook Explorer

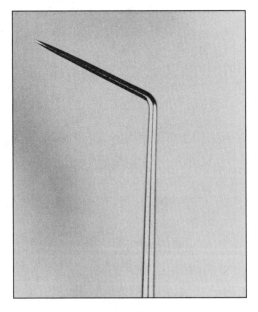

Straight Explorer

Curved and Orban-Type Explorer Designs

Curved explorers are unpaired explorers; one working-end can be used throughout the dentition. If used subgingivally, this explorer design is limited to use in normal sulci or shallow pockets. This explorer also has a sharp pointed tip that is directed toward the junctional epithelium when the working-end is used subgingivally. Curved explorers may be used for calculus detection, however, care must be taken not to injure the junctional epithelium with the pointed tip. Examples of curved explorers are the 3 and 3A.

The *Orban-type explorer* is an unpaired explorer that has several unique design characteristics. The first unique design characteristic is the tip of this explorer, which is bent at a 90-degree angle to the terminal shank. This design feature allows the back of the tip (instead the point) to be directed toward the junctional epithelium. The second unique design characteristic of the Orban-type explorer is the straight lower shank, which allows insertion in narrow, deep pockets with only slight displacement of the tissue away from the root surface. The straight shank design, however, also limits the use of this explorer since it is difficult to adapt to line-angles and proximal surfaces of posterior teeth. Orban-type explorers are used for calculus detection in narrow, deep pockets on anterior teeth or the facial and lingual surfaces of posterior teeth. Examples of Orban-type explorers are the 17, 20F, and TU17.

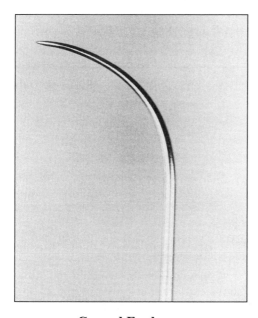

Curved Explorer

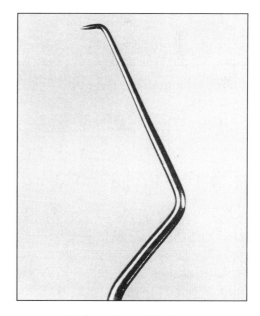

Orban-Type Explorer

Pigtail and Cowhorn Explorer Designs

The *pigtail or cowhorn explorer* is a paired universal explorer that can be adapted to all anterior and posterior surfaces. The short, broadly curved lower shank of this type of explorer causes considerable tissue displacement (stretching of the tissue wall away from the tooth). Pigtail and cowhorn explorers can be used for calculus detection in normal sulci or shallow pockets extending no deeper than the cervical-third of the root. Examples are the 3ML, 3CH, and 2A.

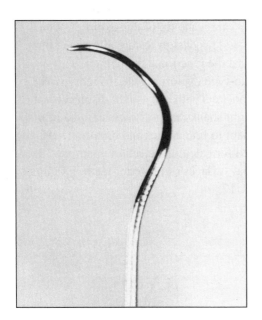

Pigtail Explorer

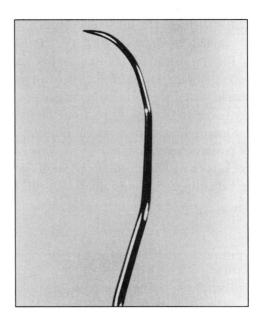

11/12-Type Explorer

11/12-Type Explorer Designs

The *11/12-type explorer* is a paired universal explorer that can be adapted to all anterior and posterior surfaces. Like the Orban-type explorer, the back of the tip can be applied to the pocket base without lacerating the junctional epithelium. The design characteristic that makes the 11/12-type explorer unique is the long functional shank design. The 11/12-type explorer is the most effective explorer design for calculus detection. It adapts well to all surfaces throughout the mouth and is equally useful when exploring a shallow sulcus or a deep periodontal pocket. Examples are the ODU 11/12 and the 11/12 AF.

Section 4: Debridement Instruments

Sickle Scalers

A **sickle scaler** is a debridement instrument with a pointed back and two cutting edges that meet in a point. Sickle scalers are confined to *supra*gingival use and should NOT be used on root surfaces. Sickle scalers are available in either anterior or posterior designs. As their name suggests, **anterior** sickle scalers are limited to use on anterior treatment sextants. Often they are single-ended instruments since only one working-end is needed to instrument the crowns of the anterior teeth. It is common, however, to combine two different anterior sickles on a double-ended instrument. **Posterior** sickle scalers are designed for use on posterior sextants, but they also may be used on anterior teeth. Usually two posterior sickles are paired on a double-ended instrument (the working-ends are mirror images of one another). For example, the Jacquette 34 is paired with the Jacquette 35 (the working-end of the Jacquette 34 is a mirror image of the working-end of the Jacquette 35).

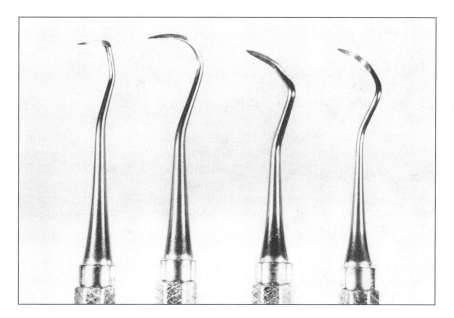

Sickle Scalers. From left to right, the first instrument is an anterior sickle scaler. The next three instruments are examples of posterior sickles.

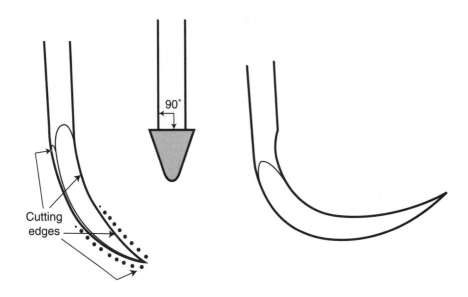

Design of Sickle Scalers

Design Highlights of Sickle Scalers:
- Pointed back
- Pointed tip
- Triangular in cross section
- Two cutting edges per working-end
- Face is perpendicular to the lower shank

Examples of Sickle Scalers:

Anterior sickle scalers—OD-1, Jacquette-30, Jacquette-33, Whiteside-2, USC-128, Towner-U15, Goldman-H6, and Goldman-H7

Posterior sickle scalers—Jacquette 34/35, Jacquette 14/15; Jacquette 31/32; Ball 2/3; Mecca 11/12; and the Catatonia 107/108

Reference Sheet: Sickle Scaler	
Cross Section	Triangular
Back	Pointed (pointed back not suited to subgingival use; may injure the sulcular epithelium)
Cutting Edges	Two cutting edges per working-end
Tip	Pointed (pointed tip and straight cutting edges do not adapt well to rounded root surfaces and concavities)
Face	Perpendicular to the lower shank so that cutting edges are level with one another (level cutting edges mean that the lower shank must be tilted slightly toward the tooth surface to establish correct angulation)
Shank	Anterior sickles—simple design Posterior sickles—complex design
Application	Anterior sickles—only one single-ended instrument is needed to instrument the crowns of the anterior teeth Posterior sickles—one double-ended instrument is needed to instrument the crowns of posterior teeth
Primary Functions	Removal of medium- to large-sized *supra*gingival calculus deposits Provides good access to the (1) proximal surfaces on anterior crowns and (2) enamel surfaces apical to contact areas of posterior teeth NOT recommended for use on root surfaces
Examples of Anterior Sickle Scalers	OD-1, Jacquette-30, Jacquette-33, Whiteside-2, USC-128, Towner-U15, Goldman-H6, and Goldman-H7
Examples of Posterior Sickle Scalers	Jacquette 34/35, Jacquette 14/15; Jacquette 31/32; Ball 2/3; Mecca 11/12; and the Catatonia 107/108

Periodontal Files

A **periodontal file** is a calculus removal instrument that has many cutting edges per working-end and is used to prepare calculus deposits before removal with another instrument. There are two instances when periodontal files can facilitate calculus removal. The first instance is the removal of a burnished calculus deposit (a deposit with a smooth outer surface). A burnished calculus deposit is difficult to remove because the cutting edge tends to slide over its smooth surface. A file is used to scratch the surface of a burnished deposit so that it can be removed with another instrument. The second instance, in which a file is useful, is in crushing a calculus deposit to facilitate its removal by another hand-activated instrument. Once the deposit has been crushed with the file, it is easier to remove with a curet.

Each file is designed for use on a single tooth surface; therefore, a set of files is needed to instrument the four tooth surfaces (facial, lingual, mesial, distal). Instruments with simple shanks work best on anterior teeth, those with complex shanks work best on posterior teeth.

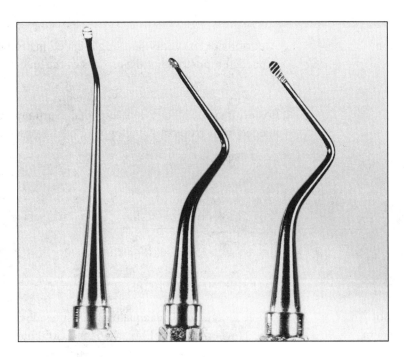

Periodontal Files

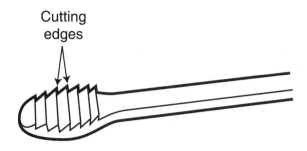

Cutting
edges

Periodontal File. The working-end of a file has multiple, straight cutting edges.

Reference Sheet: Periodontal File	
Working-End	Thin in width with large base circumference
Cutting Edges	Multiple, at a 90-105° to lower shank
Shank	Short, rigid functional shank Anterior—simple design Posterior—complex design
Application	Each working-end is designed for use on a single surface (four working-ends needed to instrument all tooth surfaces)
Primary Functions	Limited to use on enamel surfaces or application to the outer surface of calculus deposit Preparation of burnished calculus prior to removal Crushing of large calculus deposits
Examples	Orban 10/11, Orban 12/13, Hirschfeld 3/7, Hirschfeld 5/11, and Hirschfeld 9/10

Universal Curets

A **universal curet** is a debridement instrument with a rounded back and rounded toe. Universal curets have two working cutting edges per working-end. (A *working cutting edge* is a cutting edge that is used for debridement.) Usually, two curets are paired on a double-ended instrument (the paired working-ends are mirror images of one another). This type of curet is called **universal** because it can be applied to all tooth surfaces in both the anterior and posterior sextants of the mouth. In other words, this type of curet is used universally throughout the entire mouth. Universal curets are used on crown and root surfaces (supragingivally and subgingivally).

Universal curets are one of the most frequently used and versatile of all the debridement instruments. These curets can be used both supragingivally and subgingivally for removal of light- to moderate-sized calculus deposits.

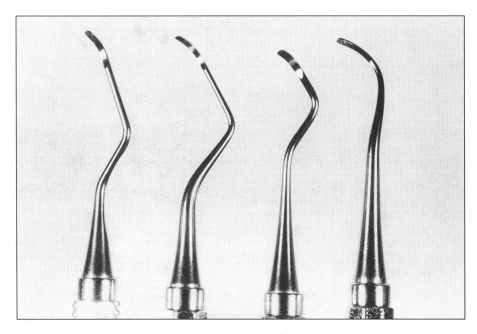

Universal Curets

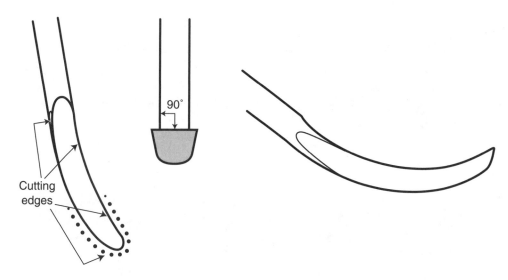

Design of Universal Curets

Design Highlights of Universal Curets:
- Rounded back
- Rounded toe
- Semicircular in cross section
- Two cutting edges per working-end
- Face is perpendicular to the lower shank

Examples of Universal Curets:
Columbia 2R/2L; Columbia 13/14; Rule 3/4; Barnhart 1/2; Barnhart 5/6; Younger-Good 7/8; Indiana University 13/14; HU 1/2; Bunting 5/6; Mallery 1/2; Langer 1/2; Langer 3/4; Langer 5/6, and Langer 17/18

Reference Sheet: Universal Curet	
Cross Section	Semi-circular
Back	Rounded (rounded back is ideal for subgingival use)
Cutting Edges	Two cutting edges per working-end Edges curve upward at the toe
Toe	Rounded (curved cutting edges and rounded toe enhance adaptation to rounded root surfaces and root concavities)
Face	Perpendicular to the lower shank so that cutting edges are level with one another (level cutting edges mean that the lower shank must be tilted slightly toward the tooth surface to establish correct angulation)
Shank	Complex design Some designs allow access to middle-third of root
Application	Universal use—one double-ended instrument can be used to instrument all tooth surfaces in the dentition
Primary Functions	Debridement of crown and root surfaces Removal of light- to medium-sized calculus deposits
Examples	Columbia 2R/2L; Columbia 13/14; Rule 3/4; Barnhart 1/2; Barnhart 5/6; Younger-Good 7/8; Indiana University 13/14; HU 1/2; Bunting 5/6; Mallery 1/2; Langer 1/2; Langer 3/4; Langer 5/6, and Langer 17/18

Selecting a Universal Curet

There are numerous universal curet designs. In selecting a universal curet for a particular task, the clinician should consider the design characteristics of the working-end and functional shank. To illustrate how the design of the shank and working-ends can influence instrument selection, the photographs below and on the following page compare a Columbia 13/14 and a Barnhart 1/2 universal curet.

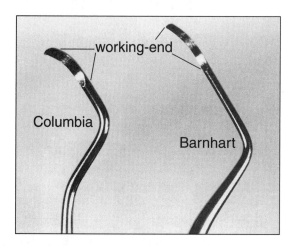

The instrument on the left, the Columbia 13/14, is an example of a universal curet with a short lower shank and a short working-end. The instrument on the right, the Barnhart 1/2, is a universal curet with a longer lower shank and a long working-end.

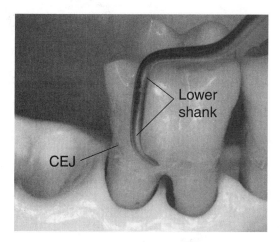

On posterior teeth, its short lower shank limits application of the Columbia 13/14 to normal sulci and shallow pockets.

The Barnhart 1/2 has a longer lower shank that makes it a better choice for instrumenting root surfaces within deeper pockets.

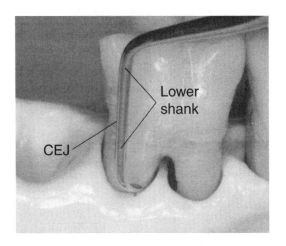

The short working-end of the Columbia 13/14 limits its reach across the proximal surfaces of posterior teeth.

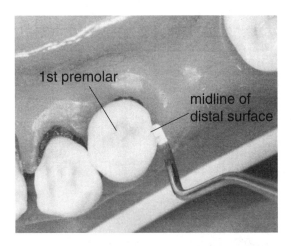

The longer working-end of the Barnhart 1/2 provides better access to the col area of posterior teeth.

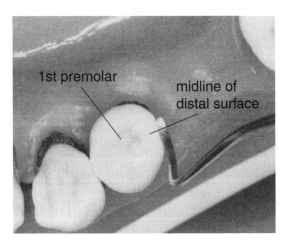

Area-Specific Curets

An **area-specific curet** is a debridement instrument with a rounded back, a rounded toe, and one *working* cutting edge (only one cutting edge per working-end is used for instrumentation). The name **area-specific** signifies that each curet can be applied only to specific surfaces and areas of the mouth. For this reason, a set of curets is needed to instrument the entire mouth. Area-specific curets are used on crown and root surfaces (supragingivally and subgingivally).

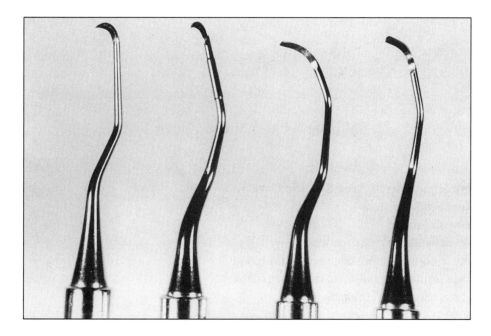

Area-Specific Curets

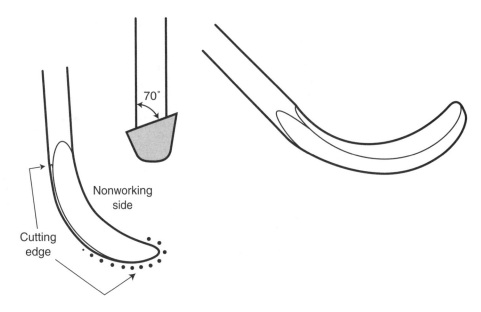

Design of Area-Specific Curets

Design Highlights of Area-Specific Curets:
- Rounded back
- Rounded toe
- Semicircular in cross section
- One working cutting edge per working-end
- Face is tilted in relation to the lower shank
- Long, very complex shank design

Examples of Universal Curets:
Gracey series, Kramer-Nevins series, Turgeon series, After Five Gracey Curette series, Mini Five Gracey Curette series, and Vision Curvette series

Reference Sheet: Area-Specific Curet	
Cross Section	Semi-circular
Back	Rounded (rounded back is ideal for subgingival use)
Cutting Edge	One *working* cutting edge per curet Edge curves upward at the toe
Toe	Rounded (curved cutting edge and rounded toe enhance adaptation to rounded root surfaces and root concavities)
Face	Tilted at a 60-to-70° angle to the lower shank (the working cutting edge is lower than the non-working edge) (This tilted relationship makes the working-end self-angulated. When positioned with the lower shank parallel to the tooth surface being instrumented, the cutting edge is automatically at the correct angulation.)
Shank	Complex design Some designs allow access to apical-third of root
Application	Area-specific, each working-end is limited to use on a specific area or specific tooth surface(s)
Primary Functions	Debridement of crown and root surfaces Removal of light calculus deposits
Examples	Gracey series, Kramer-Nevins series, Turgeon series, After Five Gracey Curette series, Mini Five Gracey Curette series, and Vision Curvette series

Identifying the Working Cutting Edge

On an area-specific curet, only one cutting edge per working-end is used for instrumentation. The second cutting edge is a nonworking edge that is tilted too close to the lower shank for use.

To identify the working cutting edge:
1. Hold your instrument so that you are looking at the toe of the working-end.
2. Raise or lower the instrument handle until the lower shank is perpendicular ($\perp$) to the floor.
3. Look closely at the working-end, note that one of the cutting edges is lower (closer to the floor) than the other.
4. The lower cutting edge is the one that is used for instrumentation (the working cutting edge).

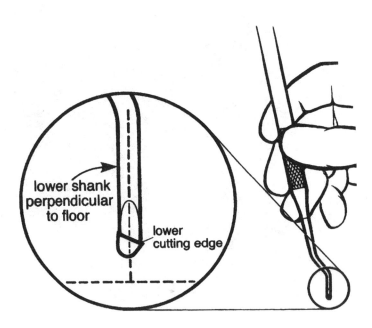

lower shank perpendicular to floor

lower cutting edge

The Gracey Curet Series

Dr. Clayton Gracey developed the first area-specific curet designs in the late 1930s. These curets represented an important breakthrough in instrument design. Dr. Gracey's curets facilitated instrumentation of root surfaces within periodontal pockets without trauma to the pocket epithelium. The Gracey instrument series continues to be popular today and is the basis for several other area-specific curets. Gracey curets are manufactured in standard, prophy, rigid, extended shank, and miniature working-end styles.

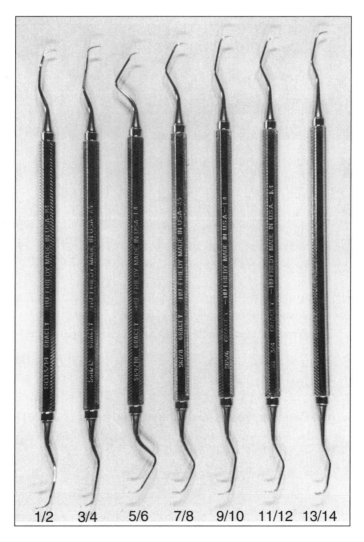

The standard (original) Gracey instrument series designed by Dr. Gracey is comprised of 7 double-ended instruments (or 14 single-ended instruments).

Application of Gracey Curets

The original Gracey series contains 14 curets, Gracey 1—14. In practice, rarely are all 14 curets used on a single patient's mouth. Over the years, clinicians have found that they are able to instrument the mouth using a fewer number of Gracey curets. A set of three Gracey curets usually is adequate to instrument the entire dentition, such as: (1) Gracey 3/4, Gracey 11/12, and Gracey 13/14, (2) Gracey 5/6, Gracey 11/14, and Gracey 12/13, or (3) Gracey 7/8, Gracey 11/12, and Gracey 13/14. Of course, you should not hesitate to use additional Gracey curets if you are having difficulty removing a piece of calculus from a particular surface.

The Gracey Instrument Series	
Curet	**Area of Application**
Gracey 1, 2, 3, and 4	Anterior teeth: all tooth surfaces [G]
Gracey 5 and 6	Anterior teeth: all tooth surfaces [G] Premolar teeth: all tooth surfaces [G] Molar teeth: facial, lingual, and mesial surfaces
Gracey 7, 8, 9, and 10	Anterior teeth: all surfaces Premolar teeth: all surfaces Posterior teeth: facial and lingual surfaces [G]
Gracey 11 and 12	Anterior teeth: mesial and distal surfaces Posterior teeth: mesial surfaces [G] Posterior teeth: facial, lingual, and mesial surfaces
Gracey 13 and 14	Anterior teeth: mesial and distal surfaces Posterior teeth: distal surfaces [G]
Gracey 15 and 16	Posterior teeth: facial, lingual, and mesial surfaces
Gracey 17 and 18	Posterior teeth: distal surfaces

KEY: The [G] symbol indicates the areas of application as originally designated by Dr. Gracey.

The O'Hehir Debridement Series

The O'Hehir Debridement curets are a new type of area-specific curet. The debridement curets are designed to remove light residual calculus deposits and bacterial contaminants from the entire root surface. These instruments are used with gentle stroke pressure with either push or pull strokes in a vertical, oblique, or horizontal direction.

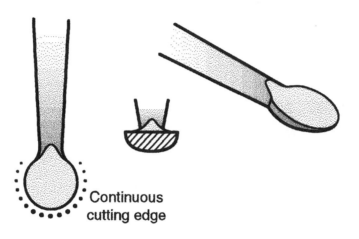

Continuous cutting edge

Characteristics of Debridement Curets	
Working-end	Disc-shaped
Cutting edge	The entire circumference of the working-end
Functional shank	Extended
Application	Area-specific
OH 1/2	Posterior teeth, facial and lingual surfaces
OH 3/4	Posterior teeth, mesial and distal surfaces
OH 5/6	Anterior teeth
OH 7/8	Anterior teeth with deep pockets

Selecting an Area-Specific Curet

Area-specific curets come in a variety of unique design configurations.

Curet	Design Characteristics
Gracey Finishing Series	Original Gracey curets designed by Dr. Clayton Gracey.
Gracey Prophy Series	Shank is shorter and more rigid for increased strength; however, working-end will not reach as far subgingivally because of shorter shank.
Rigid Gracey Series	Shank and working-end more rigid; will remove tenacious deposits. May result in excessive cementum removal if used by inexperienced clinician.
After Five Graceys and Gracey +3 Series	Extended lower shank and thinner working-end. Slim working-end is easier to insert but is not as strong. Extended shank allows access to surfaces 5 mm or more apical to CEJ.
Mini Five Graceys and Gracey +3 Deep Pocket Series	Thin miniature working-end and extended lower shank. Tiny working-end aids in access to root concavities, furcation areas, and midline regions of anterior roots. Thin working-end limited to use on light deposits.
Gracey 11/14 Curet Gracey 12/13 Curet	Changes the way that the Gracey 11, 12, 13, 14 curets are paired. The new pairings allow the clinician to complete the surfaces of an *aspect* without changing instruments. New pairings are more time efficient.
Gracey 15/16 Curet	Modification of Gracey 11/12 with an acutely angled shank for improved access to mesial surfaces of posterior teeth.
Gracey 17/18 Curet	Modification of Gracey 13/14 with an extended, acutely angled shank for improved access to distal surfaces of posterior teeth
Curvette Series	Shorter, more curved working-ends facilitate access to root concavities, furcation areas, and midlines of anterior teeth.
OH Debridement Series	Disc-shaped working-end with a continuous cutting edge; used for root surface debridement and de-plaquing.

Summary Sheet: Design Analysis of Sickle Scalers and Curets

Instruments	Characteristic:	Critique:
Sickle	Back pointed	*Advantage* = strong, "bulky" working-end *Disadvantage* = cannot be used subgingivally
Universal & Area-Specific	Back rounded	*Advantage* = used subgingivally without tissue trauma *Disadvantage* = none
Sickle	Tip (pointed)	*Advantage* = provides good access to proximal surfaces on anterior crowns and enamel surfaces apical to contact areas of posterior teeth *Disadvantage* = sharp point can gouge cemental surfaces
Universal & Area-Specific	Toe (rounded)	*Advantage* = adapts well to convex, rounded root surfaces and root concavities *Disadvantage* = is wider than a pointed tip and, therefore, more difficult to adapt to proximal surfaces of anterior crowns
Sickle	Cutting edge straight	*Advantage* = none *Disadvantage* = adapts poorly to rounded root surfaces and root concavities
Universal & Area-Specific	Cutting edge curves up at the toe	*Advantage* = enhances adaptation to rounded root surfaces and root concavities *Disadvantage* = none
Sickle & Universal	Face perpendicular to lower shank	*Advantage* = efficient, two cutting-edges per working-end both of which can be used for calculus removal *Disadvantage* = level cutting edges mean that the lower shank must be tilted slightly toward the tooth for correct angulation
Area-Specific	Face tilts in relation to lower shank	*Advantage* = working cutting edge is self-angulated *Disadvantage* = only one working cutting edge per working-end means more frequent instrument exchanges

Summary Sheet: Use of Hand-Activated Instruments

Classification	Purpose
Calibrated Probe	Measurement of pocket depths, clinical attachment level, width of attached gingiva, gingival recession, and intraoral lesions. Evaluation of gingival tissue for consistency and presence of bleeding or exudate.
Furcation Probe	Detection of furcation involvement in multirooted teeth.
Explorer	Detection of calculus deposits, tooth surface irregularities, defective margins on restorations, decalcified areas, and carious lesions.
Sickle Scaler	Removal of medium- to large-sized calculus deposits from enamel surfaces. Provides good access to proximal surfaces on anterior crowns and enamel surfaces apical to contact areas of posterior teeth. Usually confined to *supra*gingival use; should NOT be used for root surface debridement.
Periodontal File	Used to crush large calculus deposits and prepare burnished calculus prior to removal with another instrument. Should NOT be used directly on cemental surfaces.
Universal Curet	Debridement of crown and root surfaces. Removal of light- to medium-sized supra- and subgingival calculus deposits. Some designs have long functional shanks that allow access to the cervical- and middle-thirds of root surfaces.
Area-Specific Curet	Debridement of crown and root surfaces. Removal of light supra- and subgingival calculus deposits. Some designs have extended shanks that allow access to the middle-and apical-thirds of root surfaces.

Skill Evaluation: Instrument Design and Classification
(Modules 7 and 8)

Student: _____   Instrument 1 = _____

Evaluator: _____   Instrument 2 = _____

Date: _____   Instrument 3 = _____

Instrument 4 = _____

Instrument 5 = _____

DIRECTIONS: For each instrument, use **Column S** for student self-evaluation and **Column I** for instructor evaluation. For each skill evaluated, indicate the skill level as: **S** (satisfactory), **I** (improvement needed), or **U** (unsatisfactory).

CRITERIA:	1 S	1 I	2 S	2 I	3 S	3 I	4 S	4 I	5 S	5 I
Instrument: Identifies each working-end by its design name and number.										
Determines if the instrument is balanced.										
Working-End: Identifies the classification of each working-end.										
Identifies parts of working-end (face, back, lateral surfaces, tip or toe, cutting edges).										
States the shape of the working-end in cross section.										
On an area-specific curet, identifies the working and nonworking cutting edges.										
Shank: Identifies the functional shank.										
Identifies the lower shank.										
Identifies shank as simple or complex.										

Skill Evaluation: Instrument Design and Classification

Student: _____

Evaluator Comments:

_____

_____

_____

_____

_____

_____

_____

_____

_____

_____

_____

_____

_____

_____

_____

_____

Box for sketches pertaining to written comments.

9

MODULE

Adaptation and Angulation

This module introduces two principles used in positioning the instrument's working-end against the tooth surface prior to the production of an instrumentation stroke. These are the principles of adaptation and angulation.

Required Equipment:

- anterior sickle scaler
- universal curet
- typodont and manikin

Key Terms:

Adaptation   0- to 40-degree angle
Leading-third   Closed angle
Angulation   45- to-90 degree angle
Insertion   Burnished calculus

Section 1: Adaptation

Adaptation is placing the first one or two millimeters of the side of the working-end in contact with the tooth surface.

The first few millimeters of the side of the explorer working-end are adapted against the tooth surface.

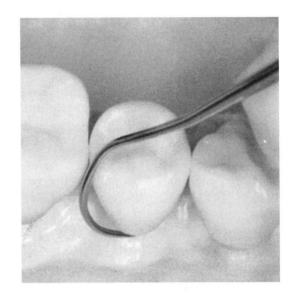

Adaptation of a sickle scaler to the tooth surface.

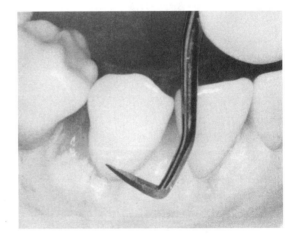

The Leading-Third of the Cutting Edge

The cutting edge has three imaginary sections the 1) leading-third, 2) middle-third, and 3) heel-third. The **leading-third** is the section of the cutting edge that is used most often during instrumentation.

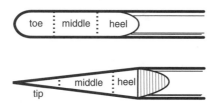

On curets, the leading-third of the cutting edge is the **toe-third**.

On sickle scalers, the leading-third of the cutting edge is the **tip-third**.

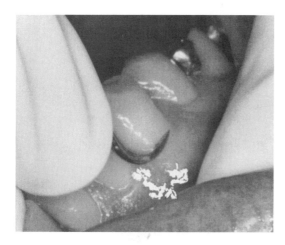

Correct Adaptation
The tip-third of the cutting edge of this sickle scaler is correctly adapted to the tooth surface.

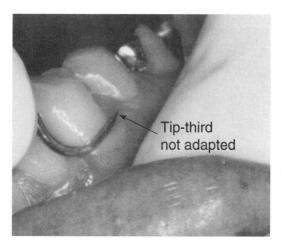

Tip-third not adapted

Incorrect Adaptation
The middle-third of the cutting edge, rather than the tip-third is adapted to the tooth. Note how the instrument tip is sticking out and could cut the soft tissue (ouch!).

Technique Practice: Adaptation

Equipment: anterior sickle scaler, dental typodont, and manikin head

1. Position yourself for the *mandibular anterior sextant, surfaces toward you.*

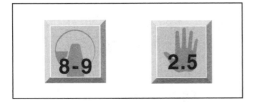
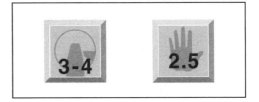

Right-Handed Clinicians   Left-Handed Clinicians

2. **Correct Adaptation**
   Adapt the tip-third of a sickle scaler at the midline of the mandibular canine. Notice that the middle- and heel-thirds of the cutting edge are not in contact with the tooth surface. (Photographs show the surfaces toward a right-handed clinician.)

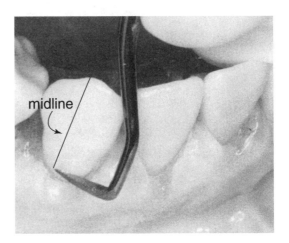

3. **Incorrect Adaptation**
   Now, adapt the middle-third of the cutting edge to the tooth. In this position, the tip-third of the cutting edge is not adapted to the tooth.

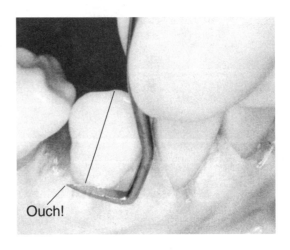

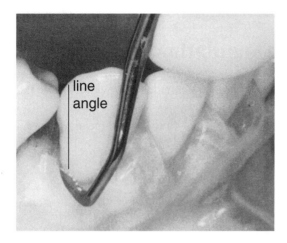

4. **Correct Adaptation**
    Adapt the tip-third of the sickle scaler on the mesiofacial line angle of the canine.

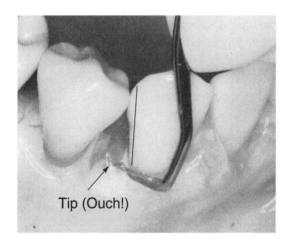

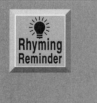

5. **Incorrect Adaptation**
    Adapt the middle-third of the sickle scaler on the mesiofacial line angle of the canine. Can you see why this is not correct technique for adaptation? OUCH!

Rhyming Reminder: Adaptation

Rhyming Reminder

If the leading-third leaves the tooth's side,
my patients just want to run and hide.

When I'm contacting the tooth , I concentrate
so I know I'm not going to lacerate.

Cause if the end of my instrument is not on the tooth,
it's somewhere in soft tissue and that's the truth!

Section 2: Angulation

Angulation is the angle formed between the face of a calculus removal instrument and the tooth surface.
1. For insertion beneath the gingival margin, the face-to-tooth surface angulation should be an angle *between 0- and 40-degrees.*
2. For calculus removal, the face-to-tooth surface angulation should be an angle *between 45-and 90-degrees.*

For Insertion Beneath the Gingival Margin

Insertion is the action of moving the working-end beneath the gingival margin into the sulcus or pocket. Care must be used during insertion when the gingival margin is closely adapted to the tooth. Curets are the primary calculus removal instruments for subgingival instrumentation. The working-end is inserted at an angle between 0- and 40-degrees. This 0-to-40° angle is referred to as a **closed angle**.

For insertion, the instrument face should be positioned in a closed angle. In this position, the curet is moved gently beneath the gingival margin down the surface of the root.

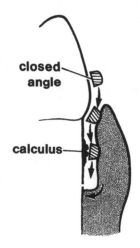

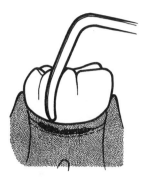

Position the working-end with the toe pointed toward the gingival margin. Keeping the face as close to the tooth as possible, slide the toe beneath the gingival margin.

For Calculus Removal

For calculus removal, it is vital to establish the correct angle between the instrument face and the tooth surface.

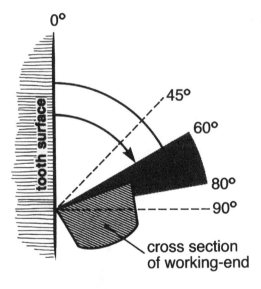

Angulation for Calculus Removal

The *face-to-tooth* angulation for calculus removal is an angle that is greater than 45-degrees and less than 90-degrees.

Incorrect Angulation—angle greater than 90-degrees

The face is tilted away from the tooth surface. In this position, calculus removal will be difficult and tissue trauma is likely.

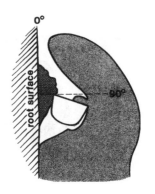

Incorrect Angulation—angle less than 45-degrees

The face is tilted too close to the tooth surface. The cutting edge will slip over the calculus deposit.

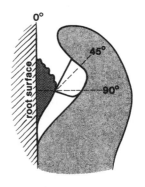

Incorrect angulation will result in a **burnished calculus deposit** (a calculus deposit that has had the outermost layer removed). A burnished deposit has a smooth outer surface and therefore, is more difficult to remove.

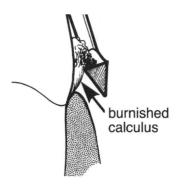

burnished calculus

Technique Practice: Angulation

Equipment: universal curet, dental typodont, and manikin head

1. If you are **right-handed**, position yourself for the *mandibular right posterior sextant, facial aspect*. If you are **left-handed**, position yourself for the *mandibular left posterior sextant, facial aspect*.

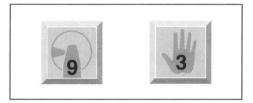

Right-Handed Clinicians

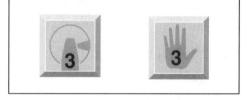

Left-Handed Clinicians

2. Ask your instructor to help you identify the correct working-end of a universal curet for use on this treatment area. (You will learn to identify the correct working-end yourself in a later module.)

3. Establish a finger rest and adapt the toe-third of the cutting edge to the facial surface of the mandibular second premolar.

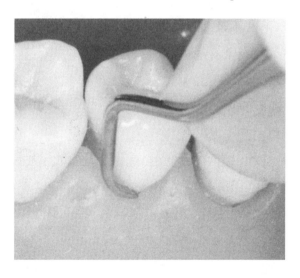

4. **Establish Angulation**
   Establish a face-to-tooth angulation that is between 45- and 90-degrees. An angulation of about 80-degrees usually is used for calculus removal. (Photographs show a right-handed clinician.)

5. **Preparation for Insertion**
   Reposition the working-end at the distofacial line angle. Position the working-end so that the toe is pointing toward the gingival margin. You will have to lower your hand and the instrument handle to obtain this position.

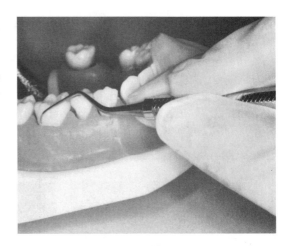

6. **Insertion**
   Maintaining your hand position, gently slide the toe of the curet beneath the gingival margin. Continue until the entire length of the working-end is beneath the gingival margin.

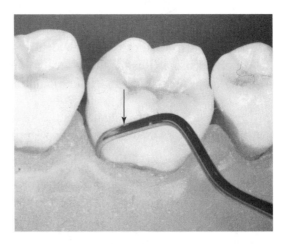

7. **Establish Adaptation and Angulation**
   Reposition your hand and re-establish your finger rest. Adapt the toe-third of the curet to the facial surface. Establish correct angulation.

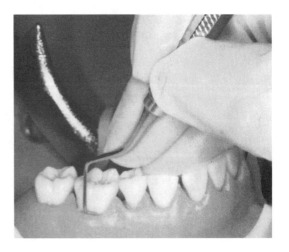

Skill Evaluation: Adaptation and Angulation

Student: _____

Evaluator: _____

Date: _____

DIRECTIONS: Use **Column S** for student self-evaluation and **Column I** for instructor evaluation. For each skill evaluated, indicate the skill level as: **S** (satisfactory), **I** (improvement needed), or **U** (unsatisfactory).

CRITERIA:	S	I
Identifies the 1) tip-third or toe-third, 2) middle-third, and 3) heel-third of the cutting edge on a sickle scaler and a universal curet.		
Using a typodont, demonstrates a face-to-tooth angulation of 0– to 40-degrees (for insertion).		
Using a typodont, demonstrates a face-to-tooth angulation of less than 45-degrees (incorrect angulation).		
Using a typodont, demonstrates a face-to-tooth angulation of 90-degrees (incorrect angulation).		
Using a typodont, demonstrates a face-to-tooth angulation between 45- and 90-degrees (correct angulation for calculus removal).		
Using a typodont and an anterior sickle scaler, adapts the tip-third of the cutting edge to a canine and establishes correct face-to-tooth angulation.		
Using a typodont and a curet, demonstrates insertion of a curet beneath the gingival margin.		

Skill Evaluation: Adaptation and Angulation

Student: _____

Evaluator Comments:

_____

_____

_____

_____

_____

_____

_____

_____

_____

_____

_____

_____

_____

_____

_____

_____

_____

Box for sketches pertaining to written comments.

10
MODULE

Activation, Pivot, and Handle Roll

This module introduces the techniques used during the production of an instrumentation stroke: motion activation, the hand pivot, and handle roll. The first section discusses how to move the instrument to produce a stroke. The second section explains how to pivot the hand and roll the instrument handle to maintain adaptation as the working-end moves around the tooth.

General recommendations for stroke production may not be suitable for everyone. If you experience any discomfort, consult a physician.

Key Terms:

Motion activation
Hand pivot
Handle roll

Section 1: Moving the Working-End

Motion activation refers to moving the instrument in order to produce an instrumentation stroke. Two types of motion activation commonly are used in periodontal instrumentation, hand-forearm motion activation and digital motion activation.

When moving (**activating**) an instrument, the weight of your hand will be supported by your fulcrum finger. Once you initiate (begin) a stroke, you should press down with your fulcrum finger against the tooth; this action allows the fulcrum to function as a "brake" to allow you to stop the stroke. If you fly off the tooth at the end of a stroke, you did not stop the stroke by pressing down on your fulcrum.

Regardless of the type of motion activation being used, it is important to remember that instrumentation strokes are tiny movements. You only move the working-end a few millimeters with each stroke. On the following pages, you will practice using hand-forearm motion activation and digital motion activation. In the technique practice, the movements you will make will be broad, large movements when compared with the actual movements used to instrument a tooth.

Hand-Forearm Motion Activation

Hand-forearm motion activation is the act of rotating the hand and forearm as a unit to provide the power for an instrumentation stroke. The movement is a rotating motion similar to the action of turning a doorknob. Hand-forearm motion activation is recommended for calculus removal with hand-activated instruments. This type of motion activation allows the clinician to use the power of the hand and arm to move the instrument. Together, the hand and arm are stronger than the fingers. You will experience less fatigue with hand-forearm activation than would occur if you used your fingers to move the instrument for calculus removal.

Technique Practice: Hand-Forearm Motion Activation

Hand-forearm motion activation is similar to the action of turning a doorknob.

1. Grasp a pencil with a modified pen grasp in your *dominant hand*. The photographs show a right-handed clinician.
2. Place your ring finger on a countertop. Your thumb, middle, and index fingers should be in a curved position and relaxed. Your ring finger is straight and acts as a support beam for your hand.
3. Grasp a pencil in a modified pen grasp and establish a finger rest on a countertop. The pencil tip should be touching the countertop and the long axis of the pencil should be perpendicular ($\perp$) to the countertop. Your wrist should be in neutral position so that the back of your hand and wrist are in straight alignment and your arm is parallel ($=$) to the countertop.
4. The photograph below shows the starting position, **Position A**, when viewed from behind.
5. Use hand-forearm motion activation to move the pencil tip off of the counter, by rotating your hand and arm away from your body into **Position B** shown below. Right-handed clinicians will rotate the hand and arm to the right in a clockwise direction. Left-handed clinicians will rotate the hand and arm to the left in a counter-clockwise direction. Your ring finger should remain motionless pressing down against the countertop.
6. Return the pencil to **Position A** by rotating your hand and arm back toward your body.

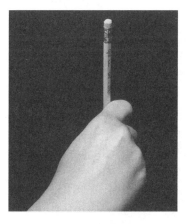

Position A. Starting position, your hand and arm as viewed from behind.

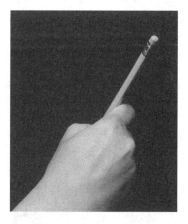

Position B. Finishing position of your hand and arm.

Digital Motion Activation

Digital motion activation is created by flexing your fingers to move the instrument. Digital motion activation is used whenever physical strength is not required during instrumentation. It may be used with periodontal probes and explorers or for calculus removal with *mechanized instruments*. With mechanized instruments, the machine, rather than the clinician, provides the force necessary for calculus removal. Digital motion activation also may be used to instrument areas where movement is restricted, such as when instrumenting furcation areas.

Technique Practice: Digital Motion Activation
Digital motion activation is made with pull-push motions of the thumb, index and middle fingers.

1. Grasp a pencil with a modified pen grasp in your *dominant hand*.
2. Assume the starting position, **Position A**. (The photographs show a right-handed clinician.)
3. Use digital motion activation to pull the pencil tip away from the countertop by pulling your thumb, index and middle fingers toward the palm of your hand into **Position B**. Your ring finger should remain motionless pressing down against the countertop.
4. Return the pencil tip to **Position A** by pushing downward with your thumb, index and middle fingers. Note that you have little strength when using this type of motion activation.

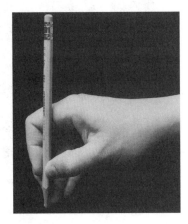
Position A. Starting position.

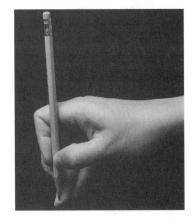
Position B. Finishing position.

Section 2: Maintaining Adaptation

Hand Pivot

Pivoting is turning the hand and arm slightly, as a unit, while resting on the fulcrum. Pivoting the hand and arm assists the clinician in maintaining adaptation as the working-end moves around the tooth. Neutral wrist position should be maintained during the pivot. Pivoting is used principally when moving around line angles and onto proximal surfaces.

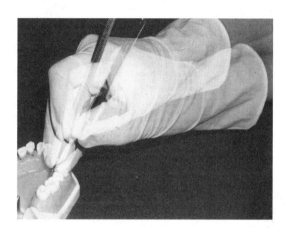

As the clinician moves from instrumenting the lingual surface and onto the proximal, he or she pivots on the fulcrum to aid in adaptation.

Technique Practice: Pivoting

RIGHT-Handed clinicians should use the illustration on the *top* of page 234 for practice. *LEFT-Handed clinicians* should use the illustration at the *bottom* of page 234 for practice.

1. Grasp a pencil in a modified pen grasp and establish a fulcrum in the circle on the illustration. Touch the pencil point to the "**X**" on the illustration.
2. Begin with your hand and arm aligned with dotted line **A**.
3. Push down lightly on your fulcrum as you pivot your hand and arm as a unit to align with dotted line **B**. Be sure to maintain neutral wrist position.

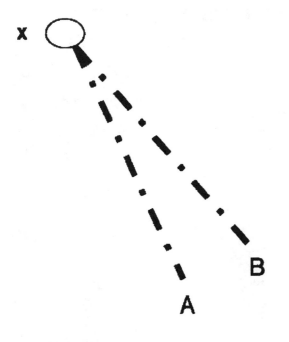

RIGHT-Handed Clinician

LEFT-Handed Clinician

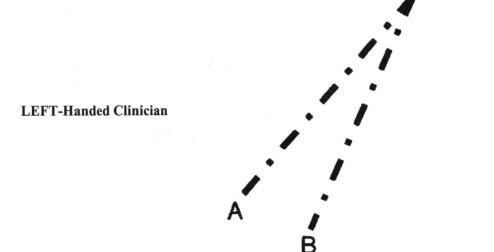

Handle Roll

As the instrumentation strokes advance around the tooth surface, the working-end constantly is readjusted to maintain adaptation with the tooth surface. These readjustments are accomplished by rolling the instrument handle between strokes. The **handle roll** is the act of turning the instrument handle slightly between the thumb and index finger to readapt the working-end to the next segment of the tooth. Either the index finger *or* the thumb acts as the **drive finger** to turn the instrument. The finger used to roll the handle determines the direction in which the working-end will turn.

Technique Practice: Handle Roll

This Technique Practice is designed to help you learn how to use your thumb and index finger to roll an instrument. Begin by using a pen or pencil which will allow you to develop muscle control without the strain of holding a heavier metal instrument. The lettering on the pen or pencil also provides a visual reference point as it turns. Do five repetitions of this activity each day until you are able to control the rolling motion in a precise manner in both clockwise and counter-clockwise directions.

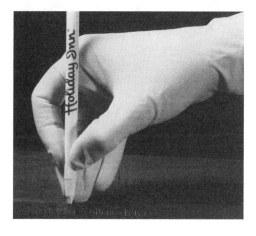

1. Establish a finger rest on a textbook and allow the tip of the pen to extend over the side of the book.

    Grasp the pen so that the lettering is visible between your index finger and thumb.

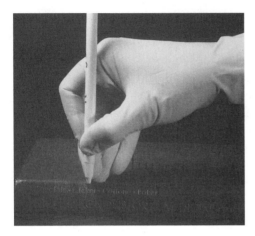

2.   Roll the pen in a clockwise direction between your index finger and thumb until the lettering is no longer visible.

Does your index finger or your thumb act as the drive finger to turn the instrument in a clockwise direction?

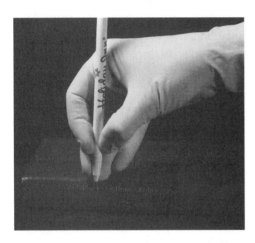

3.   Finally, turn the pen in a counter-clockwise direction, back toward the starting position. Continue rolling until the handle has returned to the original starting position.

Does your index finger or your thumb act as the drive finger to turn the instrument in a counter-clockwise direction?

Rhyming Reminder

Rhyming Reminder: Activation

When you activate you learn to move your hand
to and fro and side to side and with a special plan.
The hand functions as a unit with the arm you see,
And the wrist never moves independently.

Section 3: Activities and Evaluation

Skill Building Activity #1

Equipment: an inexpensive pen, an anterior instrument, a pad of paper

1. Draw a line around the pen about 6 mm from the top of the pen (see photographs below).
2. Sit in a comfortable seated position with your thighs parallel to the floor and feet touching the floor.
3. Lay the paper tablet on your lap. Hold the pen with your non-dominant hand as shown in the photograph below. Rest the pen point on the paper. The pen represents the tooth.
4. Grasp an anterior instrument and establish a finger rest on the edge of the pen top.

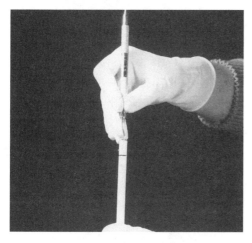 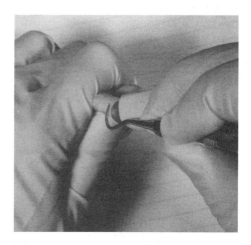

5. Adapt the leading-third of the cutting edge just above the line on the pen. Look down at the pen top and tilt the instrument face toward the pen until the face meets the pen's surface at a 70-80° angle.
6. Use hand-forearm motion to make a short stroke up the surface of the pen.
7. Make a series of strokes around the circumference of the pen, beginning each stroke near the line on pen. Roll the instrument handle in order to keep the leading-third of the cutting edge adapted to the pen.

Skill Building Activity #2

Equipment: a pencil with an eraser.

1. Use a pen to draw a *vertical line* on the eraser. The line should run vertically from the base of the eraser to the top of the eraser. In this activity you will try to adapt the vertical mark to the abstract design below.
2. Hold the pencil in a modified pen grasp. Assume that the vertical mark is the cutting edge of the instrument.
3. *Right-handed clinicians*: Establish a finger rest near the fourth dot from the letter **R**. You will be working from left to right on the design, beginning near the letter **R** and moving toward the letter **L**. *Left-handed clinicians*: Establish a finger rest near the fourth dot from the letter **L**. You will be working from right to left on the design, beginning near the letter **L** and moving toward the letter **R**.
4. Touch the vertical mark on the eraser to the first point on the line. If you are right-handed, this will be the first point beside the letter **R**. If you are left-handed, this will be the first point beside the letter **L**.
5. While maintaining your fulcrum, use hand-forearm motion activation to lift the eraser off of the paper. *Right-handed clinicians*: slide your finger rest slightly to the right. *Left-handed clinicians*: slide your finger rest slightly to the left.
6. Still holding the eraser off the paper, roll the pencil slightly between your index finger and thumb until the mark is directly above the second point on the abstract design. Return the eraser to the paper so that the mark is adapted to this point. Continue to slide your finger rest as you move along the design, adapting the mark to each point.

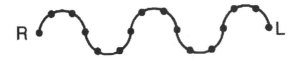

Skill Evaluation: Motion Activation and Handle Roll

Student: _____

Evaluator: _____

Date: _____

DIRECTIONS: Use **Column S** for student self-evaluation and **Column I** for instructor evaluation. For each skill evaluated, indicate the skill level as: **S** (satisfactory), **I** (improvement needed), or **U** (unsatisfactory).

CRITERIA:	S	I
Defines **motion activation**.		
States uses of hand-forearm motion activation.		
States uses of digital motion activation.		
Defines **pivoting**.		
Defines **handle roll**.		
Defines **drive finger**.		

Uses a pencil to demonstrate hand-forearm motion activation.
    Uses modified pen grasp.
    Uses ring finger as a support beam.
    Maintains neutral wrist position.		

Uses a pencil to demonstrate digital motion activation.
    Uses modified pen grasp.
    Uses ring finger as a support beam.
    Maintains neutral wrist position.		

Uses a pencil and the illustration on page 233 to demonstrate pivoting.		

Uses a pencil to demonstrate rolling the handle in clockwise and counter-clockwise directions.
    Uses modified pen grasp.
    Uses ring finger as a support beam.
    Maintains neutral wrist position.		

Skill Evaluation: Motion Activity and Handle Roll

Student: _____

Evaluator Comments:

_____

_____

_____

_____

_____

_____

_____

_____

_____

_____

_____

_____

_____

_____

_____

_____

_____

_____

Box for sketches pertaining to written comments.

Instrumentation Strokes

This module will introduce you to the instrumentation stroke and the principles employed in its production.

Key Terms:

Assessment stroke   Instrumentation zone
Calculus removal work stroke   Stabilization and lateral pressure
Root debridement work stroke   Parallelism

Section 1: Types of Instrumentation Strokes

The four types of instrumentation strokes are the placement stroke, assessment stroke, calculus removal work stroke, and root debridement work stroke. The **placement stroke** is used to position the working-end of an instrument apical to a calculus deposit or at the base of a sulcus or pocket. The placement stroke is used with light contact against the tooth surface while positioning the working-end.

Assessment strokes are used to evaluate the tooth surface for anatomic characteristics, and for the presence of calculus deposits and plaque-retentive factors. Another name for the assessment stroke is the **exploratory stroke**. Assessment strokes are used with periodontal probes to determine periodontal pocket depths and the clinical attachment level of the junctional epithelium. Assessment strokes are used with explorers and curets to locate calculus deposits or other tooth surface irregularities hidden beneath the gingival margin. An explorer provides the clinician with the best tactile information regarding the location of subgingival calculus deposits. For this reason, an explorer is recommended for the initial detection of calculus deposits. During periodontal debridement, curets are used both for calculus removal and to locate calculus deposits. Using curets in this manner is more efficient than changing back and forth between an explorer and a curet during calculus removal. When no deposits can be detected with the curet, an explorer is used to thoroughly re-assess the root surface for any remaining calculus deposits or other irregularities.

The **calculus removal work stroke** is used with sickle scalers and curets. As its name suggests, the calculus removal work stroke is used to remove calculus deposits. With hand-activated instruments, this stroke is used with moderate to firm pressure against the tooth to fracture calculus deposits from its surface.

Root debridement work strokes are used to remove residual calculus deposits, bacterial plaque and byproducts from root surfaces. Bacterial plaque and its byproducts are cytotoxic to tissue and must be removed in order for healing to occur. Bacterial byproducts adhere loosely to the root surface and may be removed with light pressure. The conservation of cementum is a goal of root surface debridement. Other terms for the "root debridement work stroke" are the **smoothing** or **finishing stroke**. Root debridement work strokes are used with curets. These strokes are applied over the entire root surface using light pressure.

Reference Sheet: Stroke Characteristics

Stroke Characteristics With Hand-Activated Instruments			
	Assessment Stroke	**Calculus Removal Work Strokes**	**Root Debridement Work Stroke**
Purpose	assess tooth anatomy/level of attachment; detect calculus and other plaque-retentive factors	remove calculus deposits	remove residual calculus; remove or disrupt bacterial plaque and byproducts
Used with	probes/explorers, curets	sickle scalers, curets, files	curets
Insertion	0° to 40°	0° to 40°	0° to 40°
Working angulation	50° to 70°	70° to 80°	60° to 70°
Lateral pressure	contacts tooth surface, but no pressure	moderate to firm; scraping	light to moderate
Character	fluid strokes of moderate length	powerful strokes; short in length	lighter strokes of moderate length
Direction	vertical, oblique, and horizontal	vertical, oblique, and horizontal	vertical, oblique and horizontal
Number	many, covering entire root surface	limited to areas where needed	many, covering entire root surface

Section 2: Stroke Direction and Pattern

Stroke Direction

Instrumentation strokes are initiated using a **pull** stroke in a coronal direction away from the junctional epithelium. Pull strokes may be made in vertical, oblique, or horizontal directions.

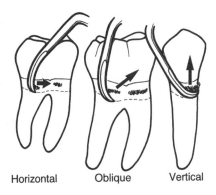

Horizontal   Oblique   Vertical

Stroke Directions. Instrumentation strokes are made in horizontal, oblique, and vertical directions.

Vertical strokes are used on the facial, lingual, and proximal surfaces of anterior teeth and on the mesial and distal surfaces of posterior teeth.

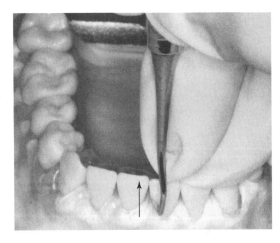

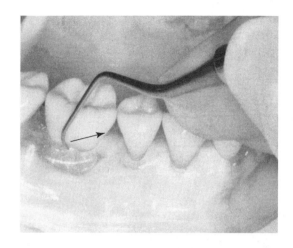

Oblique strokes are used most commonly on the *facial and lingual* surfaces of anterior and posterior teeth.

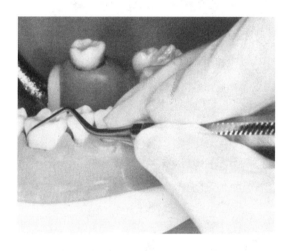

Horizontal strokes are used at the line angles of posterior teeth, furcation crotch areas, and in areas that are too narrow to allow vertical or oblique strokes. Horizontal strokes are also called "**circumferential strokes**".

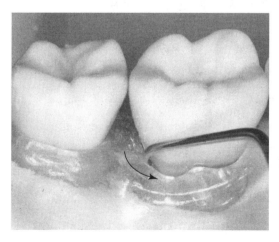

For a horizontal stroke, the handle is positioned diagonal or perpendicular to the long axis of the tooth. The working-end is oriented in a **toe-down** position with the instrument toe pointed toward the base of the sulcus or pocket.

The *facial and lingual surfaces* of anterior teeth are difficult to instrument because these teeth have a narrow mesial-distal width. Horizontal strokes are very effective in instrumenting these narrow root surfaces.

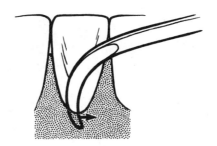

The working-end is used in a toe-down position. Short, controlled horizontal strokes are made across the tooth surface.

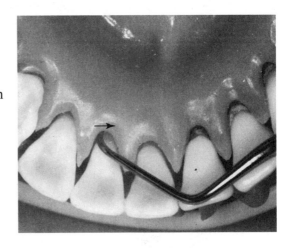

Stroke Directions on Anterior and Posterior Teeth		
Tooth Surface	**Primary**	**Secondary**
Mesial and distal surfaces	vertical	horizontal, oblique
Facial and lingual surfaces	oblique	vertical, horizontal
Line angles	horizontal	oblique, vertical
Facial or lingual root surfaces of anteriors	horizontal	vertical
Furcation crotch areas	horizontal	vertical
Narrow pockets	horizontal	vertical

Multidirectional Instrumentation Strokes

Three stroke directions should be used when assessing and instrumenting a subgingival tooth surface. Use each of the three stroke directions, one-by-one in succession, to create a multidirectional stroke pattern. For example, the clinician might begin by using vertical strokes, then oblique strokes, followed by horizontal strokes.

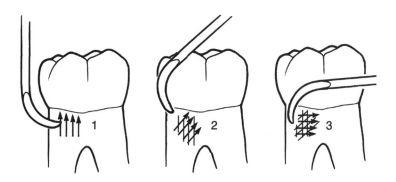

Stroke Pattern

Often a calculus deposit will be too large to be removed in one piece. Large calculus deposits should be removed in sections using a series of short, firm instrumentation strokes. The deposit should not be removed in layers since removing the outermost layer will leave the deposit with a smooth surface. A calculus deposit that has had the outermost layer removed is referred to as a **burnished deposit**. Burnished calculus is difficult to remove since the cutting edge will tend to slip over the smooth surface of the deposit.

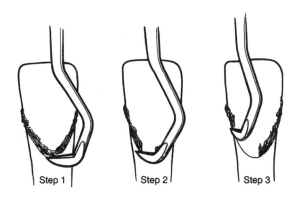

Pattern for removal of a large supragingival deposit.

Removing subgingival calculus deposits is a challenging task since the clinician is working beneath the gingival margin and cannot see the actual root surface. For this reason, the clinician must adopt a very systematic pattern of instrumentation strokes. A haphazard stroke pattern will result in sections not being instrumented and unsuccessful treatment of the root surface.

It is helpful to think of the root surface as being divided into a series of long narrow **instrumentation zones**. Each instrumentation zone is only as wide as the toe-third of the instrument's cutting edge.

The steps in employing instrumentation strokes in a series of narrow tracts is as follows:

1. Imagine that the root surface is divided into narrow tracts or instrumentation zones.
2. Begin in "instrumentation zone #1". Deposits adjacent to the junctional epithelium are removed first. Continue working in a coronal direction until all deposits in zone #1 have been removed.
3. Once you have completed zone #1, repeat the process in zone #2. Continue instrumenting each narrow zone in a similar manner until all zones on this aspect of the tooth have been completed.

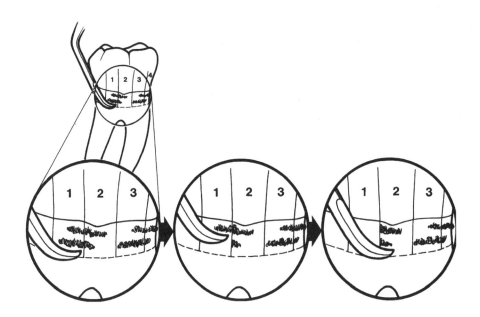

Pattern for subgingival calculus removal.

Section 3: Stabilization and Lateral Pressure

Two techniques used during the production of an instrumentation stroke are stabilization and lateral pressure. **Stabilization** is the act of preparing the ring finger for an instrumentation stroke. Stabilization provides the control necessary for calculus removal. **Lateral pressure** is the act of using the thumb and index finger to engage (press) the cutting edge against the tooth surface or calculus deposit prior to and throughout an instrumentation stroke.

Preparation for Instrumentation Stroke

Fulcrum finger held straight, supporting weight of hand

↓

Fulcrum finger presses against occlusal or incisal surface

↓

Index finger and thumb apply pressure inward against handle

↓

Cutting edge is engaged against tooth surface

Technique

A combination of stabilization and lateral pressure is used to produce a stroke that is at once effective and controlled, yet, comfortable for the patient. This combination is accomplished by using these steps:

1. The grasp is **stabilized** prior to the instrumentation stroke by:
    (a) locking the joints of the fulcrum finger and supporting the weight of the hand on the tip of the fulcrum finger (fulcrum finger acting as a support beam), and
    (b) pressing the tip of the fulcrum finger against the tooth surface. The extent of this pressure ranges from light to firm depending upon the type of stroke

used. If the working-end flies off the tooth at the end of a stroke, the clinician is not pressing down against the tooth with the fulcrum finger as the stroke is finished.

2. **Lateral pressure** is created by:
   (a) applying pressure with the *index finger and thumb* inward against the instrument handle. Both fingers must apply pressure equally against the handle or the instrument will be difficult to control, and by
   (b) maintaining pressure against the tooth surface throughout the stroke.

Amount of Pressure

The instrument classification and instrumentation task will determine the amount of pressure needed during instrumentation. More pressure applied by the fulcrum finger against the tooth results in more pressure against the tooth surface or calculus deposit. Pressure with the fulcrum finger against the tooth surface will range from light to firm; however, heavy pressure is never recommended.

Stabilization and Lateral Pressure Related to Task		
Task	**Stroke Against Tooth**	**Against Handle**
Assessment	Light	Very light
Deplaquing	Light	Light
Calculus removal	Firm , but not heavy	Moderate (not "choking")

Relaxing Between Strokes

The techniques of stabilization and lateral pressure are used only immediately prior to beginning a work stroke and during the production of a work stroke. The finger muscles should be relaxed between work strokes and when using a placement stroke to return the working-end to the base of the sulcus or pocket. Maintaining constant pressure with the fulcrum finger or when grasping the handle is very stressful to the muscles of the hand and wrist.

Rhyming Reminders

Stabilized Fulcrum

When I instrument I have a finger rest.
If you do not use it, you fail the test.

If I fail the test, it is easy to see why,
when I try to work, off the tooth I fly.

I've learned to use the finger rest as a brake.
It offsets the pressure when I activate.

I call it "my support beam", it is where I lean.
It keeps me from slipping, if you know what I mean!

Parallelism

To be parallel to a tooth, not everyone knows,
that you really line up the way the tooth grows.

If you cuddle the shank close against the tooth face,
your cutting edge surely won't be in the right place!

Some people head right for the gums I heard.
First, I line up for parallelism at the middle third.

I take parallelism seriously as it does dictate
where the cutting edge is when you activate

Section 4: Parallelism and Shank Position

Parallelism is the technique of positioning the lower shank so that it is parallel to the tooth surface being instrumented.

This illustration shows a molar, looking at the *mesial surface*. The height of contour on the lingual surface is labeled.

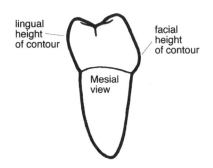

Note that the height on contour on the lingual surface is in the middle-third of the crown. The middle-third of the crown protrudes out over the cervical-third of the crown and the root surface.

The lower shank should be positioned parallel to an imaginary line drawn from the height of contour to the root surface

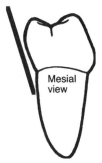

Alignment for lingual surface.

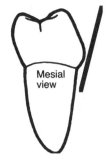

Alignment for facial surface.

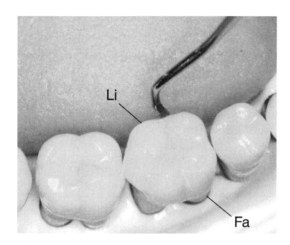

Li

Fa

Occlusal view

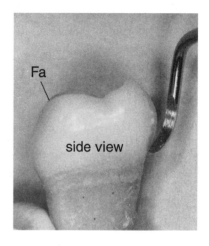

Fa

side view

Proximal view

Correct shank position. The instrument is correctly positioned with the lower shank parallel to the lingual surface of the molar. Note that the lower shank does NOT touch the lingual surface.

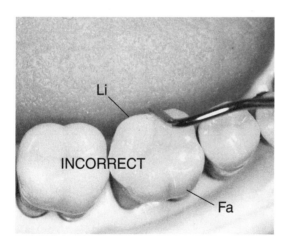

Li

INCORRECT

Fa

Occlusal view

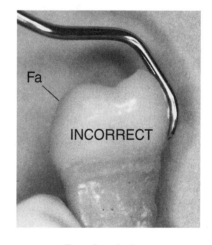

Fa

INCORRECT

Proximal view

Incorrect shank position. The instrument is incorrectly positioned so that the lower shank is touching the lingual surface and tilted toward the occlusal surface. In this position it is not possible to make an effective instrumentation stroke, in fact the instrument face rather than the cutting edge is in contact with the lingual surface.

Section 5: Stroke Production

The skills discussed in Modules 9 to 11 are combined to produce an instrumentation stroke. Those skills include adaptation, angulation, activation, pivot, handle roll, stabilization, lateral pressure, and parallelism.

Reference Sheet: Basic Steps in Stroke Production

Establish a FINGER REST (finger acting as a support beam)

↓

Position lower shank PARALLEL to the tooth surface

↓

INSERT working-end to the junctional epithelium

↓

ADAPT the toe-third of the cutting edge

↓

Establish ANGULATION between 45-to-90 degrees

↓

FINE-TUNE your position, grasp, and finger rest

↓

STABILIZE your grasp and apply LATERAL PRESSURE

↓

ACTIVATE a pull stroke away from the junctional epithelium

↓

At end of stroke, PAUSE BRIEFLY and RELAX muscles

Skill Evaluation: Instrumentation Strokes

Student: _____

Evaluator: _____

Date: _____

DIRECTIONS: Use **Column S** for student self-evaluation and **Column I** for instructor evaluation. For each skill evaluated, indicate the skill level as: **S** (satisfactory), **I** (improvement needed), or **U** (unsatisfactory).

CRITERIA:	S	I
States the characteristics and function of a **placement** stroke.		
States the characteristics and function of an **assessment** stroke.		
States the characteristics and function of a **calculus removal work stroke**.		
States the characteristics and function of a **root debridement work stroke**.		
Using a typodont and an anterior instrument demonstrates **vertical** strokes.		
Using a typodont and an anterior instrument demonstrates **oblique** strokes.		
Using a typodont and an anterior instrument demonstrates **horizontal** strokes.		
Describes the use of **multidirectional instrumentation strokes** and their importance in subgingival instrumentation.		
Using a typodont and an anterior instrument demonstrates **stabilization** in preparation for an instrumentation stroke.		
Using a typodont and an anterior instrument demonstrates **lateral pressure** during an instrumentation stroke.		
Using a typodont and a posterior instrument demonstrates **parallelism** of the lower shank to the lingual surface of a mandibular molar.		

Skill Evaluation: Instrumentation Strokes

Student: _____

Evaluator Comments:

_____

_____

_____

_____

_____

_____

_____

_____

_____

_____

_____

_____

_____

_____

_____

_____

_____

Box for sketches pertaining to written comments.

12

MODULE

Periodontal Probes

This module contains step-by-step instructions for probing and describes the types of assessments that are made using periodontal probes. The design characteristics of periodontal probes were presented in Module 8, Classification of Hand-Activated Instruments. Refer to this module if you need to review this information.

Required Equipment:

- dental mirror, calibrated and furcation probes
- protective attire, meeting OSHA Standards for the clinician and patient

Key Terms:

Calibrated probe
Furcation probe
Clinical finding
Junctional epithelium
Biologic width
Col
Sulcus
Periodontal pocket

Gingival recession
Probing
Walking stroke
Probing depth
Clinical attachment level
PSR
Mobility

Section 1: Introduction to Probing

Terminology

This section contains terminology used in this module. Some of the terms will be familiar while others may be new to you.

A **calibrated probe** is a type of periodontal probe that is marked in millimeter increments and is used in assessing the periodontal health of the tissues.

A **furcation probe** is a type of periodontal probe used to evaluate bone support in the furcation areas of multirooted teeth.

A **line angle** is the angle formed by the junction of two tooth surfaces (where two tooth surfaces meet). Line angles are designated by combining the names of the surfaces that form the angle. For example, the line angle formed by the junction of the mesial and facial surfaces is called the *mesiofacial* line angle.

The **proximal surfaces** of a tooth are the mesial and distal surfaces of the tooth. Instead of saying: "*probe the mesial and distal surfaces of the anterior teeth*", you could say: "*probe the proximal surfaces of the anterior teeth*".

The **facial aspect** is the cheek- or lip-side of a tooth. The facial aspect includes half of the distal surface, the facial surface, and half of the mesial surface.

The **lingual aspect** is the tongue-side of a tooth. The lingual aspect includes half of the distal surface, the lingual surface, and half of the mesial surface.

A **clinical finding** refers to the visual observation or measurement of a condition in the mouth.

The **junctional epithelium** is a thin layer of epithelium that forms the base of a sulcus or periodontal pocket and provides the epithelial attachment to the tooth surface.

The **biologic width** of the gingival attachment is the distance from the base of a sulcus or pocket to the crest of the alveolar bone. This distance is approximately 1.7 mm in width.

The **col** is the nonkeratinized interdental tissue that lies beneath (apical to) the interproximal contact area of two adjacent teeth.

The **sulcus** is the shallow space between the inner aspect of the free gingiva and the tooth. Sulci, by definition, have probing depths that measure from 0.5 to 3 mm in depth.

A **periodontal pocket** is a diseased sulcus that has been deepened by the apical migration of the junctional epithelium along the root surface and destruction of the periodontal ligament and alveolar bone. Periodontal pockets have probing depths measuring 4 mm or greater in depth.

Gingival recession exists when the gingival margin is located *apical to* the cementoenamel junction (CEJ). The presence of recession indicates apical migration of the junctional epithelium.

Probing is the act of activating a calibrated probe within a sulcus or periodontal pocket for the purpose of assessing the health status of the tissue.

A **walking stroke** is the movement of a calibrated probe within a sulcus or pocket. Walking strokes are used to cover the entire circumference of the junctional epithelium. These strokes are short, 1-2 mm in length, and only 1 mm apart.

A **probing depth** is a measurement of the depth of a sulcus or periodontal pocket. It is determined by measuring the distance from the gingival margin to the base of the sulcus or pocket with a calibrated probe.

The **clinical attachment level** is a measurement of the apical migration of the epithelial attachment. It is determined by measuring the distance from the cementoenamel junction (CEJ) to the base of the sulcus or pocket with a calibrated probe.

The **Periodontal Screening and Recording System (PSR)** is an efficient easy-to-use system for the detection of periodontal disease.

Mobility is the movement of a tooth within its socket.

Uses of Periodontal Probes

The periodontal probe is the most important clinical tool for obtaining information about the health status of the periodontium. Calibrated periodontal probes are used to gather information about the health of the gingival tissues, bone loss, and to measure the size of intraoral lesions. Furcation probes are used to obtain information regarding bone loss in furcation areas.

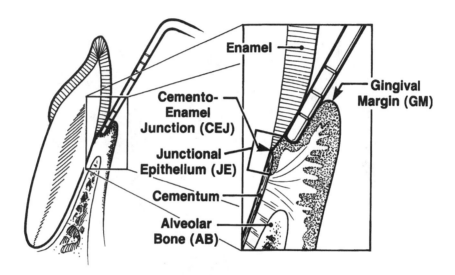

The periodontal tissues in cross-section

Probing Accuracy

Probing is the act of walking the tip of a probe along the junctional epithelium within the sulcus or pocket for the purpose of determining the presence of past disease activity. Good probing technique is essential, for although a probe is a most valuable assessment tool, it does have limitations. The accuracy of the measurements obtained by probing can vary significantly depending on the clinician's skill, size and design of the probe, probing technique, and tissue health.

1. Tissue Health and Related Factors. The probe is inserted in an apical direction until it meets the physical resistance of the base of the sulcus (or pocket).
   a. In Health. The probe encounters physical resistance when it comes in contact with the junctional epithelium.
   b. In Disease. The probe passes through the junctional epithelium and encounters physical resistance when it reaches the underlying connective tissue.
   c. Calculus Deposits. Large calculus deposits can hinder placement of the probe.

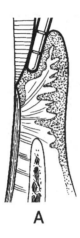

A

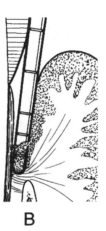

B

Probe Penetration. **A**, if the tissues are healthy, the probe tip will stop at the "outermost layers" of the junctional epithelium. **B**, when the tissues are inflamed, the probe tip may pass through the junctional epithelium and be stopped by the connective tissue.

2. Clinician Technique. Limitations of clinician technique include improper adaptation of the probe tip, poor stroke control, and excessive pressure against the junctional epithelium.
   a. Adaptation. The probe tip is placed in contact with the tooth surface and the length of the probe is positioned as parallel as possible to the tooth surface being probed. To assess the col region, the probe is angled to reach under the contact area.

    b.   Stroke Technique. Probing strokes must be close to each other (in 1 mm steps) to assess the entire circumference of the junctional epithelium.

    c.   Probing Pressure. Use a scale to standardize probing pressure. Sensitive scales are available from scientific supply companies that will measure weight in grams. Calibrate your probing pressure so that it is between 10 and 20 grams. (See the Skill Building Activities on page 297 for two activities for calibrating probing force.)

3.   Probe Design. Use a thin probe (no more than 0.5 mm in diameter) with easily readable millimeter markings. Be knowledgeable about the millimeter increments indicated on the probe that you are using. If you are uncertain of the increments, use a millimeter ruler to determine them!

Basic Concepts of Probing Technique

    Careful probing technique is essential if the information obtained with a periodontal probe is to be accurate. Technique concerns include the correct positioning of the probe, adaptation, and walking stroke.

1.   **Parallelism**. The probe is positioned as *parallel as possible to the tooth surface*. The probe must be parallel in a mesial-distal dimension and in facial-lingual dimension.

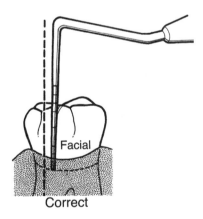

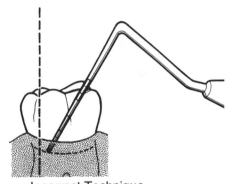

Correct Technique. This probe is positioned with the working-end parallel to the long axis of the tooth.

Technique Error. Here the probe is incorrectly positioned at an angle to the long axis of the tooth.

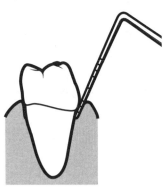

Proximal View

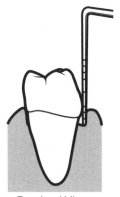

Proximal View

Correct Technique. The probe should be positioned parallel to an imaginary line drawn from the height of contour to the root surface.

Technique Error. Here the probe is not parallel to the root surface. This position will result in inaccurate measurement readings.

2. **Probing Interproximally**. When a tooth is in contact with an adjacent tooth, a special technique is used to probe the area directly beneath the contact area.

A two-step technique is used:

(a) Step 1: The probe is positioned parallel to the proximal surface until it touches the contact area. The area beneath the contact area cannot be probed directly because the probe will not fit between the contact areas of the adjacent teeth.

(b) Step 2: Slant the probe slightly so that the tip reaches under the contact area. The tip of the probe extends under the contact area while the upper portion touches the contact area. With the probe in this position, gently press downward to touch the junctional epithelium.

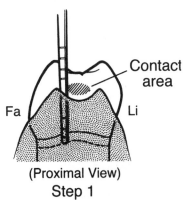

Contact area

Fa   Li

(Proximal View)
Step 1

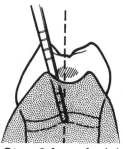

Step 2 from facial

In this illustration you are viewing the *mesial surface* of a molar tooth. The probe is positioned in a parallel position until it encounters the contact area.

This illustration shows correct technique for assessing the tissue apical to the contact area (from the facial aspect of the tooth).

3. **Handle Position for Distal Surfaces of Maxillary Molars**. When probing the distal surfaces of the maxillary molars, it is often difficult to position the probe parallel to the distal surface (because the patient's lower arch is in the way). This problem can be overcome by repositioning the instrument handle to the side of the patient's face. Using an advanced fulcrum also can be helpful; advanced fulcruming techniques are presented in Module 25.

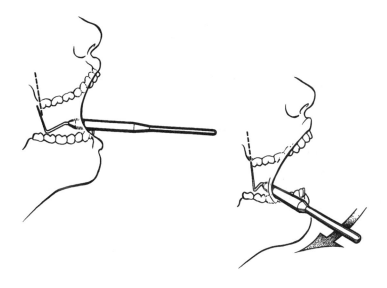

4. **Adaptation**. The side of the probe tip should be kept in contact with the tooth surface.

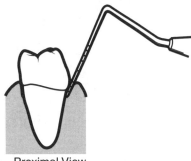

Proximal View

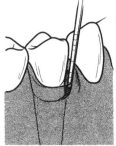

Incorrect Technique

Correct Adaptation. The side of the probe tip is *held in contact with the tooth surface.*

Incorrect Adaptation. The probe tip should not be held away from the tooth surface.

5. **The Walking Stroke**. The entire circumference of the sulcus or pocket base must be covered with a series of probing strokes. It is essential to evaluate the entire "length" of the pocket base because the junctional epithelium is not necessarily at a uniform level around the tooth. In fact, differences in the depths of two neighboring areas along the pocket base are common.

   To accomplish a thorough evaluation of the junctional epithelium, a special walking stroke is used with the probe. Walking strokes are a series of bobbing strokes that are made within the sulcus or pocket while *keeping the probe tip against the tooth surface*. The probe is NOT removed from the sulcus after each measurement.
   a. The stroke begins when the probe is inserted into the sulcus or pocket until the tip encounters the resistance of the junctional epithelium. The junctional epithelium will feel soft and resilient when touched by the probe.
   b. The walking stroke is created by moving the probe up and down (↕) in short bobbing strokes and forward in 1 mm increments (↔). With each down stroke, the probe returns to touch the junctional epithelium.

    c. Digital (finger) activation may be used with the probe because only light pressure is used when probing.

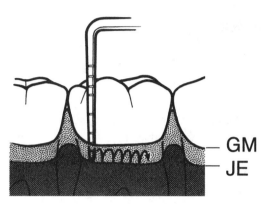

The Walking Stroke. The probe is moved up and down within the sulcus in a series of short, bobbing strokes along the junctional epithelium (JE). Each up-and-down stroke should be approximately 1- to 2-mm in length (↕). The strokes must be very close together, about 1 mm apart (↔).

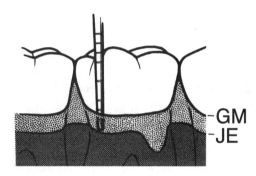

Stroke Technique. It is common for the depth of the pocket base to vary considerably from one spot to the next.

What would happen if only one or two probing strokes were made on the facial surface of the tooth illustrated here?

6. **Recording Probing Depths**. For the purpose of documentation, each tooth is divided into six areas. Only six periodontal probing depths are recorded on the chart for each tooth (three readings from the facial aspect and three from the lingual aspect of the tooth).

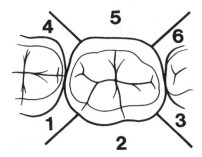

For the purpose of probing, each tooth is divided into six areas:
1: distofacial line angle to the midline of the distal surface
2: facial surface
3: mesiofacial line angle to the midline of the mesial surface
4: distolingual line angle to the midline of the distal surface
5: lingual surface
6: mesiolingual line angle to the midline of the mesial surface

Only one reading per area is recorded. If the probing depths vary within an area, the deepest reading obtained in that area is recorded. For example, if the probing depths in an area ranged from 2 mm to 6 mm, only the 6 mm reading would be entered on the chart for that area. Depths are recorded to the nearest full millimeter. A reading of 5.5 mm should be rounded up and recorded as a 6 mm reading.

Record the Deepest Reading. The depth of the pocket base shown in this illustration varies considerably at spots A, B. and C. Since only a single reading can be recorded for the facial surface, the deepest reading at point C is recorded.

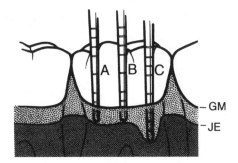

Section 2: Step-by-Step Technique on Posteriors

Example: Mandibular Right First Molar, Facial Aspect

RIGHT-Handed Clinician				

LEFT-Handed Clinician				

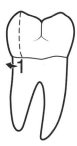

1. Insert the probe into the sulcus near the distofacial line angle of the *first* molar. Keep the side of the tip in contact with the tooth surface as you gently slide the probe to the sulcus base. (Illustration shows the facial view.)

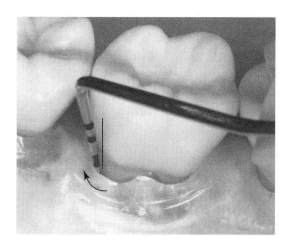

2. Your probe is now positioned to evaluate Area 1 of this tooth. Keeping the tip in contact with the tooth, initiate a series of short, bobbing strokes *toward the distal* surface. Use a walking stroke, keeping your strokes close together.

3. Walk the probe onto the proximal surface. Keep it as parallel as possible to the distal surface. Walk the probe across the distal surface until it touches the contact area.

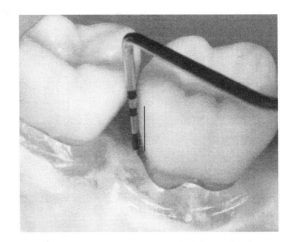

4. Tilt the probe so that the tip reaches beneath the contact area (the upper portion of the probe touches the contact area).

Gently press downward to touch the junctional epithelium.

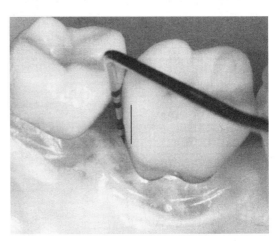

5. Technique check. (Distal View) In this photo, the adjacent tooth has been removed to show the correct probe position for assessing the col area from the facial aspect.

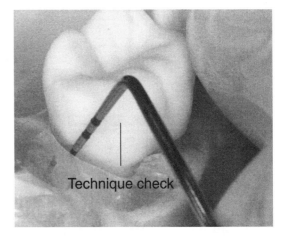

Technique check

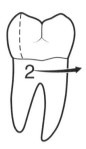

6. Remove the probe from the sulcus and reinsert it at the distofacial line angle. You are now in position to probe the facial surface.

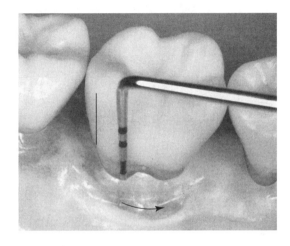

7. Make a series of tiny walking strokes across the facial surface, moving in a forward direction toward the mesial surface.

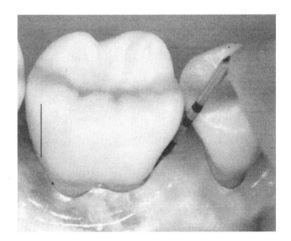

8. Walk the probe across the mesial surface until it touches the contact area. The probe should be parallel to the mesial surface.

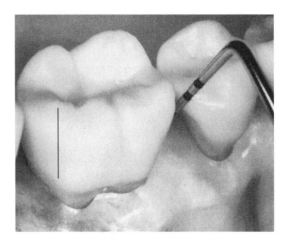

9. Tilt the probe and extend the tip beneath the contact area. Press down gently to touch the junctional epithelium.

10. This illustration shows the sequence for probing the entire mandibular right posterior sextant. This sequence allows you to probe the sextant in the most efficient manner.

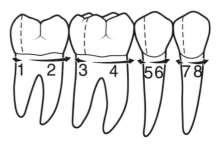

11. Practice probing the facial and lingual aspects of the four posterior sextants using the sequence shown in the illustration above.

RIGHT-Handed Clinicians: Begin your practice with the mandibular right posterior sextant.

LEFT-Handed Clinicians: Begin your practice with the mandibular left posterior sextant.

Section 3: Step-by-Step Technique on Anteriors

Example: Mandibular Left Canine, Facial Aspect

RIGHT-Handed Clinician		8-9	↕ST	2.5
LEFT-Handed Clinician		3-4	ST↕	2.5

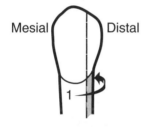

Mesial   Distal

1

1. Begin by inserting the probe at the distofacial line angle of the left canine. You are now in position to assess the distal surface of the canine.

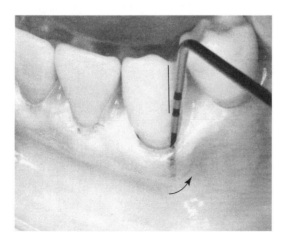

2. Walk the probe across the distal surface until it touches the contact area.

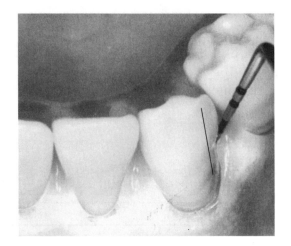

3. Tilt the probe and extend the tip beneath the contact area. Press down gently to touch the junctional epithelium.

4. Remove the probe from the sulcus and reinsert it at the distofacial line angle. You are now in position to probe the facial surface of the canine.

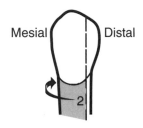

Mesial   Distal

2

5. Make a series of walking strokes across the facial surface.

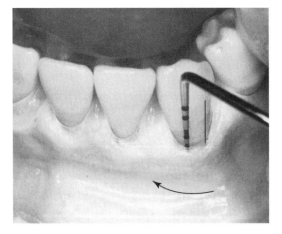

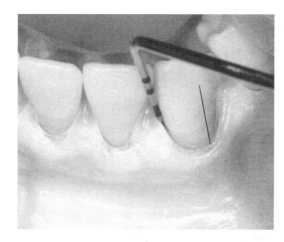

6. Walk across the mesial surface until the probe touches the contact area.

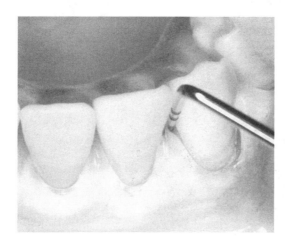

7. On adjacent *anterior* teeth, only a slight tilt is needed to probe the col area. Gently probe the col area.

8. Practice probing the facial and lingual aspects of the mandibular and maxillary anterior sextants. When probing all the teeth in an anterior sextant, you should begin on the distofacial or distolingual line angle of the canine farthest from you and work toward yourself. For example, right-handed clinicians should begin on the left canine and work across to the right canine. Refer to the appropriate sequence shown below.

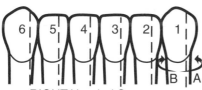

RIGHT-Handed Sequence

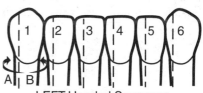

LEFT-Handed Sequence

Section 4: Assessments with Probes

Measurement of Gingival Recession

Gingival recession is the movement of the gingival margin from its normal position slightly coronal to the CEJ to a position apical to the CEJ (leading to exposure of a portion of the root surface). Gingival recession is an indication of the apical migration of the junctional epithelium.

The extent of recession is measured in millimeters from the CEJ to the gingival margin with a calibrated periodontal probe.

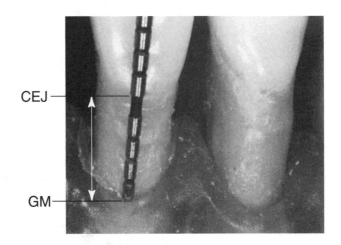

Probing Depths

A probing depth is the measurement in millimeters of the depth of a sulcus or pocket. A probing depth alone is not a reliable indication of the loss of attachment or level of bone support to the tooth. Gingival recession is common in periodontally involved teeth and in such cases the probing depth does not accurately describe the extent of apical migration of the junctional epithelium. Probing depths are helpful in calculating clinical attachment levels (refer to the next section of module), prescribing patient self care regimens and educating patients in plaque control procedures. For purposes of supportive periodontal therapy and patient self care, the patient needs to understand that a pocket is more difficult to deplaque and know the location of pockets in the mouth.

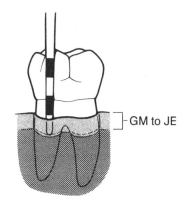

The probing depth is determined by measuring from the gingival margin (GM) to the junctional epithelium (JE). The probing depth for this tooth is 2 mm.

The 2 mm reading, however, is NOT an accurate indication of the extent of bone loss because gingival recession is present.

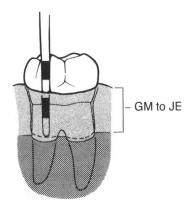

The probing depth for this tooth is 7 mm.

The 7 mm reading, however, is NOT an accurate indication of the extent of bone loss because the gingival margin is coronal to the CEJ.

A probing depth is the distance in millimeters from *the gingival margin* to the base of the sulcus or periodontal pocket as measured with a calibrated probe.

Biologic Width and Estimated Bone Level

The crest of the alveolar bone is approximately 1.7 mm apical to (beneath) the junctional epithelium. This 1.7 mm distance from the base of the sulcus or periodontal pocket is known as the **biologic width**. The biologic width is the same in healthy sulci and diseased periodontal pockets. Therefore, the measurement of the clinical attachment level provides an estimate of the bone support for the tooth. The clinical attachment level (CAL) + biologic width (BW) = distance that the alveolar bone crest is apical to the CEJ in millimeters. For example, if the CAL is 5 mm; then, the approximate bone level is about 6.7 mm apical to the CEJ (5 mm CAL + 1.7 mm BW = 6.7 mm).

Clinical Attachment Level (CAL)

The clinical attachment level (CAL) is determined by measuring the distance in millimeters from a fixed point on the tooth (usually the CEJ) to the base of the sulcus or periodontal pocket with a calibrated probe. This measurement is a means of estimating the level of the junctional epithelium and the approximate position of the crest of the alveolar bone. (The clinical attachment level is the visual estimation of the attachment level as measured with a probe. It is only an estimation of the actual histologic level of attachment.)

> The clinical attachment level is the distance in millimeters from the *cementoenamel junction* to the base of the gingival sulcus or pocket as measured with a calibrated periodontal probe.

Usually, two measurements are made with the periodontal probe in order to determine the clinical attachment level. The two measurements are recorded and then used to mathematically calculate the clinical attachment level.
1. The first measurement is the probing depth. (The distance from the gingival margin to the junctional epithelium.)
2. The second is the distance from the CEJ to the gingival margin.

Three possible relationships exist between the CEJ and the gingival margin:
1. gingival recession—the gingival margin is apical to the CEJ,
2. the gingival margin is coronal to the CEJ—seen in gingival edema, hyperplasia, and sometimes in fibrotic tissue, and
3. the gingival margin is approximately level with the CEJ.

The clinician must understand the procedure for determining the clinical attachment level in each of these three relationships.

Gingival Recession

When recession is present, the clinical attachment level is calculated by ADDING the probing depth to the measurement of gingival recession.

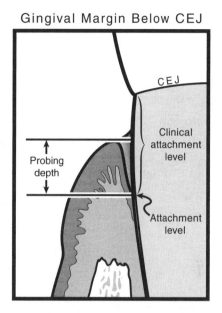

Gingival Margin Below CEJ

Step 1. Measure the probing depth from the gingival margin (GM) to the junctional epithelium (JE). In this example, the probing depth is 2 mm.

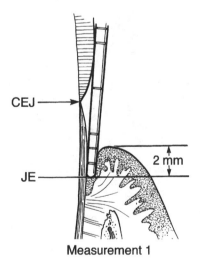

Measurement 1

Step 2. Measure the amount of recession from the CEJ to the gingival margin (GM). In this example, the measurement of recession is 3 mm.

Step 3. Calculate the CAL.
GM to JE = 2 mm (probing depth)
CEJ to GM = 3 mm (recession)

2 mm + 3 mm = 5 mm CAL

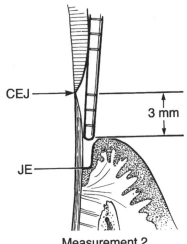

Measurement 2

Gingival Margin Covers the CEJ

Gingival Margin Above CEJ

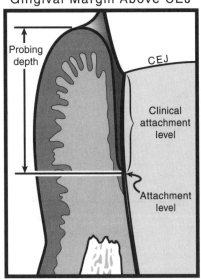

When the gingival margin is coronal to the CEJ, the clinical attachment level is calculated by SUBTRACTING *the measurement from the gingival margin to the CEJ* from the probing depth.

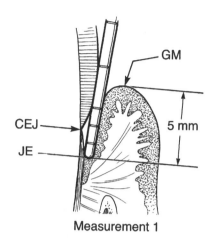

Measurement 1

Step 1. Measure the probing depth from the gingival margin (GM) to the junctional epithelium (JE). In this example, the probing depth is 5 mm.

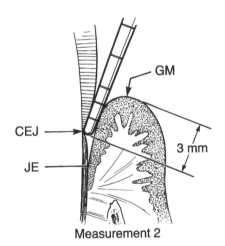

Measurement 2

Step 2. Measure from the gingival margin (GM) to the CEJ. In this example, this measurement is 3 mm.

Step 3. Calculate the CAL.
GM to JE = 5 mm (probing depth)
GM to CEJ = 3 mm (recession)

5 mm—3 mm = 2 mm CAL

Gingival Margin Level With CEJ

The probing depth and the clinical attachment level are equal when the gingival margin is level with the CEJ. The probing depth (from GM to JE) and the clinical attachment level (from the CEJ to JE) are identical measurements.

Only one measurement is needed to determine the clinical attachment level when the gingival margin is level with the CEJ—the probing depth.

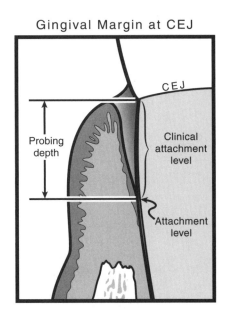

Gingival Margin at CEJ

The probing depth (GM to JE) and the clinical attachment level (CEJ to JE) are identical when the gingival margin is level with the CEJ. (Both are 5 mm in this example.)

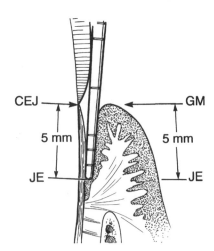

Mucogingival Examination

The purpose of the mucogingival examination is to determine the width of the attached gingiva. The **attached gingiva** extends from the base of the sulcus to the mucogingival junction and is attached to the cementum of the tooth and the alveolar bone by a network of collagenous fibers. The function of the attached gingiva is to keep the free gingiva from being pulled away from the tooth. The width of the attached gingiva on the facial aspect varies in different areas of the mouth. It is widest in the anterior teeth (3.5–4.5 mm in the maxilla and 3.3–3.9 mm in the mandible) and narrowest on the premolar teeth (1.9 in the maxilla and 1.8 in the mandible). The **alveolar mucosa** is located apical to the mucogingival junction. This tissue is a deeper red in color than the attached gingiva; it is shiny in appearance and is loosely attached to the underlying bone.

To calculate the width of the attached gingiva, you will need to take two measurements: (1) the distance in millimeters from the gingival margin to the mucogingival junction on the external (outer) surface of the gingiva and (2) the probing depth of the sulcus or periodontal pocket. *The width of the attached gingiva is calculated by SUBTRACTING the probing depth FROM the measurement from the gingival margin to the mucogingival junction.*

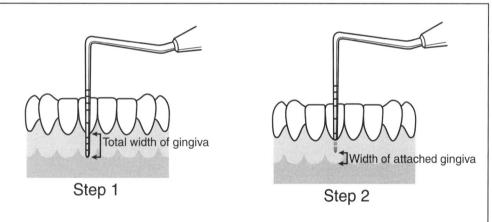

Measuring the width of the attached gingiva:
1. On the external surface of the gingiva, measure from the gingival margin to the mucogingival junction.
2. Insert the probe into the sulcus or pocket and measure the probing depth.
3. SUBTRACT the *probing depth* FROM the *distance from the gingival margin to the mucogingival junction.*

Furcation Involvement

Furcation involvement occurs when periodontal infection invades the area between and around the roots of bifurcated or trifurcated teeth.

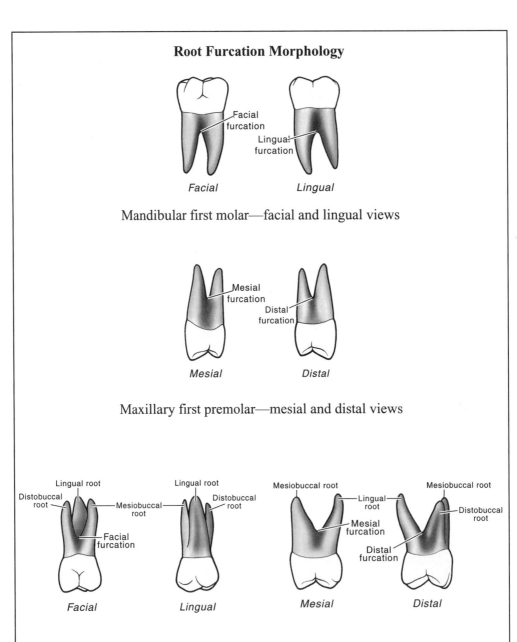

Root Furcation Morphology

Mandibular first molar—facial and lingual views

Maxillary first premolar—mesial and distal views

Maxillary first molar—facial, lingual, mesial, and distal views

Furcation probes have mirror-image, paired working-ends. The correct working-end of the probe has been selected if the lower (terminal) shank is positioned parallel to the tooth surface being examined. The incorrect working-end has been selected if the lower shank is perpendicular to the tooth surface being examined.

Access to Furcation Area

Mandibular molars (bifurcated: mesial and distal roots)—the furcation area can be examined from the facial and lingual surfaces.

Maxillary first premolars (bifurcated: buccal and palatal roots)—the furcation area can be examined from the mesial and distal surfaces apical to the contact areas.

Maxillary molars (trifurcated: mesiobuccal, distobuccal and palatal roots)—the furcation area can be examined from the facial, mesial, and distal surfaces.

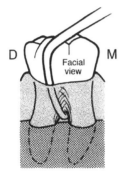

Mandibular molar—facial view. The probe is inserted between the mesial and distal roots from the facial and lingual aspects of the tooth.

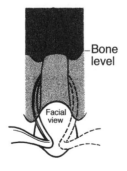

Maxillary first premolar—facial view. The probe is inserted between the buccal and palatal roots from the mesial and distal surfaces apical to the contact areas.

Maxillary molars—facial view. The probe is inserted between the mesiobuccal root and distobuccal root from the facial aspect (the probe will contact the palatal root if a through and through furcation is present).

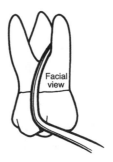

Maxillary molars—lingual view. The probe is inserted between the mesiobuccal root and palatal root, or between the distobuccal root and palatal root, from the mesial or distal surface.

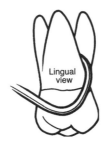

Classification of Furcation Involvement

Furcation involvement is classified according to the *extent* of bone loss.

Class I: Curvature of concavity can be felt with the probe tip; however, the furcation probe cannot enter the furcation area.

Class II: The probe is able to partially enter the furcation, extending approximately 1/3 of the width of the tooth (but NOT able to pass completely through the furcation).

Class III: Probe will pass completely through the furcation. In mandibular molars, the probe passes completely through the furcation between the roots. In maxillary molars, the probe passes between the mesiobuccal and distobuccal roots and will touch the palatal root.

Class IV: Same as the Class III except that the entrance to the furca is visible clinically because of the presence of gingival recession.

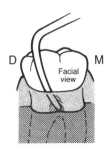

Class I

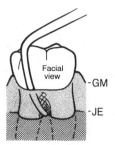

Class II

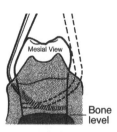

Class III

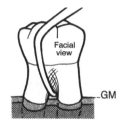

Class IV

Evaluation of Oral Deviations

When an oral lesion or deviation is observed in a patient's mouth, this finding should be recorded in the patient's chart. Information recorded should include the date, size, location, color, and character of the lesion, as well as, any information provided by the patient (e.g., duration, sensation, or oral habits).

A calibrated probe is used in determining the size of the lesion or deviation. It is best to use anatomic references, rather than "length" or "width", to document your measurements (e.g., as the anterior-posterior measurement and the superior-inferior measurement).

Sample chart entry:
January 12, 2000: a soft, red, papillary lesion located on the buccal mucosa opposite the maxillary left first premolar; measuring 5 mm in an anterior-posterior direction and 6 mm in a superior-inferior direction.

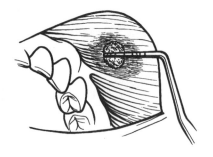

To determine the height of a raised deviation, place the probe tip on normal tissue alongside of the deviation. Imagine a line at the highest part of the deviation, and record this measurement as the height.

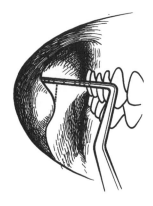

To determine the depth of a sunken deviation, carefully place the probe tip in the deepest part. Imagine a line running from edge to edge of the deviation. The depth is the distance from this imaginary line to the base of the deviation.

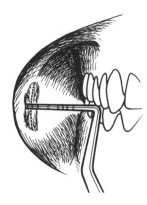

Mobility

Mobility refers to the movement of a tooth in its socket. All teeth exhibit slight mobility due to the presence of the periodontal ligament. The handles of two single-ended instruments are needed to assess tooth mobility.

Technique for Assessing Mobility

1. Dry the tooth to be examined with compressed air. Place the ends of the handles on opposite sides of the tooth (facial and lingual aspects).
2. Apply alternating pressure with the handles, first from the facial aspect, then from the lingual. Pathologic mobility is most often evident in a facial-lingual direction.
3. Finally, check for vertical mobility by using the end of handle to exert vertical pressure on the occlusal surface or incisal edge of the tooth. **Vertical mobility** refers to the ability to depress the tooth in its socket.

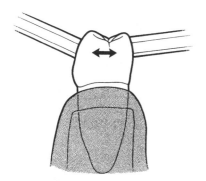

Horizontal Mobility. Using the ends of two handles, apply alternating pressure, first from the facial and then, from the lingual aspects of the tooth.

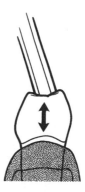

Vertical Mobility. Use the end of an instrument handle to exert pressure against the occlusal surface or incisal edge of the tooth.

Mobility Scale

N = normal physiologic mobility

Grade I = slight mobility, up to 1 mm movement in a facial-lingual direction

Grade II = greater than 1 mm movement in a facial-lingual direction

Grade III = greater than 1 mm movement in all directions (horizontal and vertical mobility)

Reference Sheet: Probing and Clinical Attachment Level

Probing Technique

1. *Posterior sextants*: Insert probe at the distofacial or distolingual line angle. Begin with the posterior-most tooth in the sextant.
   Anterior sextants: Insert probe at the distofacial or distolingual line angle of the tooth farthest from the clinician.
2. Position the probe as parallel as possible to the long axis of the tooth surface being probed.
3. Adapt the tip of the probe to the tooth surface as you activate short up and down strokes within the sulcus or pocket. Touch the junctional epithelium with each down stroke.
4. Assess the col area by tilting the probe and extending the tip beneath the contact area. Press down gently to touch the junctional epithelium.
5. Walk the probe around the entire circumference of the junctional epithelium using strokes that are about 1 mm apart.
6. Use light stroke pressure, between 10 and 20 grams.
7. Record 6 measurements per tooth (the deepest measurement in each of the 6 areas is recorded).

Clinical Attachment Level (CAL)

Gingival Recession Present: Calculate the CAL by ADDING the *probing depth* to the *measurement of gingival recession*.

Gingival Margin Covering CEJ: Calculate the CAL by SUBTRACTING the *measurement from the CEJ to the gingival margin* from the *probing depth*.

Gingival Margin Level with CEJ: Measure the probing depth. The probing depth and the CAL are identical.

Section 5: Documentation of Measurements

The information gathered with a periodontal probe is recorded on a periodontal assessment form that becomes a permanent part of the patient chart.

Lingual Aspect	32	31	30	29	28
Probing depth (initial)	546	545	444	434	434
Gingival Recession					
Clinical attachment level					
Facial Aspect					
Probing depth (initial)	556	656	646	434	434
Gingival Recession					
Clinical attachment level					

In this example, the probing depths for the *lingual aspect* of tooth #32 are:
- 5 mm distal reading
- 4 mm lingual reading
- 6 mm mesial reading

Lingual Aspect	32	31	30	29	28
Probing depth (initial)	546	545	444	434	434
Gingival Recession				222	222
Clinical attachment level					
Facial Aspect					
Probing depth (initial)	556	656	646	434	434
Gingival Recession	112	222	233	333	333
Clinical attachment level					

The presence of gingival recession also is recorded on the form. In this example, recession on the *facial aspect* of tooth #32 is:
- 1 mm on the distal
- 1 mm on the facial
- 2 mm on the mesial

Lingual Aspect	32	31	30	29	28
Probing depth (initial)	546	545	444	434	434
Gingival Recession				222	222
Clinical attachment level	546	545	444	656	656
Facial Aspect					
Probing depth (initial)	556	656	646	434	434
Gingival Recession	112	222	233	333	333
Clinical attachment level	668	878	879	767	767

The clinical attachment level is calculated by adding the probing depth to the recession measurement. In this example, recession on the *facial aspect* of tooth #32 is:
- 6 mm on the distal
- 6 mm on the facial
- 8 mm on the mesial

Section 6: Periodontal Screening and Recording

The American Dental Association and the American Academy of Periodontology suggest that routine dental examinations include the Periodontal Screening and Recording system (PSR). The PSR is an efficient, easy to use system for the detection of periodontal disease.

A specially designed periodontal probe is used with the PSR. The probe has the following design features:
- a 0.5 ball-tipped end.
- a **color-coded band** located 3.5 to 5.5 mm from the tip.

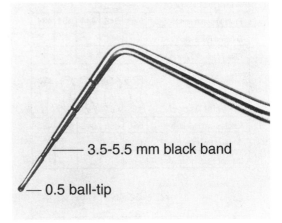

The periodontal probe is inserted into the sulcus or pocket and gently walked around the circumference of each tooth using the same probing technique as for a comprehensive periodontal examination.

The unique aspects of the PSR screening are the manner in which the probe is read and the minimal amount of information recorded. Instead of reading and recording 6 readings per tooth, the clinician only needs to observe the position of the color-coded band in relation to the gingival margin and the presence of furcation invasion, mobility, mucogingival problems or recession.

Only one score is recorded for each sextant in the mouth. In each sextant, only the highest code obtained is recorded. An "X" is recorded if a sextant is edentulous.

> For the PSR, the clinician only needs to observe the position of the color-coded band in relation to the gingival margin and the presence of furcation invasion, mobility, mucogingival problems or recession.

PSR Codes

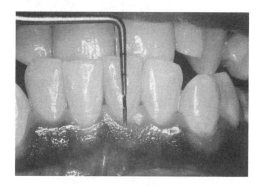

CODE 0:
- **Colored band** is completely visible in the deepest sulcus or pocket in the sextant.
- No calculus or defective margins.
- Gingival tissues are healthy with no bleeding evident upon gentle probing.

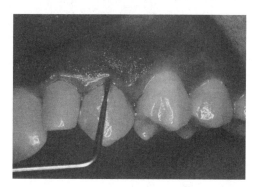

CODE 1:
- **Colored band** is completely visible in the deepest sulcus or pocket in the sextant.
- No calculus or defective margins are detected.
- Bleeding *IS* event on probing.

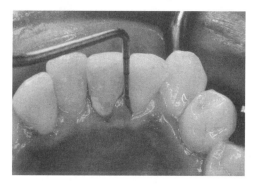

CODE 2:
- **Colored band** is completely visible in the deepest sulcus or pocket in the sextant.
- Supra- or subgingival calculus and/or defective margins are detected.

CODE 3:
Colored band is **partially** visible in the
deepest sulcus or pocket in the sextant.

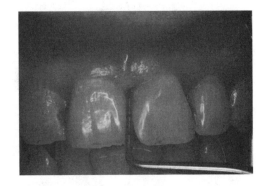

CODE 4:
Colored band **is not visible** in the
deepest sulcus or pocket in the sextant.
This indicates a probing depth of greater
than 5.5 mm.

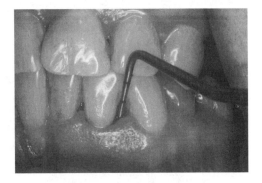

CODE ✱ :
The ✱ symbol is added to any sextant exhibiting any of the following
abnormalities:
- furcation invasion
- mobility
- mucogingival problems
- recession extending into the colored area of the probe (3.5 mm or greater)

Use of the ✻ Symbol:

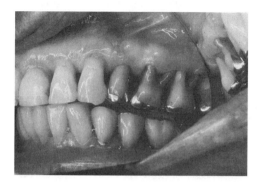

This sextant exhibits furcation involvement and, therefore, should include the ✻ symbol next to the sextant code.

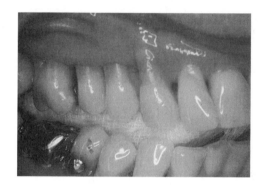

This sextant exhibits gingival recession and mucogingival problem and, therefore, should include the ✻ symbol next to the sextant code.

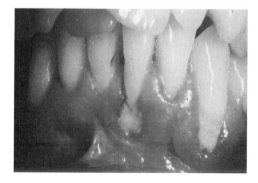

This sextant exhibits mucogingival problems and calculus and, therefore, should include the ✻ symbol next to the sextant code.

Recording PSR Codes

The PSR code is recorded in a box chart. For example, the box chart would look like the one below, for a PSR completed on May 14, 2001 with the following scores:

Max. rt. posteriors = Code 3
Max. anteriors = Code 2
Max. lt. posteriors = Code 1

Mand. rt. posteriors = Code 3
Mand. anteriors = Code 3
Mand. lt. posteriors = Code 4 + mobility

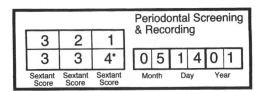

Implications of PSR Codes for Patient Management

CODE 0: Reinforce daily plaque control habits.

CODE 1: Reinforce daily plaque control habits. Provide appropriate treatment.

CODE 2: Reinforce daily plaque control habits. Provide appropriate treatment.

CODE 3: If a single sextant scores a **Code 3**, a comprehensive periodontal examination is indicated for that *sextant*. If two or more sextants score **Code 3**, a comprehensive periodontal examination is indicated for the *entire mouth*.

CODE 4: Do a comprehensive periodontal examination and charting of the *entire mouth*.

CODE ✳: If an abnormality is present in a sextant with a **Code 0, 1, or 2** score—note the abnormality. If an abnormality is present in a sextant with a **Code 3 or 4** score—do a comprehensive periodontal examination and charting of the *entire mouth*.

Section 7: Activities and Evaluation

Skill Building Activities

1. **Calibrate probing pressure with a scale.** Obtain a scale calibrated in grams from a scientific supply company. Prepare the scale by padding the top of the scale platform with a *thin* sponge (like the kind sold to wipe kitchen countertops). Cover the sponge with a piece of rubber dam material and seal the rubber dam around the bottom edges of the scale platform. Grasp a calibrated probe in a modified pen grasp. Apply pressure against the scale platform with the tip of the probe. Calibrate your pressure to between 10 and 20 grams.

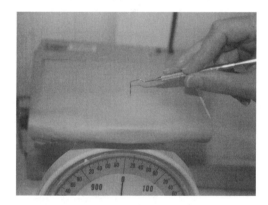

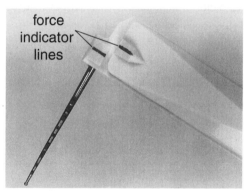

Scientific scale used to measure probing force.

Vivacare TPS Probe from Vivadent with force indicator lines.

2. **Use a probe with force indicator lines.** Obtain a probe like the one pictured above that has force indicator lines. According to the manufacturer when the force indicator lines on the TPS Probe are aligned, a probing force of 20 grams is being exerted. Try the probe on the scientific scale and see if the gram measurement is around 20 grams.

3. **Assessing furcation areas.** Mount the following extracted or synthetic teeth in plaster: mandibular 1st molar, bifurcated maxillary 1st premolar, and maxillary 1st molar. Place only the tips of the roots in plaster, so that the furcation areas are exposed. Use a furcation probe to examine the furcation area of each tooth.

Skill Evaluation: Periodontal Probes

Student: _____   Area 1 = _____

Evaluator: _____   Area 2 = _____

Date: _____   Area 3 = _____

Area 4 = _____

Area 5 = _____

Area 6 = _____

DIRECTIONS: For each area, use **Column S** for student self-evaluation and **Column I** for instructor evaluation. For each skill evaluated, indicate the skill level as: **S** (satisfactory), **I** (improvement needed), or **U** (unsatisfactory).

CRITERIA:	Area 1		Area 2		Area 3		Area 4		Area 5		Area 6	
	S	I	S	I	S	I	S	I	S	I	S	I
Positioned correctly in relation to the patient, equipment, and treatment area												
Uses correct patient head position												
Uses all criteria for mirror												
Uses all criteria for correct grasp												
Holds ring finger straight to act as a "support beam" for the hand												
Fulcrums on same arch, near tooth being instrumented												
Positions probe parallel to tooth surface												
Keeps tip in contact with tooth surface												
Uses small walking strokes within sulcus												
Tilts probe and extends beneath contact area; assesses col												
Covers entire circumference of tooth												
Uses furcation probe on bifurcated and trifurcated teeth												

Skill Evaluation: Assessment Skills

Student: _____   Evaluator: _____

Date: _____

DIRECTIONS—Complete this assessment on a classmate.
PART 1: For each skill, use **Column S** for student self-evaluation and **Column I** for instructor evaluation. For each skill evaluated, indicate the skill level as: **S** (satisfactory), **I** (improvement needed), or **U** (unsatisfactory).

Competency:	S	I
Maintains aseptic technique throughout the procedure.		
Explains assessment procedure to patient.		
Identifies the free gingiva, attached gingiva, and mucogingival junction.		
Documents probing depths, measurement of recession, and clinical attachment levels for one sextant of the mouth.		
Demonstrates technique for assessing mobility.		

DIRECTIONS—PART 2: As the evaluator calls out a tooth number in each quadrant, the student: (1) assumes correct clock and patient positioning, (2) demonstrates correct probing technique, and (3) obtains probing depth reading within 1 mm of the evaluator's finding.

Quadrant	Tooth #	Positioning	Student Reading	Evaluator Reading
1, facial	#			
1, lingual	#			
2, facial	#			
2, lingual	#			
3, facial	#			
3, lingual	#			
4, facial	#			
4, lingual	#			

Skill Evaluation: Periodonal Probes and Assessment Skills

Student: _____

Evaluator Comments:

_____

_____

_____

_____

_____

_____

_____

_____

_____

_____

_____

_____

_____

_____

_____

_____

_____

_____

Box for sketches pertaining to written comments.

13

MODULE

Explorers

This module contains step-by-step instructions for using an explorer for the detection of root surface irregularities, calculus deposits, and dental caries. The design characteristics of explorers were presented in Module 8, Classification of Hand-Activated Instruments. Refer to this module if you need to review this information.

Required Equipment:

- dental mirror
- explorers
- protective attire for the clinician and patient

Key Terms:

Tactile sensitivity
Explorer tip
Functional shank
Lower shank
Inner side of explorer tip
Outer side of explorer tip

Supragingival calculus deposit
Subgingival calculus deposit
Calculus spicule
Calculus ledge
Calculus ring

Section 1: Concepts of Exploring Technique

Tactile Sensitivity

During subgingival instrumentation, the clinician relies on his or her sense of touch to locate calculus deposits hidden beneath the gingival margin. **Tactile sensitivity** is the ability to detect tooth irregularities by feeling vibrations transferred from the instrument tip to the handle. Vibrations are created as the explorer tip quivers slightly as it travels over rough calculus deposits on the tooth surface. These vibrations are transmitted from the tip, through the shank, and into the handle. The clinician feels the vibrations with his or her fingertips resting on the handle and instrument shank.

The fine working-end and flexible shank of an explorer are used to enhance tactile information to the clinician's fingers. The superior tactile conduction of an explorer makes it the instrument of choice for *locating calculus deposits* and for *re-evaluating tooth surfaces* following debridement with a hand-activated instrument or ultrasonic tip. *While removing calculus* from the teeth in a sextant, you should use a curet or an ultrasonic tip for calculus detection. When all deposits detectable with the debridement instrument have been removed, you should make a definitive evaluation of the tooth surface with an explorer. Because the explorer provides superior tactile information, it is likely that you will detect some roughness with the explorer that you could not detect with the debridement instrument.

Grasp

Successful exploring technique demands a relaxed modified pen grasp. The index finger and thumb should effortlessly grasp the handle. The middle finger should rest lightly on the instrument shank. A tense, "death-grip" on the handle severely limits the clinician's ability to detect tactile sensations with the fingers.

Activation

Either hand-forearm or digital motion activation may be used with an explorer. Digital motion activation is permissible with an explorer because physical strength is not required for assessment strokes. A smooth rhythmic activation style is used when exploring.

Adaptation

One to two millimeters of the side of the explorer is adapted to the tooth for detection of tooth surface irregularities. This portion of the explorer is referred to as the **explorer tip**. The actual <u>point</u> of the explorer is never used for detection of calculus.

Shank Design

The **functional shank** of an explorer extends from the first bend in the shank (nearest the handle) up to the working-end. Explorers with long functional shanks are ideal for subgingival use.

The **lower shank** is the section of the shank nearest to the tip. It begins below the working-end and extends to the first shank bend. The lower shank is also known as the **terminal shank**. Some instrument manufacturers make explorers with extended lower shanks that are 3 millimeters longer than usual. Explorers with extended lower shanks are ideal for working in deep periodontal pockets. An example of an explorer with an extended lower shank is the After Five 11/12 Explorer.

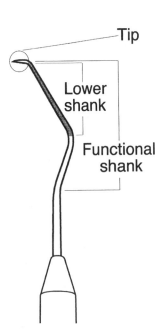

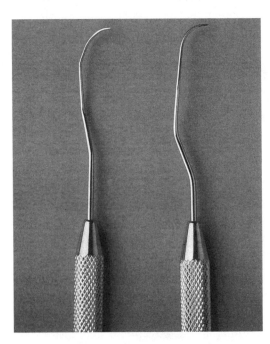

The explorer tip, functional shank, and lower shank.

The explorer on the *left* has a long functional shank. The explorer on the *right* has an extended lower shank.

Reference Sheet: Assessment Strokes

Assessment strokes require a high degree of subtlety and precision. The proper use of an explorer requires light, controlled strokes. The assessment stroke is slightly longer than a calculus removal stroke. Assessment strokes should be multidirectional and overlap one another.

Assessment Stroke With an Explorer	
Purpose	Detection of calculus deposits and other tooth surface irregularities
Grasp	Relaxed grasp; middle finger rests lightly on shank
Lateral Pressure	Light pressure with working-end against tooth
Characteristics	Fluid, sweeping strokes
Stroke Direction	A pull stroke, beginning at the base of the sulcus or periodontal pocket and moving away from the junctional epithelium. AVOID push strokes toward the sulcus or pocket base that could damage the junctional epithelium
Number	Many, overlapping strokes are used to cover every square millimeter of the root surface
Common errors to AVOID	AVOID a tight, tense "death grip" on handle AVOID applying pressure with the middle finger against the instrument shank as this will reduce tactile information to the finger

Inner and Outer Side of the Explorer Tip

Many explorer designs have paired, mirror-image working-ends. These double-ended explorers have universal application (one double-ended instrument is needed to instrument all tooth surfaces in the dentition).

Each of the two working-ends of a universal explorer has two sides, an inner side and an outer side. The **outer side** of the explorer tip is the side that is *farther* from the instrument handle. The **inner side** of the explorer tip is the side that is *closer* to the instrument handle.

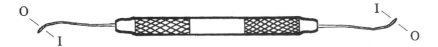

Each of the two working-ends of a universal explorer has two sides, an inner (I) and an outer (O) side.

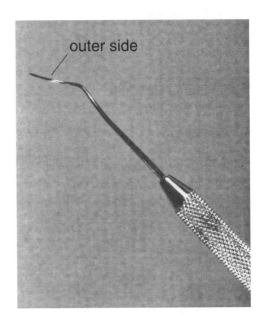

outer side

To identify the outer side of an explorer tip, hold the instrument so that you are looking at the face of the explorer working-end.

The **outer side** is the side of the explorer tip that is farthest from the instrument handle.

Section 2: Step-by-Step Technique on Anteriors

Selecting the Correct Working-End for Anteriors

Several visual clues can be used to select the correct working-end of a universal explorer. With experience, you will learn which visual clue is easiest for you to recognize. Some individuals may use one visual clue; others will find another visual clue to be most helpful. It doesn't matter which visual clue you use, as long as it works well for you.

When using a universal explorer on an <u>anterior</u> tooth:
- only the outer side of the tips are used (inner sides are not used)
- the face should curve toward the tooth surface
- the lower shank goes across the tooth

Visual Clues for Anterior Teeth

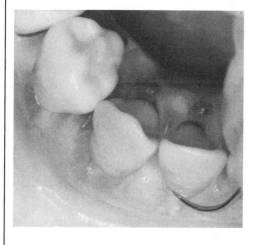   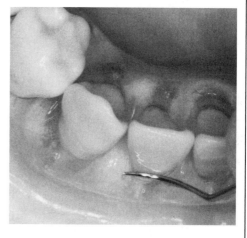

Correct Working-End   Incorrect Working-End

Use the following visual clues to identify the correct working-end:

- **Outer side** of working-end is adapted to the tooth surface.

- **Face** of working-end curves toward the tooth surface.

- **Lower shank** reaches across the tooth surface. (Think "anterior across".)

Practice in Selecting the Working-End for Anteriors

Can you apply the visual clues to each of these photographs? The answers to the questions can be found at the bottom of page 316.

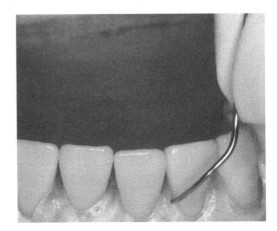

This photograph shows a pigtail explorer. Is this the correct working-end for use on the mesial surface of the mandibular left lateral incisor?

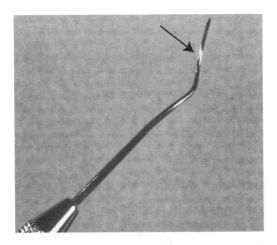

This photograph shows a pigtail explorer. Is the arrow pointing to the outer or inner side of the tip? Would this side of the tip be used on anterior teeth?

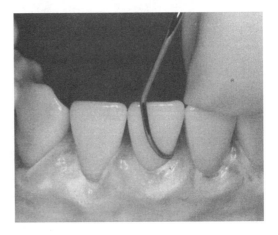

This photograph shows an 11/12-Type explorer. Is this the correct working-end for use on the mesial surface of the mandibular right central incisor?

Use of a Universal Explorer on Anterior Teeth

Example: Mandibular Left Canine, Facial Aspect

RIGHT-Handed Clinician				

LEFT-Handed Clinician				

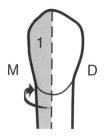

1. Begin by exploring the mesial-half of the mandibular left canine, facial aspect. If you are <u>right-handed</u>, this is the *surface toward you*. If you are <u>left-handed</u>, this is the *surface away from you*.

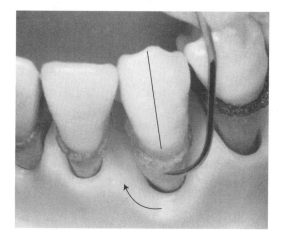

2. Position the tip slightly to the right of the midline so that your strokes will overlap at the midline. Activate feather-light assessment strokes.

3. Continue strokes until you have explored at least halfway across the mesial proximal surface of the canine. (The other half of the mesial surface will be reached from the lingual aspect of the tooth.)

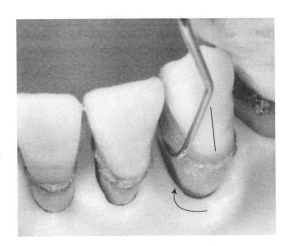

4. Use the sequence shown in this illustration to complete the shaded tooth surfaces, ending with the distal surface of the <u>right</u> canine.

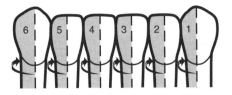

5. When you have completed these surfaces, change your clock position and complete the remaining facial surfaces, beginning with the mesial surface of the <u>right canine</u>. Remember to use the correct clock positions: sit at 8-9:00 for surfaces toward you and 12:00 for surfaces away from you.

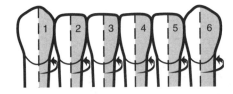

Section 3: Step-by-Step Technique on Posteriors

Selecting the Correct Working-End for Posteriors

When using a universal explorer on a posterior tooth:
- the inner side of the tip adapts to the distal surfaces
- the outer side of the tip adapts to the facial, lingual, and mesial surfaces.

In addition, the **lower shank** should be **parallel** to the tooth surface being explored.

Visual Clues for Posterior Teeth

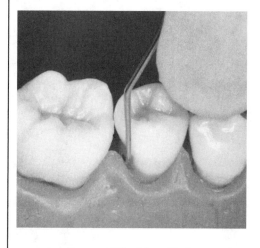

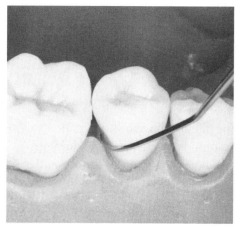

Correct Working-End   Incorrect Working-End

Use the following visual clues to identify the correct working-end:

- **Outer side** of tip adapts to the facial, lingual, and mesial surfaces.

- **Inner side** of tip adapts to the distal surface of posterior teeth.

- **Lower shank** is *parallel* to the tooth surface being instrumented. (Think "posterior parallel".)

Practice in Selecting the Working-End for Posteriors

Can you apply the visual clues to each of these photographs? The answers to the questions can be found at the bottom of page 316.

This photograph shows a pigtail explorer. Is this the correct working-end for use on the distal surface of this mandibular molar?

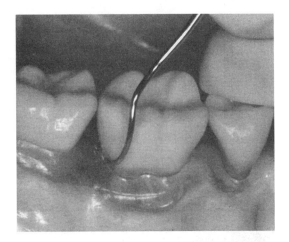

This photograph shows a pigtail explorer. Is this the correct working-end for use on the distal surface of this mandibular molar?

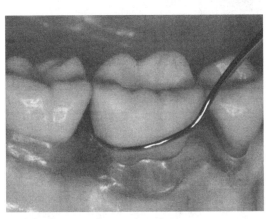

This photograph shows an 11/12-Type explorer. Is this the correct working-end for use on the facial surface of this mandibular molar?

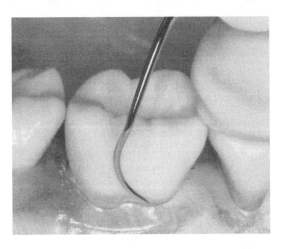

Use of a Universal Explorer on Posterior Teeth

Example: Mandibular Right Mandibular First Molar, Facial Aspect

| **RIGHT-Handed Clinician** | | | | |

| **LEFT-Handed Clinician** | | | | |

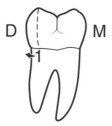

1. As an introduction to exploring posterior teeth, first practice on the **mandibular right first molar**. The distal surface is completed first, beginning at the distofacial line angle and working onto the distal surface.

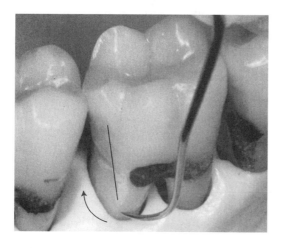

2. Adapt the tip to the right of the distofacial line angle so that your strokes will overlap slightly at the line angle. The tip should aim toward the back of the mouth because this is the direction in which you are working.

3. Roll the instrument handle slightly to adapt to the distal surface. Explore at least halfway across the distal surface from the facial aspect. Keep the tip adapted to the tooth surface at all times.

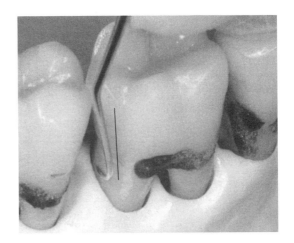

4. You are now ready to explore the facial and mesial surfaces of the tooth, beginning at the distofacial line angle.

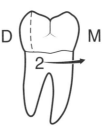

5. While maintaining your fulcrum, remove the tip from the sulcus and turn it so that it aims toward the front of the mouth. Reinsert the tip and reposition it just to the left of the distofacial line angle.

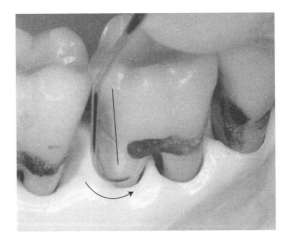

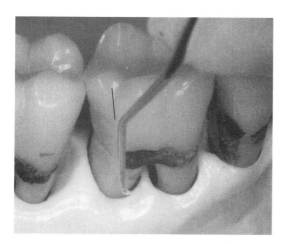

6. If there is bone loss present in the furcation area, you will need to explore the root branches on either side of the furcation. Roll the instrument handle to adapt the tip to the *mesial surface of the distal root*. Explore the mesial half of the distal root.

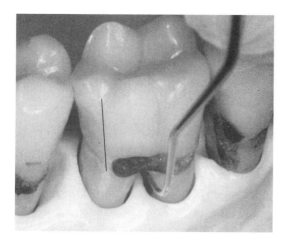

7. While maintaining your fulcrum, move the tip from the furcation and turn it to adapt to the *distal surface of the mesial root*. Explore the distal half of the mesial root.

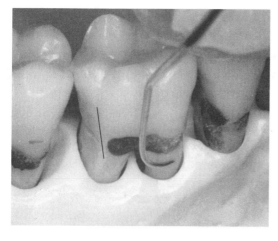

8. Continue working across the facial surface. Remember to use a relaxed grasp and maintain adaptation at all times.

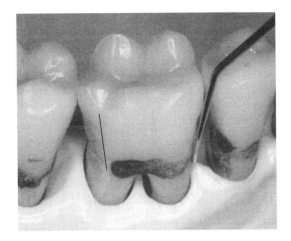

9. Explore at least halfway across the mesial surface from the facial aspect. (The other half will be explored from the lingual aspect.)

10. Next, use the sequence shown in this illustration to explore the facial aspect of the sextant, beginning with the posterior-most molar. This sequence allows you to explore the sextant in the most efficient manner.

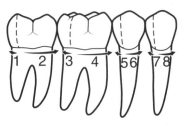

When you have completed the facial aspect, change your clock position and explore the lingual aspect of the sextant. The remaining three posterior sextants are explored in a similar manner.

Answers to questions on page 308. The top photograph shows the correct working-end. The arrow on the middle photograph points to the inner side of the tip; the inner side is not used on anterior teeth. The bottom photograph shows the correct working-end for this tooth surface.

Answers to questions on page 312. The top photograph shows the correct working-end. The middle photograph shows the incorrect working-end. The bottom photograph shows the incorrect working-end for this tooth surface.

Reference Sheet: Explorers

General Technique
1. Use relaxed grasp and rest middle finger lightly on shank.
2. Light, flowing strokes should cover every mm of root surface.

Anterior Teeth

1. For surfaces toward, sit at 8-9:00 if you are a right-handed clinician or at 4-3:00 if you are a left-handed clinician. For surfaces away, sit at 12:00.

2. Selection of correct working-end:
   - Use the outer side of the tip.
   - The face should curve toward the tooth surface to be instrumented.
   - The lower shank reaches across the tooth surface (*"anterior across"*).

3. Sequence: Begin with the surfaces toward you. Start on the canine on opposite side of the mouth and work toward yourself. (Right-handed: left canine, mesial surface; Left-handed: right canine, mesial surface)

4. For each tooth, position the tip so that the strokes on *the surfaces toward* will overlap your *strokes for the surfaces away* at the midline. Explorer tip is aimed in the direction in which you are working.

Posterior Teeth

1. For aspects toward, sit at 9:00 (or 3:00). For aspects away, sit at 10-11:00 (or 2-1:00).

2. Selection of correct working-end:
   - Use outer side of tip for facial, lingual, and mesial surfaces. Use inner side of tip for distal surfaces.
   - The lower shank is parallel to tooth surface (*"posterior parallel"*)

3. Sequence: Begin with the posterior-most tooth in the sextant. On each tooth, do the distal surface first, followed by facial and mesial (or lingual and mesial) surfaces.

4. For each tooth: (1) Distal surface: Begin slightly mesial to the distofacial line angle using inner side of tip—tip aimed toward distal surface. (2) Mesial and Facial (or Lingual) Surfaces: Begin slightly distal to the distofacial line angle using outer side of tip—tip aimed toward the front of mouth.

Section 4: Calculus Detection

Types and Characteristics

Supragingival calculus deposits are located coronal to the gingival margin (above the gingival margin) and can be detected visually. These deposits can usually be detected using compressed air and a dental mirror. A supragingival deposit is difficult to detect when it is wet with saliva; the wet surface reflects light and blends in with the wet tooth surface. Dry supragingival calculus, however, has a rough, chalky appearance and contrasts visually with the smooth enamel surfaces.

Subgingival calculus deposits are hidden beneath the gingival margin within the gingival sulcus or periodontal pocket. (Think "*sub*marines travel beneath the surface of the water".)

Comparison of Supragingival and Subgingival Calculus		
	Supragingival Deposits	**Subgingival Deposits**
Location	Above the gingival margin; detected visually	Beneath the gingival margin; detected by tactile means
Color	White, beige; may be discolored from food, beverages, or tobacco	Brown, black
Occurrence	Lingual aspect of mandibular anteriors; Facial surfaces of maxillary molars; crowded or poorly aligned teeth	Heaviest on mesial and distal surfaces
Attachment	On enamel—attached by acquired pellicle or cuticle On cementum—direct contact with tooth surface or locked into microscopic irregularities in cemental surface	

The Nature of Calculus Formation

When attempting to imagine the nature of subgingival deposits, remember that the deposits are built up layer by layer slowly over time. It may be helpful to imagine that you have taken a bucket of wet cement into your classroom! Once there, everyone takes turns throwing handfuls of cement against a plywood wall. Some individuals fling large globs of cement; some throw small handfuls. One aims at a new spot on the wall each time, another tries to hit the same area over and over. Now, imagine how the wall will appear when the cement has hardened. The cement mounds will be irregular and randomly spread over the wall. If you can imagine this absurd wall in your mind's eye, you have a fairly accurate concept of what subgingival calculus deposits look like on the root surface. To develop your ability to form a mental picture of the deposits that you detect, it is helpful to diagram what you are feeling and get feedback on your performance. Refer to the Skill Building Activity on page 324 for an activity designed to develop your abilities.

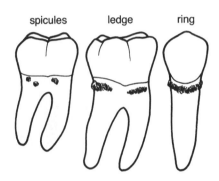

Three common types of calculus formations are spicules, a calculus ledge, and a calculus ring.

Common Calculus Formations	
Spicule	Isolated, minute particle or speck of calculus Common under contact areas, at line angles, and at midlines Feels like a slight "catch" as explorer tip moves along the tooth
Ledge	Ridge of calculus Common on all tooth surfaces, running parallel to gingival margin Feels like a distinct bump, causes a definite quiver of explorer tip
Ring	Ridge of calculus that encircles the tooth Feels like a large protuberance jutting out from tooth surface

Interpretation of Subgingival Conditions

The ability to recognize what you are feeling beneath the gingival margin is an important skill that takes time and concentration to develop. The following descriptions should aid you in interpreting what you feel. (From Trott, J.R.: The cross subgingival calculus explorer. Dental Digest 67: 481-483, 1961.)

Normal Conditions. Your fingers do not feel any interruptions in the path of the explorer as it moves from the junctional epithelium to the gingival margin.

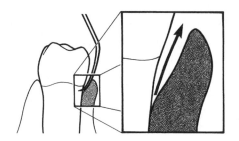

Spicules of Subgingival Calculus. The explorer tip transmits a gritty sensation to the clinician's fingers as it passes over fine, granular deposits. This can be compared to the sensation experienced when skating over a few pieces of gravel scattered on one area of a paved surface.

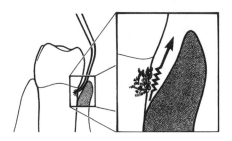

Ledge of Subgingival Calculus. As the explorer tip moves along the tooth surface, it moves out and around the raised bump, and returns back to the tooth surface. This is similar to the sensation of skating over speed bumps in a parking lot or over a cobblestone surface.

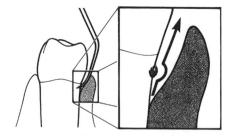

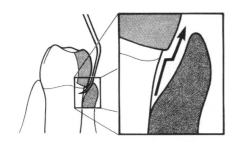

Restoration With Overhanging Margin. The explorer's path is blocked by the overhang and must move away from the tooth surface and over the restoration. This is similar to encountering the edge of a section of pavement that is higher than the surrounding pavement. Your skates must move up and over the higher section of pavement.

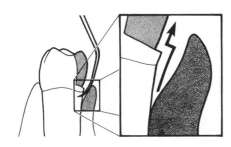

Restoration With Deficient Margin. The explorer passes over the surface of the tooth and then dips in to trace the surface of the restoration. This is similar to encountering the edge of a section of pavement that is lower than the surrounding pavement. Your skates must move down onto this section of pavement.

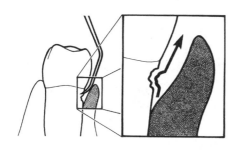

Carious Lesion (Decay). The explorer dips in and then comes out again as it travels along the tooth surface. This would be like skating into a pothole, across the pothole, and then back onto the pavement.

Reference Sheet: Common Causes of Undetected Calculus

Errors in exploring technique are the most common cause of a failure to detect subgingival calculus deposits. As this reference sheet shows, often a small change in technique makes a big difference in the ability to detect calculus deposits. Calculus detection is the most difficult of all skills for new clinicians to develop. Attention to instrumentation basics will aid you in acquiring this skill.

Causes of Undetected Calculus Deposits	
Location	Technique Error
No particular pattern to the location of the undetected deposits	• Use of inappropriate explorer for task • "Death-grip" on instrument handle • Middle finger not on shank (fewer vibrations can be felt through handle than through the shank) • Middle finger applying pressure against shank, reducing tactile information • Strokes too far apart (not overlapping)
Undetected deposits at midlines of anteriors, or line angles of posteriors	• Failure to overlap strokes in these areas • Failure to maintain constant adaptation to surface • Not using horizontal strokes in these areas
Undetected deposits on mesial or distal surfaces	• Strokes not extended apical to contact area so that at least one-half of surface is explored from both the facial and lingual aspects
Undetected deposits at base of sulcus or pocket on any surface of tooth	• Failure to insert explorer to junctional epithelium before initiating stroke

Section 5: Caries Detection

It is not a good idea to use the same explorer for both calculus and caries detection. The tip of an 11/12-type or a pigtail explorer can be damaged if used for caries detection. Once damaged, the burred working-end will not provide accurate tactile information to the clinician's fingers for detection of calculus. A straight or Shepherd Hook explorer is a good choice for caries detection.

Technique for Caries Detection

Enamel caries often can be detected visually by changes in the appearance of the enamel. The lesion may appear chalky-white, gray, brown, or black in color. When the walls of the lesion are explored, the surface will feel soft, tacky, or leathery in consistency. Subgingivally, a smooth surface lesion will be detected as a rough, concave area on the surface of the root.

The general technique for caries detection is to apply pressure with the point of the explorer against the region of suspected caries. Light pressure should be exerted with the explorer tip against the tooth surface. Firm pressure should not be used to force the explorer tip to penetrate the tooth surface. An obvious carious lesion that can be detected visually should not be explored.

1. *Pit and Fissure Caries:* Direct the point straight into the pit or fissure using light pressure. Trace the entire length of a fissure with the explorer while applying light pressure downward into the developmental depression. If caries is present, the tip will "catch" in the surface of the enamel.

2. *Smooth Surface Caries:* Move the tip of the explorer over the enamel surface, be alert for roughness, discontinuity, or change in hardness of the tooth surface. Visually, check for discoloration of enamel surfaces.

3. *Root Surface Caries:* While assessing the root surface, you will feel the explorer dip in and then come out again as it proceeds along the surface of the root. The depressed area of caries may feel rough or leathery.

4. *Recurrent Decay:* Trace the margin of the restoration with the explorer. Be careful to check for overhanging margins on restorations that extend over the incisal or occlusal surface of a tooth.

Section 6: Activity and Evaluation

Skill Building Activity: Diagramming Calculus Deposits

This activity will help you to develop tactile detection skills and the ability to form a mental picture of the deposits you detect.

Begin by creating some objects to represent roots and calculus. If possible, locate some discarded pieces of old copper tubing. The maintenance department at your college or university might be able to supply some. Use synthetic calculus to create "ledges and spicules of calculus" on the surface of the copper tubes. The "calculus deposits" should have a random pattern and each copper tube should have a unique pattern of "deposits". Allow the "calculus" to dry overnight. Obtain a small *opaque* trash bag.

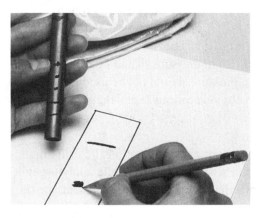

Compare the actual deposits on the copper tube with your diagram.

Directions for Activity:

1. Put an explorer, a copper tube and both of your hands inside the trash bag. Use your mirror hand to hold the copper tube. Grasp the explorer in your other hand and establish a finger rest on the side of the copper tube. Initiate assessment strokes along the surface of the tube. As you form a mental picture of the "calculus deposits" diagram them on a piece of paper on which you have drawn a rectangle representing the copper tube. Indicate the location and relative size of the "calculus deposits" on the tube.

2. Finally, remove the copper tube from the bag. Compare the actual "calculus deposits" to your drawing. How did you do? Repeat this activity with different copper tubes to improve your detection and visualization skills.

Skill Evaluation: Explorers

Student: _____   Area 1 = _____

Evaluator: _____   Area 2 = _____

Date: _____   Area 3 = _____

Area 4 = _____

Area 5 = _____

Area 6 = _____

DIRECTIONS: For each area, use **Column S** for student self-evaluation and **Column I** for instructor evaluation. For each skill evaluated, indicate the skill level as: **S** (satisfactory), **I** (improvement needed), or **U** (unsatisfactory)

CRITERIA:	Area 1		Area 2		Area 3		Area 4		Area 5		Area 6	
	S	I	S	I	S	I	S	I	S	I	S	I
Positioned correctly in relation to the patient, equipment, and treatment area												
Uses correct patient head position												
Index finger & thumb are across from one another and not touching; middle finger rests lightly on shank												
Ring finger acts as "support beam" ; finger rest is on a stable tooth surface												
Hand in correct palm-down or palm-up position; handle placement against hand is correct												
Selects correct side of explorer tip												
Inserts tip to junctional epithelium												
Uses mirror appropriately												
Maintains adaptation												
Uses appropriate motion activation												
Uses light, overlapping strokes												
Uses correct sequence												
Completely assesses the midlines on proximal surfaces, midlines of facial/lingual surfaces on anteriors, and line angles on posteriors												

Skill Evaluation: Explorers

Student: _____

Evaluator Comments:

_____

_____

_____

_____

_____

_____

_____

_____

_____

_____

_____

_____

_____

_____

_____

_____

_____

_____

Box for sketches pertaining to written comments.

14

MODULE

Anterior Sickle Scalers

This module contains step-by-step instructions for using a sickle scaler to remove medium-sized or heavy calculus deposits from the anterior sextants. The design characteristics of sickle scalers were presented in Module 8, Classification of Hand-Activated Instruments. Refer to this module if you need to review this information.

Required Equipment:

- dental mirror
- anterior sickle scaler (s)
- protective attire for the clinician and patient
- a manikin and typodont and/or a classmate

Section 1: Basic Concepts

Characteristics of the Calculus Removal Work Stroke

Before beginning the step-by-step technique practice with anterior sickle scalers, you should review the characteristics of the work stroke as used with an anterior sickle scaler and the steps in supragingival stroke production.

Calculus Removal Work Stroke With Anterior Sickles	
Application	One single-ended instrument is needed to instrument the crowns of anterior teeth
Stabilization	Apply pressure with the <u>index finger and thumb</u> inward against the instrument handle and press the tip of the fulcrum finger against the tooth surface
Adaptation	Tip-third of cutting edge
Angulation	70- to 80-degrees: the lower shank must be tilted slightly toward the tooth surface
Lateral Pressure	Moderate to firm pressure against the tooth surface is maintained throughout the pull stroke (Note: lateral pressure is NOT used with the placement stroke when positioning the working-end beneath a calculus deposit)
Characteristics	Powerful controlled strokes, short in length
Stroke Direction	Vertical strokes are most commonly used on anteriors
Number	Limited to areas where calculus is present and to the minimum number of strokes needed to remove deposits

Production of a Calculus Removal Work Stroke

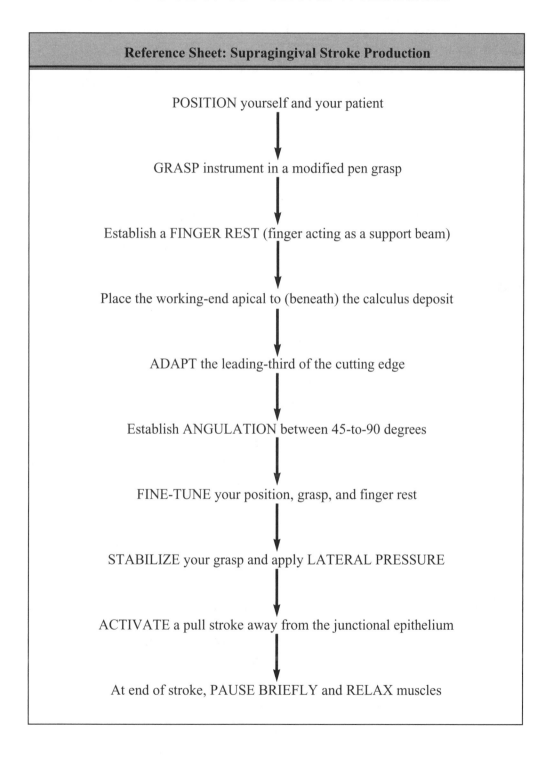

Reference Sheet: Supragingival Stroke Production

POSITION yourself and your patient

GRASP instrument in a modified pen grasp

Establish a FINGER REST (finger acting as a support beam)

Place the working-end apical to (beneath) the calculus deposit

ADAPT the leading-third of the cutting edge

Establish ANGULATION between 45-to-90 degrees

FINE-TUNE your position, grasp, and finger rest

STABILIZE your grasp and apply LATERAL PRESSURE

ACTIVATE a pull stroke away from the junctional epithelium

At end of stroke, PAUSE BRIEFLY and RELAX muscles

Application of Cutting Edges

An anterior sickle scaler may be a single-ended instrument because one working-end can be used to instrument the mesial, distal, facial, and lingual surfaces of the crowns in anterior sextants. It is common, however, for two anterior sickles to be combined on a double-ended instrument. Sickle scalers are limited to *supra*gingival use and should NOT be used on root surfaces.

The working-end of an anterior sickle scaler has two cutting edges (C1 and C2).

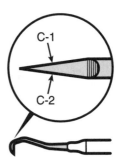

Application to anterior tooth surfaces. This illustration shows how the two cutting edges are applied to the coronal surfaces of anterior teeth.

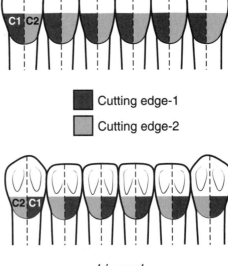

Facial

■ Cutting edge-1
▧ Cutting edge-2

Lingual

Section 1: Step-by-Step Technique

Example: Mandibular Left Canine, Facial Aspect

RIGHT-Handed Clinician				
		8-9	ST	2.5

LEFT-Handed Clinician				
		12	SA	2.1

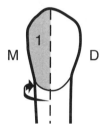

1. Begin by instrumenting the mesial-half of the mandibular left canine, facial aspect. If you are <u>right-handed</u>, this is the *surface toward you*. If you are <u>left-handed</u>, this is the *surface away from you*.

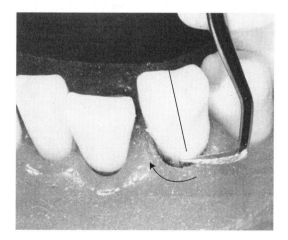

2. Position the tip-third of the cutting edge slightly to the right of the midline. The tip should be aimed toward the mesial surface.

Establish a 70° to 80° instrument face-to-tooth surface angulation.

3. As you approach the line angle, you will need to roll the instrument handle to maintain adaptation of the tip-third of the working-end.

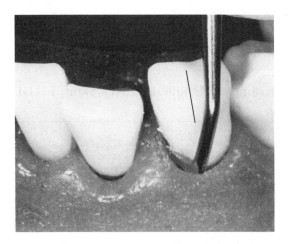

4. Roll the instrument handle to adapt to the mesial surface. Adapt the cutting edge.

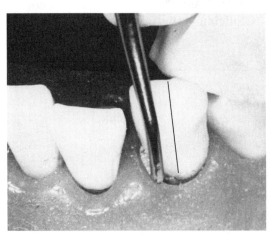

5. Continue strokes until you work at least halfway across the mesial surface. (The other half of the mesial surface will be instrumented from the lingual aspect of the tooth.)

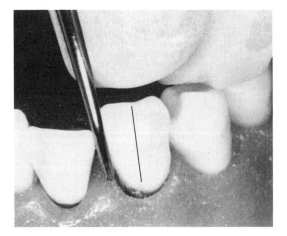

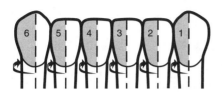

6. Use the sequence shown here to instrument the shaded tooth surfaces.

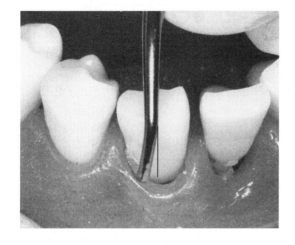

7. You will end with the <u>distal surface</u> of the <u>right</u> canine.

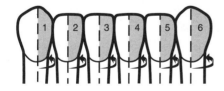

8. Change your clock position and complete the remaining facial surfaces, beginning with the mesial surface of the <u>right canine</u>. Remember to use the correct clock positions: sit at 8-9:00 (or 1-2:00) for surfaces toward you and 12:00 for surfaces away from you.

Reference Sheet: Anterior Sickle Scalers

Use:
Anterior sickle scalers are used to remove medium-sized and heavy calculus deposits from the crowns of anterior teeth. The pointed tip provides good access to the mesial and distal surfaces on anterior crowns. Sickle scalers are NOT recommended for use on root surfaces.

Anterior Teeth:

1. For surfaces toward, sit at 8-9:00 if you are a right-handed clinician or at 4-3:00 if you are a left-handed clinician. For surfaces away, sit at 12:00.

2. Sequence: Begin with the facial aspect, surfaces toward you. Start on the canine on opposite side of the mouth and work toward yourself. (Right-handed: facial aspect of left canine, mesial surface; Left-handed: facial aspect of right canine, mesial surface)

3. For each tooth, position the tip so that the strokes on *the surfaces toward* and *the surfaces away* will overlap at the midline. Aim the tip in the direction in which you are working.

4. Maintain adaptation of the tip-third of the cutting edge to the tooth surface.

5. Press down with your fulcrum finger and apply pressure against the instrument handle with the index finger and thumb to create lateral pressure against the tooth surface during the calculus removal work stroke.

6. Use hand-forearm motion activation.

7. Relax your fingers in between work strokes.

Skill Evaluation: Anterior Sickles

Student: _____ Area 1 = _____

Evaluator: _____ Area 2 = _____

Date: _____ Area 3 = _____

Area 4 = _____

DIRECTIONS: For each area, use **Column S** for student self-evaluation and **Column I** for instructor evaluation. For each skill evaluated, indicate the skill level as: **S** (satisfactory), **I** (improvement needed), or **U** (unsatisfactory).

CRITERIA:	Area 1 S	Area 1 I	Area 2 S	Area 2 I	Area 3 S	Area 3 I	Area 4 S	Area 4 I
Positioned correctly in relation to the patient, equipment, and treatment area								
Uses correct patient head position								
Index finger & thumb are across from one another and not touching; middle finger rests lightly on shank								
Ring finger acts as "support beam"; finger rest is on a stable tooth surface								
Handle placement correct (Mandibular toward—2.5; Maxillary toward—V; all surfaces away—2.1)								
Uses mirror appropriately								
Uses appropriate motion activation								
Maintains adaptation of tip-third of cutting edge								
Maintains correct face-to-tooth surface angulation								
Uses controlled work strokes								
Applies stroke pressure in a coronal direction only								
Uses correct sequence								
Completely instruments the midlines on proximal surfaces and midlines on facial or lingual surfaces								

Skill Evaluation: Anterior Sickles

Student: _____

Evaluator Comments:

_____

_____

_____

_____

_____

_____

_____

_____

_____

_____

_____

_____

_____

_____

_____

_____

_____

Box for sketches pertaining to written comments.

15

MODULE

Posterior Sickle Scalers

This module contains step-by-step instructions for using a sickle scaler to remove medium-sized or heavy calculus deposits from the posterior sextants. The design characteristics of sickle scalers were presented in Module 8, Classification of Hand-Activated Instruments. Refer to this module if you need to review this information.

Required Equipment:

- dental mirror
- posterior sickle scaler
- a manikin and typodont and/or a classmate
- protective attire for the clinician and patient, if working on a classmate

Section 1: Basic Concepts

Characteristics of the Calculus Removal Work Stroke

Before beginning the step-by-step technique practice, review the characteristics of the calculus removal work stroke as used with a posterior sickle scaler.

Calculus Removal Work Stroke With Posterior Sickles	
Application	One *double-ended instrument* is needed to instrument the crowns of posterior teeth
Stabilization	Apply pressure with the index finger and thumb inward against the instrument handle and press the tip of the fulcrum finger against the tooth surface
Adaptation	Tip-third of cutting edge
Angulation	70- to 80-degrees: the lower shank must be tilted slightly toward the tooth surface
Lateral Pressure	Moderate to firm pressure against the tooth surface is maintained throughout the pull stroke (Note: lateral pressure is NOT used with the placement stroke when positioning the working-end beneath a calculus deposit)
Characteristics	Powerful controlled strokes, short in length
Stroke Direction	Vertical on proximal surfaces, oblique on facial and lingual surfaces, and horizontal at line angles
Number	Limited to areas where calculus is present and to the minimum number of strokes needed to remove deposits

Inner and Outer Cutting Edges

Each of the two working-ends of a posterior sickle scaler has two cutting edges, an inner cutting edge and an outer cutting edge. The **outer cutting edges** are the ones that are *farther* from the instrument handle. The **inner cutting edges** are the ones that are *closer* to the instrument handle.

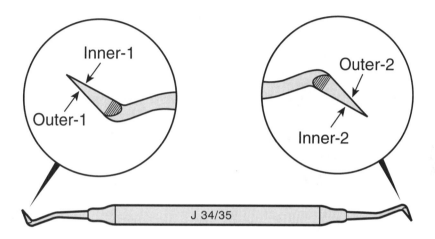

Each of the two working-ends of a posterior sickle scaler has two cutting edges, an inner (I) and an outer (O) cutting edge.

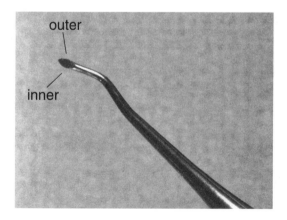

The inner (I) and outer (O) cutting edges of a posterior sickle. To identify the cutting edges, hold the instrument so that you are looking at the face of the working-end.

Selecting the Correct Cutting Edge for Posteriors

- When using a posterior sickle scaler on the <u>facial aspect</u> of a posterior tooth, one of inner cutting edges adapts to the distal surface. On the same working-end, the outer cutting edge adapts to the facial and mesial surfaces of the tooth crown.

- The cutting edges of the other working-end will adapt to the lingual aspect of the same tooth (inner edge for distal, outer for lingual and mesial).

- The **lower shank** should be **parallel** to the tooth surface being instrumented.

Visual Clues for Posterior Teeth

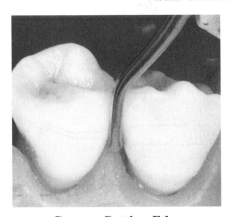
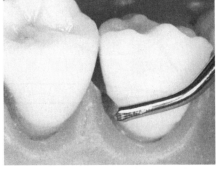

       Correct Cutting Edge   **Incorrect Cutting Edge**

Use the following visual clues to identify the correct cutting edge for <u>supragingival</u> use on the <u>crowns</u> of posterior teeth:

- **Inner cutting edges** adapt to the distal surfaces of posterior teeth.

- **Outer cutting edges** adapt to the facial, lingual, and mesial surfaces.

- **Lower shank** is *parallel* to the tooth surface being instrumented. (Think "posterior parallel".)

Practice in Selecting the Correct Cutting Edge

Can you apply the visual clues to each of these photographs? The answers to the questions can be found at the bottom of page 342.

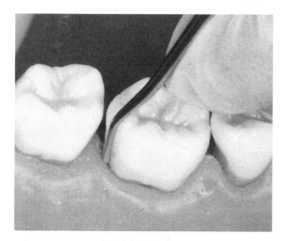

Is this the correct cutting edge for use on the distal surface of this mandibular molar?

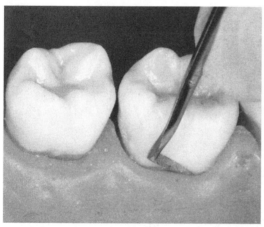

Is this the correct cutting edge for use on the facial surface of this mandibular molar?

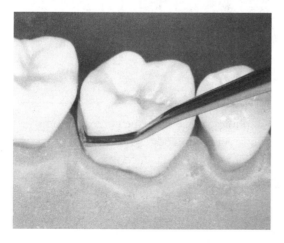

Is this the correct cutting edge for use on the distal surface of this mandibular molar?

Application of Cutting Edges

Application to posterior teeth.

The inner cutting edges (Inner-1 and Inner-2) adapt to the distal surfaces of posterior crowns.

The outer cutting edges (Outer-1 and Outer-2) adapt to the facial, lingual, and mesial surfaces of the crowns on posterior teeth.

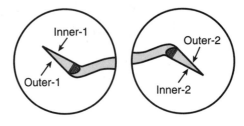

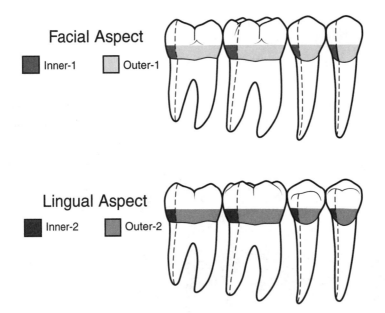

Facial Aspect

■ Inner-1   □ Outer-1

Lingual Aspect

■ Inner-2   ▨ Outer-2

Answers to questions on page 341. The top photograph shows the correct cutting edge. The middle photograph shows the incorrect cutting edge. The bottom photograph shows the incorrect cutting edge for this tooth surface.

Section 2: Step-by-Step Technique

Example: Mandibular Right Posteriors, Facial Aspect

RIGHT-Handed Clinician				

LEFT-Handed Clinician				

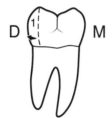

1. Begin with the last molar in the sextant. The distal surface is completed first, beginning at the distofacial line angle and working onto the distal surface.

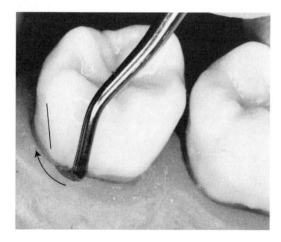

2. Adapt the cutting edge to the right of the distofacial line angle so that your strokes will overlap slightly at the line angle. The tip should aim toward the back of the mouth because this is the direction in which you are working.

3. Roll the instrument handle slightly to adapt to distal surface. Work at least halfway across the distal surface from the facial aspect. Keep the cutting edge adapted to the tooth surface at all times.

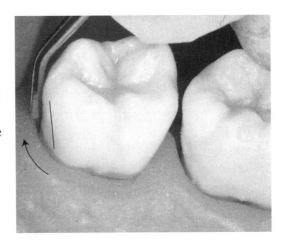

4. You are now ready to instrument the facial and mesial surfaces of the tooth, beginning at the distofacial line angle.

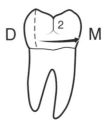

5. While maintaining your fulcrum, lift the working-end away from the tooth and turn it so that it aims toward the front of the mouth. Reposition the working-end at the distofacial line angle.

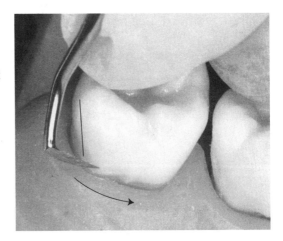

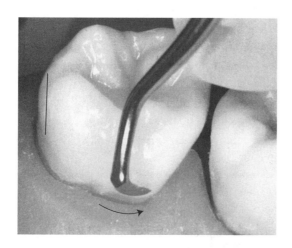

6. Continue working across the facial surface. Remember to maintain adaptation at all times.

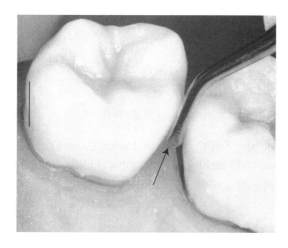

7. Work at least halfway across the mesial surface from the facial aspect. (The other half will be instrumented from the lingual aspect.)

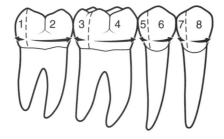

8. Use the sequence shown in this illustration to instrument the facial aspect of the remaining teeth in the sextant. This sequence allows you to instrument the sextant in the most efficient manner.

When you have completed the facial aspect, change your clock position and instrument the lingual aspect of the sextant. The remaining three posterior sextants are instrumented in a similar manner.

Reference Sheet: Posterior Sickle Scalers

Use:
Posterior sickle scalers are used to remove medium- and large-size supragingival calculus deposits from the crowns of posterior teeth. The pointed tip provides good access to the proximal surfaces apical to the contact areas on posterior teeth. Sickle scalers are NOT recommended for use on root surfaces.

Posterior Teeth:

1. For aspects toward, sit at 9:00 (or 3:00). For aspects away, sit at 10-11:00 (or 2-1:00).

2. Posterior sickle scalers are limited to use on enamel surfaces above the gingival margin (coronal to the gingival margin).

3. The **inner** cutting edges are used on the distal surfaces.

   The **outer** cutting edges are used on the facial, lingual, and mesial surfaces.

4. Sequence: Begin at the distofacial line angle of the tooth and work toward the distal surface. Reposition at the distofacial line angle and complete the facial (or lingual) and mesial surfaces of the tooth, working toward the front of the mouth.

5. For each tooth, position the working end so that the strokes will overlap at the distofacial line angle. Aim the tip in the direction in which you are working.

6. Maintain adaptation of the tip-third of the cutting edge to the tooth surface.

7. Press down with your fulcrum finger and apply pressure against the instrument handle with the index finger and thumb to create lateral pressure against the tooth surface during the calculus removal work stroke.

8. Use hand-forearm motion activation.

9. Relax your fingers in between work strokes.

Skill Evaluation: Posterior Sickles

Student: _____   Area 1 = _____

Evaluator: _____   Area 2 = _____

Date: _____   Area 3 = _____

Area 4 = _____

DIRECTIONS: For each area, use **Column S** for student self-evaluation and **Column I** for instructor evaluation. For each skill evaluated, indicate the skill level as: **S** (satisfactory), **I** (improvement needed), or **U** (unsatisfactory).

CRITERIA:	Area 1		Area 2		Area 3		Area 4	
	S	I	S	I	S	I	S	I
Positioned correctly in relation to the patient, equipment, and treatment area								
Uses correct patient head position								
Index finger & thumb are across from one another and not touching; middle finger rests lightly on shank								
Ring finger acts as "support beam"; finger rest is on a stable tooth surface								
Handle placement correct (Mandibular arch—at or near position 3; Maxillary arch—2.5 to 3.5)								
Uses mirror appropriately								
Uses appropriate motion activation								
Maintains adaptation of tip-third of cutting edge								
Maintains correct face-to-tooth surface angulation								
Uses controlled work strokes								
Applies stroke pressure in a coronal direction only								
Uses correct sequence								
Completely instruments the midlines on proximal surfaces and distofacial line angle on facial or lingual surfaces								

Skill Evaluation: Posterior Sickles

Student: _____
Evaluator Comments:

_____

_____

_____

_____

_____

_____

_____

_____

_____

_____

_____

_____

_____

_____

_____

_____

Box for sketches pertaining to written comments.

16
MODULE

Universal Curets

This module contains step-by-step instructions for using a universal curet to remove small- or medium-sized calculus deposits. The design characteristics of universal curets were presented in Module 8, Classification of Hand-Activated Instruments. Refer to this module if you need to review this information.

Required Equipment:

1. dental mirror and universal curet(s)
2. a manikin and typodont and/or a classmate

Section 1: Basic Concepts

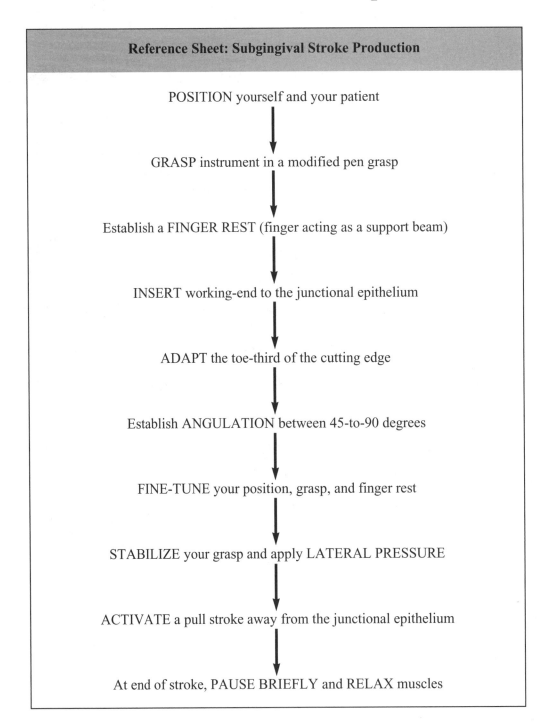

Reference Sheet: Subgingival Stroke Production

POSITION yourself and your patient

GRASP instrument in a modified pen grasp

Establish a FINGER REST (finger acting as a support beam)

INSERT working-end to the junctional epithelium

ADAPT the toe-third of the cutting edge

Establish ANGULATION between 45-to-90 degrees

FINE-TUNE your position, grasp, and finger rest

STABILIZE your grasp and apply LATERAL PRESSURE

ACTIVATE a pull stroke away from the junctional epithelium

At end of stroke, PAUSE BRIEFLY and RELAX muscles

Inner and Outer Cutting Edges

Each of the two working-ends of a universal curet has two cutting edges, an inner cutting edge and an outer cutting edge. The **outer cutting edges** are the ones that are *farther* from the instrument handle. The **inner cutting edges** are the ones that are *closer* to the instrument handle.

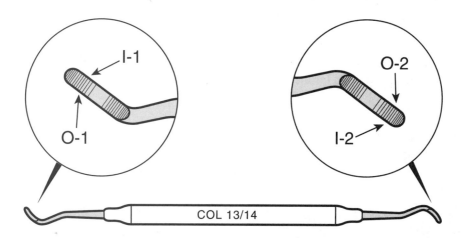

Each of the two working-ends of a universal curet has two cutting edges, an inner (I) and an outer (O) cutting edge.

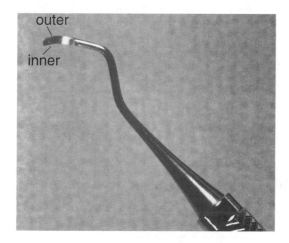

The inner (I) and outer (O) cutting edges of a universal curet. To identify the cutting edges, hold the instrument so that you are looking at the face of the working-end.

Section 2: Technique on Posterior Sextants

Selecting the Correct Cutting Edge for Posteriors

- When using a universal curet on the <u>facial aspect</u> of a posterior tooth, one of **inner** cutting edges adapts to the distal surface. The **outer** cutting edge (on the same working-end) adapts to the facial and mesial surfaces.

- The cutting edges of the other working-end will adapt to the lingual aspect of the same tooth (inner edge for distal, outer for lingual and mesial).

- The **lower shank** should be **parallel** to the tooth surface being instrumented.

Visual Clues for Posterior Teeth

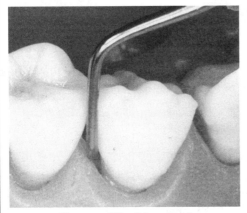

Correct Working-End

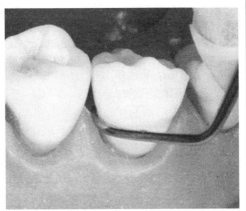

Incorrect Working-End

Use the following visual clues to identify the correct working-end for use on the posterior teeth:

- **Inner cutting edges** adapt to the distal surfaces of posterior teeth.

- **Outer cutting edges** adapt to the facial, lingual, and mesial surfaces.

- **Lower shank** is *parallel* to the tooth surface being instrumented. (Think "posterior parallel".)

Practice in Selecting the Correct Cutting Edge

Can you apply the visual clues to each of these photographs? The answers to the questions can be found at the bottom of page 354.

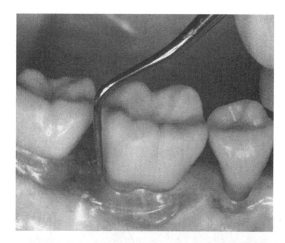

Is this the correct cutting edge for use on the distal surface of this mandibular molar?

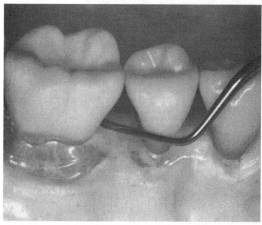

Is this the correct cutting edge for use on the mesial surface of this mandibular molar?

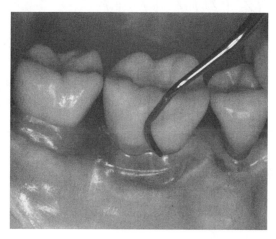

Is this the correct cutting edge for use on the facial surface of this mandibular molar?

Application of Cutting Edges

Application to posterior teeth

The inner cutting edges (Inner-1 and Inner-2) adapt to the distal surfaces of posterior crowns and roots.

The outer cutting edges (Outer-1 and Outer-2) adapt to the facial, lingual, and mesial surfaces of the crowns and roots of posterior teeth.

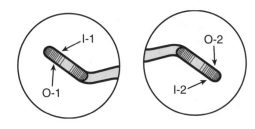

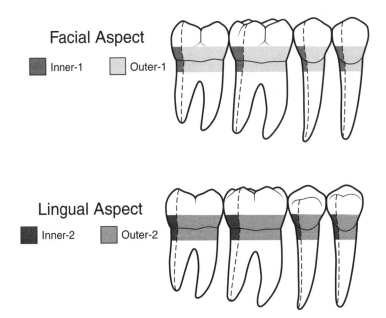

These illustrations show how the four cutting edges of a universal curet are applied to the surfaces of a posterior sextant.

Answers to questions on page 353. The top photograph shows the correct cutting edge. The middle photograph shows the incorrect cutting edge. The bottom photograph shows the incorrect cutting edge for this tooth surface.

Step-by-Step Technique on Posteriors

Example: Mandibular Right Posteriors, Facial Aspect

RIGHT-Handed Clinician

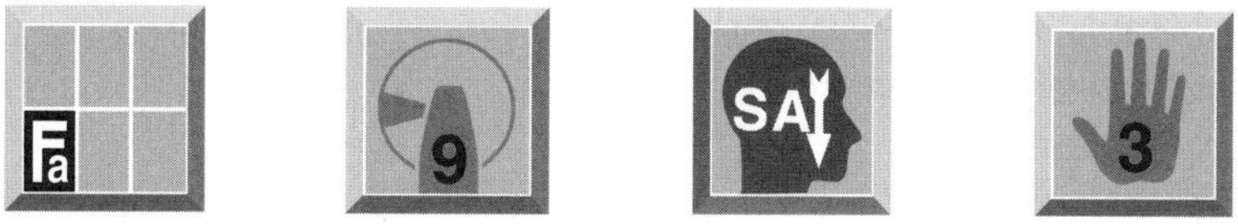

LEFT-Handed Clinician

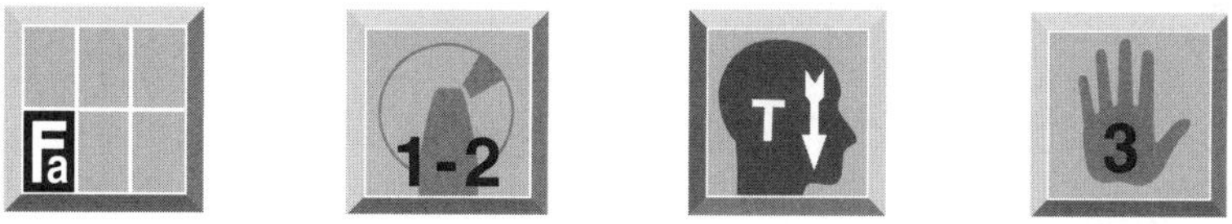

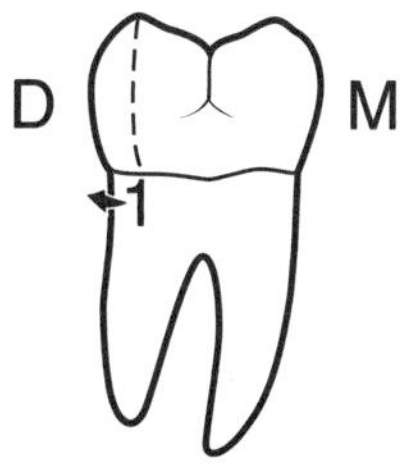

1. Begin with the last molar in the sextant. The distal surface is completed first, beginning at the distofacial line angle and working onto the distal surface.

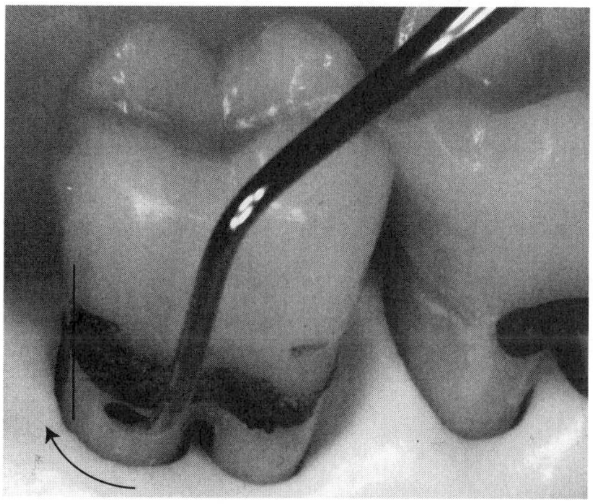

2. Insert the working-end beneath the gingival margin at a 0°-to-40° angle. Adapt the cutting edge to the right of the distofacial line angle; the toe should aim toward the back of the mouth because this is the direction in which you are working.

3. Roll the instrument handle slightly to adapt to distal surface. Work at least halfway across the distal surface from the facial aspect. Keep the cutting edge adapted to the tooth surface at all times.

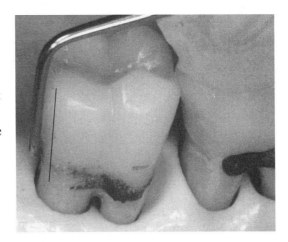

4. You are now ready to instrument the facial and mesial surfaces of the tooth, beginning at the distofacial line angle.

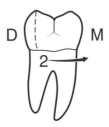

5. While maintaining your fulcrum, lift the working-end away from the tooth and turn it so that it aims toward the front of the mouth. Reposition the working-end at the distofacial line angle with the toe aiming forward.

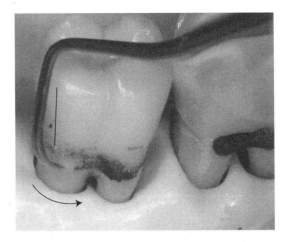

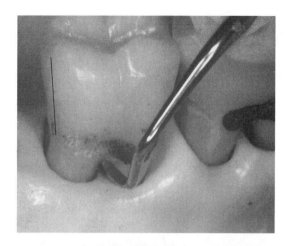

6. If there is bone loss present in the furcation area, you will need to instrument the root branches on either side of the furcation.

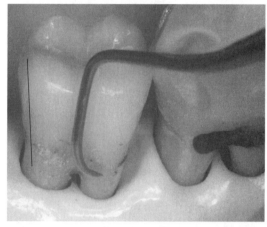

7. While maintaining your fulcrum, move the working-end from the furcation and turn it to adapt to the facial surface. Continue making strokes across the facial surface.

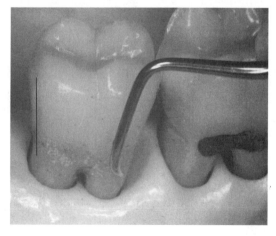

8. At the mesiofacial line angle, roll the instrument handle to readapt the toe-third of the cutting edge to the mesial surface.

9. Work at least halfway across the mesial surface from the facial aspect. (The other half will be instrumented from the lingual aspect.)

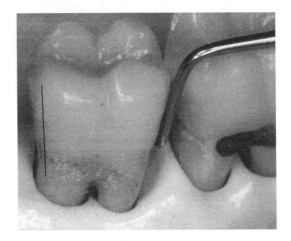

10. Use the sequence shown in this illustration to instrument the facial aspect of the remaining teeth in the sextant. This sequence allows you to scale the sextant in the most efficient manner.

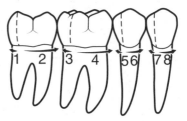

When you have completed the facial aspect, change your clock position and instrument the lingual aspect of this sextant.

The remaining three posterior sextants are instrumented in a similar manner.

Section 3: Technique on Anterior Sextants

Selecting the Correct Working-End for Anteriors

When using a universal curet on anterior teeth:
- only the **outer cutting edges** are used.

- the face should tilt toward the tooth surface

- the lower shank reaches across the tooth surface.

Visual Clues for Anterior Teeth

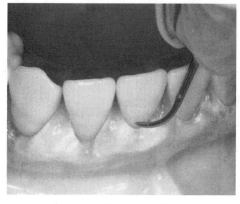 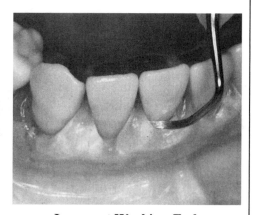

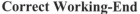

| **Correct Working-End** | **Incorrect Working-End** |

Use the following visual clues to identify the correct working-end:

- **Outer side** of cutting edge is adapted to the tooth surface.

- **Face** of working-end tilts toward the tooth surface.

- **Lower shank** reaches across the tooth surface. (Think "anterior across".)

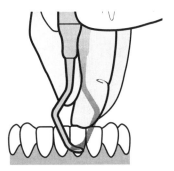

Visual Clue—Shank Position. When using a universal curet on anterior teeth, the lower shank reaches across the tooth surface. To help you remember this, think *"anterior across"*.

(Adapted from Genco, R.J., Goldman, H.M., Cohen, D.W.: *Contemporary Periodontics*. St. Louis, C.V. Mosby, 1990.)

Practice in Selecting the Correct Cutting Edge

Can you apply the visual clues to these photographs? (Answers on page 361.)

Is this the correct cutting-edge for use on the mesial surface of the mandibular left central incisor?

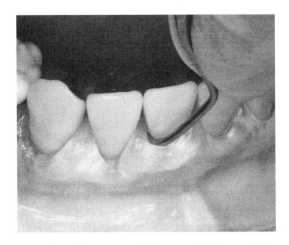

Is the arrow pointing to the outer or inner cutting edge? Would this cutting edge be used on anterior teeth?

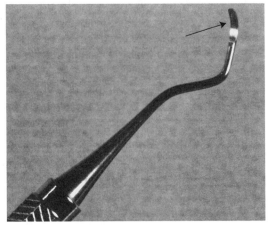

Application of Cutting Edges

Application to anterior teeth

Only the two outer cutting edges (Outer-1 and Outer-2) of a universal curet are used to instrument the anterior teeth.

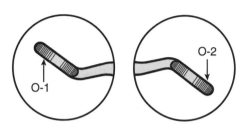

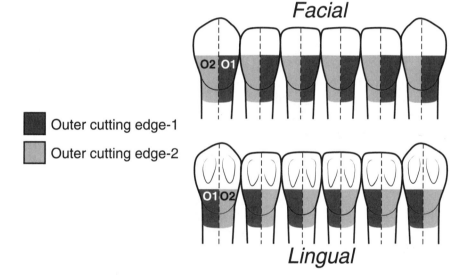

Facial

■ Outer cutting edge-1
▨ Outer cutting edge-2

Lingual

These illustrations show how the outer cutting edges of a universal curet are applied to the surfaces of an anterior sextant.

Answers to questions on page 360. The photograph shows the correct cutting edge for use on the mesial surface of the mandibular left central incisor. The arrow points to the inner cutting edge; the inner cutting edges are not used on anterior teeth.

Step-by-Step Technique on Anteriors

Example: Mandibular Left Canine, Facial Aspect

RIGHT-Handed Clinician				

LEFT-Handed Clinician				

1. Begin by instrumenting the mesial-half of the mandibular left canine, facial aspect. If you are <u>right-handed</u>, this is the *surface toward you*. If you are <u>left-handed</u>, this is the *surface away from you*.

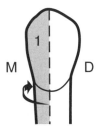

2. Begin with the left canine. Gently insert the working-end beneath the gingival margin at 0°-to-40°.

Establish the correct instrument face-to-tooth surface angulation by tilting the lower shank slightly toward the facial surface.

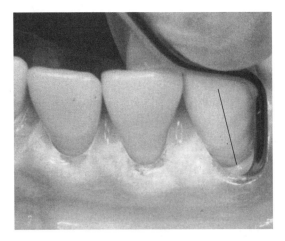

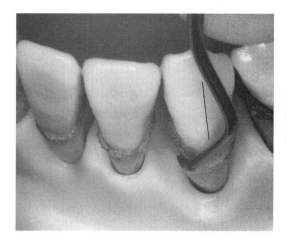

3. Roll the instrument handle to maintain adaptation of the toe-third of the working-end to the mesial surface.

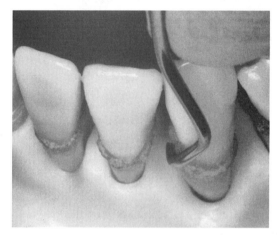

4. Continue strokes until you have instrumented at least halfway across the mesial proximal surface. (The other half of the mesial surface will be reached from the lingual aspect of the tooth.)

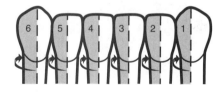

5. Use the sequence shown here to instrument the shaded tooth surfaces of the sextant.

Change your clock position and complete the remaining facial surfaces, beginning with the mesial surface of the right canine. Sit at 8-9:00 (or 1-2:00) for surfaces toward you and 12:00 for surfaces away from you.

Section 4: Refining Your Technique

Instrumenting Proximal Surfaces

Proximal surfaces of posterior teeth: Beginning clinicians often miss calculus deposits located beneath the contact areas of posterior teeth.

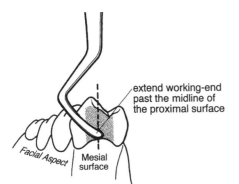

extend working-end past the midline of the proximal surface

Facial Aspect | Mesial surface

Be sure to extend working strokes under the contact area on the proximal surfaces of posterior teeth from both the facial and lingual aspects.

Proximal surfaces of anterior teeth: The working-end must be positioned <u>between</u> the papilla and the tooth surface. Many beginning clinicians "trace" the rising contours of the papilla and fail to insert the working-end subgingivally on the proximal surface.

CORRECT: Facial view. Here the working-end is positioned correctly between the papilla and the tooth surface. In this position, the working-end can be inserted to the base of the sulcus or pocket on the proximal surface.

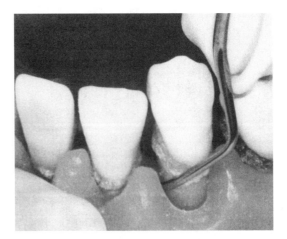

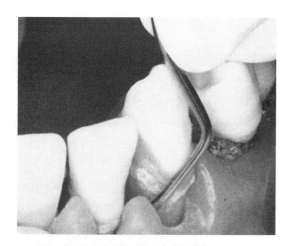

CORRECT: This photograph shows the proximal view of the working-end placement between the papilla and the tooth surface.

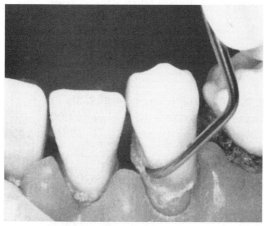

INCORRECT: Facial view. The clinician is "tracing" the rising contours of the papilla. In this position, the portion of the tooth from the gingival margin to the junctional epithelium is not instrumented.

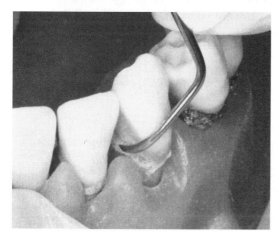

INCORRECT: Proximal view. In this position, only the portion of the proximal surface above the papilla is instrumented. Subgingival calculus on the proximal surface is not removed.

Reference Sheet: Universal Curets

Use:
Universal curets are used to remove small- and medium-size calculus deposits from the crowns and roots of the teeth.

Basic Concepts:
1. Insert the working-end beneath the gingival margin at a 0-to 40-degree angle.

2. Maintain adaptation of the toe-third of the cutting edge to the tooth surface.

3. Press down with your fulcrum finger and apply pressure against the instrument handle with the index finger and thumb to create lateral pressure against the tooth surface during the calculus removal work stroke.

4. Use hand-forearm motion activation.

5. Relax your fingers in between work strokes.

Anterior Teeth:
1. For surfaces toward, sit at 8-9:00 if you are a right-handed clinician or at 3-4:00 if you are a left-handed clinician. For surfaces away, sit at 12:00.

2. Selection of correct working-end:
    • Only the outer cutting edges are used on anterior teeth
    • The face should tilt toward the tooth surface to be instrumented.
    • The lower shank reaches across the tooth surface (*"anterior across"*).

3. Sequence: Begin with the surfaces toward you. Start on the canine on opposite side of the mouth and work toward yourself. (Right-handed: left canine, mesial surface; Left-handed: right canine, mesial surface)

Posterior Teeth:
1. For aspects toward, sit at 9:00 (or 3:00). For aspects away, sit at 10-11:00 (or 1-2:00).

2. The **inner** cutting edges are used on the distal surfaces.
    The **outer** cutting edges are used on the facial, lingual, and mesial surfaces.
    The lower shank is parallel to the tooth surface (*"posterior parallel"*)

3. Sequence: Begin at the distofacial line angle of the tooth and work toward the distal surface. Reposition at the distofacial line angle and complete the facial (or lingual) and mesial surfaces of the tooth, working toward the front of the mouth.

Skill Evaluation #1: Universal Curets, Anterior Sextants

Student: _____   Area 1 = _____

Evaluator: _____   Area 2 = _____

Date: _____   Area 3 = _____

Area 4 = _____

DIRECTIONS: For each area, use **Column S** for student self-evaluation and **Column I** for instructor evaluation. For each skill evaluated, indicate the skill level as: **S** (satisfactory), **I** (improvement needed), or **U** (unsatisfactory).

CRITERIA:	Area 1 S	Area 1 I	Area 2 S	Area 2 I	Area 3 S	Area 3 I	Area 4 S	Area 4 I
Positioned correctly in relation to the patient, equipment, and treatment area								
Uses correct patient head position								
Index finger & thumb are across from one another and not touching; middle finger rests lightly on shank								
Ring finger acts as "support beam"; finger rest is on a stable tooth surface								
Handle placement correct								
Uses mirror appropriately								
Gently inserts working-end beneath gingival margin								
Maintains adaptation of toe-third of cutting edge								
Maintains correct face-to-tooth surface angulation								
Uses controlled work strokes								
Applies stroke pressure in a coronal direction only								
Uses appropriate motion activation								
Uses correct sequence								

Skill Evaluation #1: Universal Curets, Anterior Sextants

Student: _____

Evaluator Comments:

_____

_____

_____

_____

_____

_____

_____

_____

_____

_____

_____

_____

_____

_____

_____

_____

_____

Box for sketches pertaining to written comments.

Skill Evaluation #2: Universal Curets, Posterior Sextants

Student: _____   Area 1 = _____

Evaluator: _____   Area 2 = _____

Date: _____   Area 3 = _____

Area 4 = _____

DIRECTIONS: For each area, use **Column S** for student self-evaluation and **Column I** for instructor evaluation. For each skill evaluated, indicate the skill level as: **S** (satisfactory), **I** (improvement needed), or **U** (unsatisfactory).

CRITERIA:	Area 1		Area 2		Area 3		Area 4	
	S	I	S	I	S	I	S	I
Positioned correctly in relation to the patient, equipment, and treatment area								
Uses correct patient head position								
Index finger & thumb are across from one another and not touching; middle finger rests lightly on shank								
Ring finger acts as "support beam"; finger rest is on a stable tooth surface								
Handle placement correct								
Uses mirror appropriately								
Gently inserts working-end beneath gingival margin								
Maintains adaptation of toe-third of cutting edge								
Maintains correct face-to-tooth surface angulation								
Uses controlled work strokes								
Applies stroke pressure in a coronal direction only								
Uses appropriate motion activation								
Uses correct sequence								

Skill Evaluation #2: Universal Curets, Posterior Sextants

Student: _____

Evaluator Comments:

_____

_____

_____

_____

_____

_____

_____

_____

_____

_____

_____

_____

_____

_____

_____

_____

_____

_____

Box for sketches pertaining to written comments.

Area-Specific Curets

This module contains step-by-step instructions for using area-specific curets to remove small-sized calculus deposits and for root surface debridement. The design characteristics of area-specific curets were presented in Module 8, Classification of Hand-Activated Instruments. Refer to this module if you need to review this information.

Required Equipment:

- dental mirror and area-specific curets
- a manikin and typodont and/or a classmate
- protective attire for patient and clinician, if working on a classmate

Key Terms:

Self-angulated curet
Working cutting edge
Mini working-end
Root concavity

Section 1: Basic Concepts

Terminology

Self-angulated curet—in area-specific curets, the face of working-end is tilted at a 70° angle in relation to the terminal shank. This design feature positions the lower cutting edge in correct angulation to the root surface while the opposite cutting is angled away from the soft tissue wall of the pocket.

The **working cutting edge** is the cutting edge on an area-specific curet that is used for instrumentation. An area-specific curet only has one working cutting edge per working-end.

Mini-working-end—area-specific curet with a working-end that is 50 percent shorter in length than the working-end of a standard Gracey curet.

Root concavity—a linear developmental depression in the root surface; commonly occurring on the proximal surfaces of the root.

Identifying the Working Cutting Edge

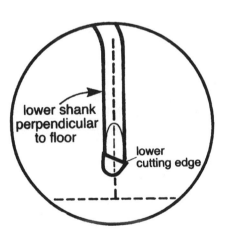

To identify the working cutting edge:
1. Hold your instrument so that you are looking at the toe of the working-end.
2. Raise or lower the instrument handle until the lower shank is perpendicular (⊥) to the floor.
3. Look closely at the working-end, note that one of the cutting edges is lower (closer to the floor) than the other.
4. The lower cutting edge is the one that is used for instrumentation (the working cutting edge).

Section 2: Technique on Anterior Sextants

Visual Clues for Anterior Teeth

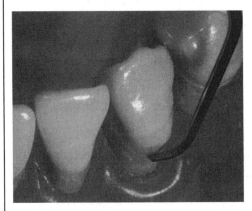 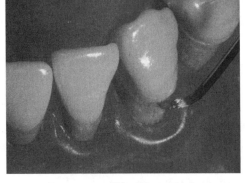

Correct Working-End   **Incorrect Working-End**

Use the following visual clues to identify the correct working-end for use on the anterior teeth:

- **Lower cutting edge** is the working cutting edge. (Only one cutting edge per working-end is used for instrumentation.)

- **Instrument face** tilts toward the tooth surface.

- **Lower shank** is *parallel* to the tooth surface being instrumented.

Refer to page 210 to review the areas of application for each of the curets in the Gracey series. For example, the Gracey 1, 2, 3, and 4 are used on anterior teeth.

Application of Cutting Edges

You will need two area-specific curets to debride the anterior tooth surfaces. For example, you might select a Gracey 3 and a Gracey 4. Usually these curets are combined on a double-ended instrument.

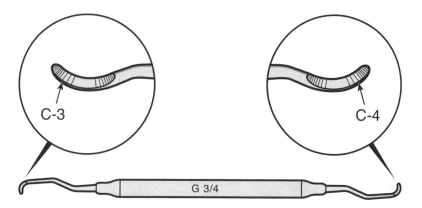

The Gracey 3 and the Gracey 4 curets are commonly paired on a double-ended instrument for use on anterior tooth surfaces.

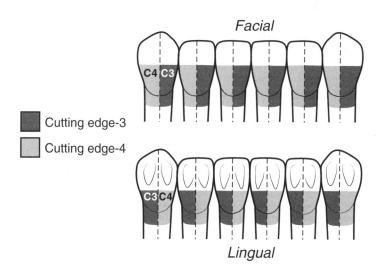

Use of the Gracey 3/4 on the mandibular anteriors. This illustration shows application of the G 3/4 to the "surfaces toward" and "surfaces away" on the mandibular anteriors.

Step-by-Step Technique on Anteriors

Example: Mandibular Anteriors, Facial Aspect

RIGHT-Handed Clinician

LEFT-Handed Clinician

1. The shaded tooth surfaces on the facial aspect should be completed in the order shown in this illustration.

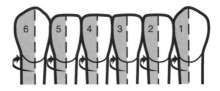

2. Begin with the left canine. Gently insert the working-end at a 0°-to-40° angle. Position the lower shank parallel to the facial surface to establish the correct instrument face-to-tooth surface angulation.

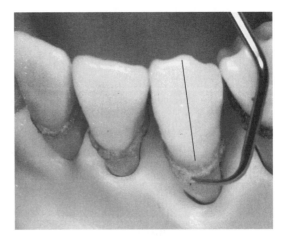

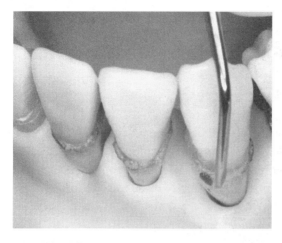

3. Roll the instrument handle to adapt to the mesial surface.

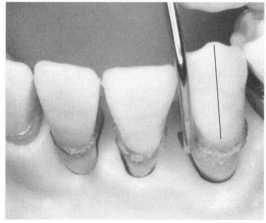

4. Continue strokes until you have instrumented at least halfway across the mesial proximal surface. (The other half of the mesial surface will be reached from the lingual aspect of the tooth.)

5. Work across the sextant, ending with the distal surface of the right canine.

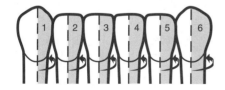

6. Next, complete the shaded surfaces in the sequence shown in this illustration. Change your clock position and begin with the mesial surface of the right canine.

When you have completed the facial aspect, instrument the lingual aspect of the mandibular anteriors. Remember to use the correct clock positions: sit at 8-9:00 (or 1-2:00) for surfaces toward you and 12:00 for surfaces away from you.

Section 3: Root Surface Debridement—Anteriors

Instrumentation of Root Concavities

In order to debride the root surfaces effectively, it is important to have a good understanding of root morphology. The majority of instrumentation on root surfaces is done beneath the gingival margin. A clear mental picture of root anatomy and a keen tactile sense are necessary for periodontal instrumentation to be successful.

A **root concavity** is a linear developmental depression in the root surface. Root concavities commonly occur on the proximal surfaces of anterior and posterior teeth. Removing dental calculus from root concavities demands careful adaptation to the working-end to the concavity.

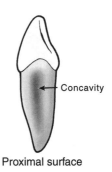

Concavity

Proximal surface

In cross section, the root of this canine is seen to have two root concavities, one concavity on the mesial root surface and one on the distal root surface.

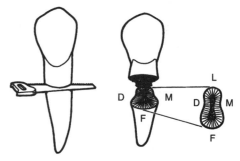

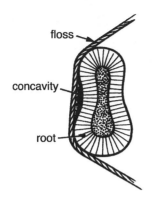

A piece of floss stretched around a <u>root surface</u> will not disrupt bacterial plaque in a proximal root concavity.

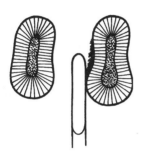

The same problem occurs when the clinician does not consider root morphology during instrumentation. The length of the cutting edge spans the depression leaving calculus deposits undisturbed.

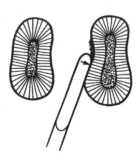

The clinician should roll the instrument handle to direct the toe-third of the cutting edge into the root concavity.

Notice that the middle- and heel-thirds of the cutting edge are rotated toward the adjacent tooth.

Root Morphology: Anterior Teeth

Tooth	Root Morphology
Mandibular Arch Central Incisor • Deep linear proximal root concavities	Mesial — Deep concavity — Distal
Lateral Incisor • Deep linear proximal root concavities	Mesial — Concavity — Distal
Canine • Deep linear proximal root concavities	Mesial — Concavity — Distal

Root Morphology: Anterior Teeth *Continued*

Tooth	Root Morphology
Maxillary Arch Central Incisor • Usually no root concavities present	*Mesial*　　　*Distal*
Lateral Incisor • May have proximal root concavities • If a palatal groove is present on the cingulum, it may extend onto the cervical third of the lingual surface	Concavity *Distal*　　　*Lingual*
Canine • May have proximal root concavities	Concavity *Mesial*　　　*Distal*

Section 4: Technique on Posterior Sextants

Visual Clues for Posterior Teeth

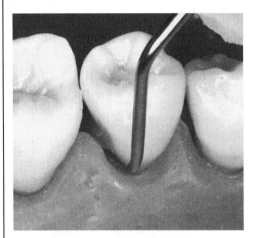

Correct Working-End

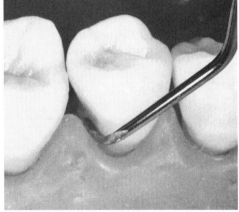

Incorrect Working-End

Use the following visual clues to identify the correct working-end for use on the posterior teeth:

- **Lower cutting edge** is the working cutting edge. (Only one cutting edge per working-end is used for instrumentation.)
- **Lower shank** is *parallel* to the tooth surface being instrumented.

Memory Helpers

When selecting the working-end, place the curet on a proximal surface and observe the relationship of the instrument shank to the tooth. Ask yourself, *"does the shank go up and over the tooth or does the shank go down and around the tooth?"*

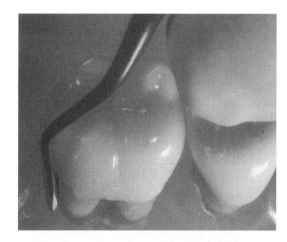

CORRECT working-end—lower shank is parallel to tooth surface. Think *"the shank goes up and over"*.

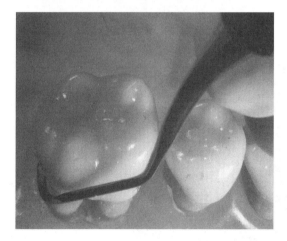

INCORRECT working-end—lower shank is not parallel. Think *"shank is down and around"*.

Application of Cutting Edges

You will use a minimum of four area-specific curets to debride the posterior teeth. For example, when using Gracey curets, you might select a Gracey 11, 12, 13, and 14. (The G13 and G14 are used on distal surfaces; the G11 and G12 are used on facial, lingual, and mesial surfaces.)

Traditional Pairing: The Gracey 11/12 and the Gracey 13/14 Instruments

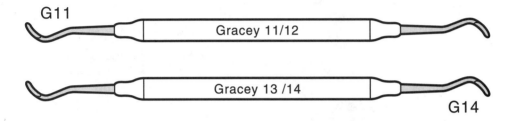

The Gracey 11, 12, 13, and 14 curets traditionally have been combined on two double-ended instruments: the Gracey 11/12 and Gracey 13/14.

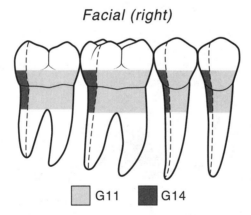

Use of the Gracey 11/12 and 13/14 instruments on the facial aspect of the mandibular right sextant. First, the clinician uses the G14 on the distal surfaces. Next, the clinician must change instruments to use the G11 on the facial and mesial surfaces of the facial aspect. (The G12 and G13 curets are used on the lingual aspect of this sextant.)

Modified Pairing: The Gracey 11/14 and Gracey 12/13 Instruments

The Gracey 11, 12, 13, and 14 curets also are available in a modified combination as the Gracey 11/14 and Gracey 12/14. These modified combinations allow the clinician to complete the surfaces of either the facial aspect or the lingual aspect without changing instruments.

G11

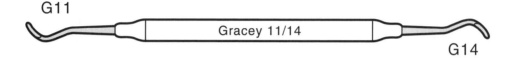

Gracey 11/14

G14

The Gracey 11/14 instrument pairs a Gracey 11 (for facial and mesial surfaces [or lingual and mesial surfaces] and a Gracey 14 (for distal surfaces) on a double-ended instrument.

Facial (right)

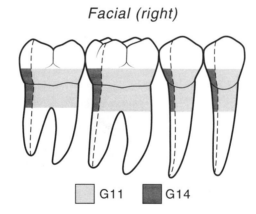

☐ G11   ■ G14

Use of the Gracey 11/14 instrument on the facial aspect of the mandibular right sextant. The clinician is able to instrument the facial aspect of the mandibular right sextant without changing instruments. (The Gracey 12/13 instrument is used to instrument the lingual aspect of this sextant.)

Step-by-Step Technique on Posteriors

Example: Mandibular Right Posteriors, Facial Aspect

RIGHT-Handed Clinician

LEFT-Handed Clinician

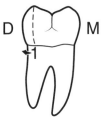

Distal Surfaces:
1. Begin with the last molar in the sextant. Start at the distofacial line angle and work onto the distal surface.

2. Insert the working-end beneath the gingival margin at a 0°-40° angle. Adapt the cutting edge to the right of the distofacial line angle; the toe should aim toward the back of the mouth because this is the direction in which you are working.

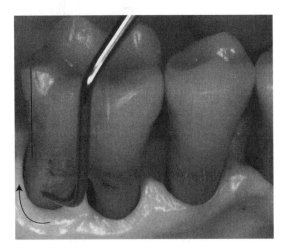

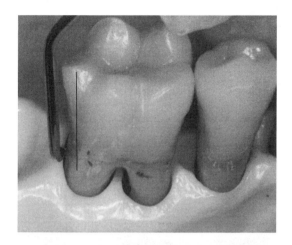

3. Roll the instrument handle slightly to adapt to distal surface. Work at least halfway across the distal surface from the facial aspect. Keep the cutting edge adapted to the tooth surface at all times.

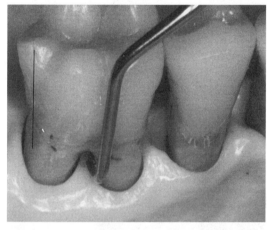

4. For multirooted tooth with furcation involvement, debride the <u>distal surface of the mesial root</u> with the distal curet.

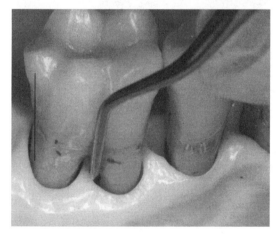

5. Extend the working-end as far into the furcation as possible. Digital (finger) activation often works well in furcation areas.

6. The distal surfaces for this sextant should be completed in the order shown in this illustration. It is easier to begin with the posterior-most molar and move forward toward the first premolar because of the pressure exerted against your hand by the patient's cheek.

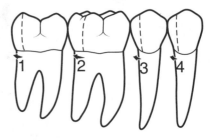

Facial & Mesial Surfaces:

7. Now you are ready to instrument the facial and mesial surfaces of the sextant beginning at the distofacial line angle.

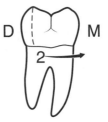

8. Select the correct curet for use on the facial and mesial surfaces. Position the curet at the distofacial line angle with the toe aiming forward. Instrument the facial surface.

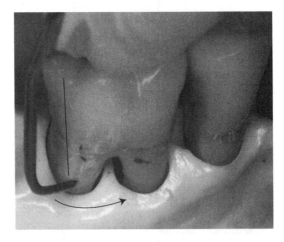

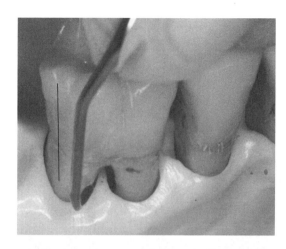

9. For multirooted teeth with furcation involvement, use the mesial curet on the <u>mesial surface of the distal root.</u>

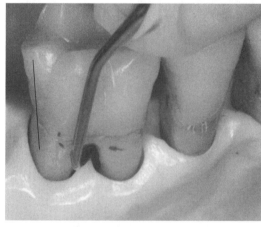

10. Extend the working-end as far into the furcation as possible.

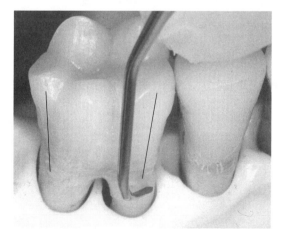

11. At the mesiofacial line angle, roll the instrument handle to adapt the toe-third of the cutting edge.

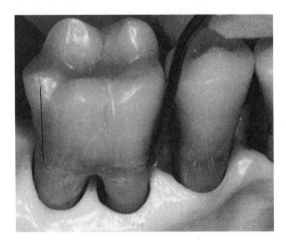

12. Complete at least half of the mesial surface from the facial aspect.

13. Complete the facial aspect of the facial and mesial surfaces in the order shown in this illustration.

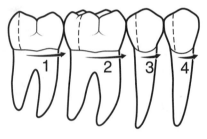

When you have completed the facial aspect, change your clock position and instrument the lingual aspect of the sextant.

The remaining three posterior sextants are instrumented in a similar manner.

Reference Sheet: Area-Specific Curets

Use:
Area-specific curets are used to remove small-size calculus deposits, and for root surface debridement and deplaquing of root surfaces.

Basic Concepts:
1. Insert the working-end beneath the gingival margin at a 0-to 40-degree angle.

2. Maintain adaptation of the toe-third of the cutting edge to the tooth surface.

3. Press down with your fulcrum finger and apply pressure against the instrument handle with the index finger and thumb to create lateral pressure against the tooth surface during work strokes.

4. Use hand-forearm motion activation. Digital activation is used in areas where movement is restricted, such as furcation areas and narrow, deep pockets.

5. Relax your fingers in between work strokes.

Anterior Teeth:
1. For surfaces toward, sit at 8-9:00 if you are a right-handed clinician or at 3-4:00 if you are a left-handed clinician. For surfaces away, sit at 12:00.

2. Selection of correct working-end:
   - Use the lower cutting edges.
   - The face should tilt toward the tooth surface to be instrumented.
   - The lower shank is parallel to the tooth surface.

3. Sequence: Begin with the surfaces toward you. Start with the canine on opposite side of the mouth from the clinician and work toward yourself.

Posterior Teeth:
1. For aspects toward, sit at 9:00 (or 3:00). For aspects away, sit at 10-11:00 (or 1-2:00).

   2. Use the lower cutting edges.
   The lower shank is parallel to the tooth surface (*"shank up and over"*).
   Use Gracey 13 or Gracey 14 for distal surfaces.
   Use Gracey 11 or Gracey 12 for mesial, facial and lingual surfaces.
   (The Gracey 7 or Gracey 8 also is used for facial and lingual surfaces.)

3. Sequence: Complete all distal surfaces first, then instrument the facial and mesial surfaces (or the lingual and mesial surfaces).

Section 5: Root Surface Debridement—Posteriors

Instrumenting Multirooted Teeth

When instrumenting a multirooted tooth, treat each root as if it was that of a single-rooted tooth. (Imagine that the roots of a mandibular molar are the roots of two premolar teeth.)

1. Begin by instrumenting the root trunk.

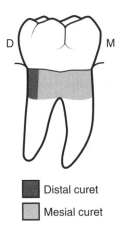

■ Distal curet

□ Mesial curet

2. Instrument each root as if it was a separate tooth.

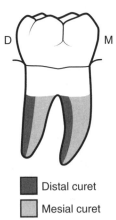

■ Distal curet

□ Mesial curet

Root Morphology: Posterior Teeth

Positioned correctly in relation to the patient, equipment, and treatment area

Tooth	**Root Morphology**

Mandibular First Premolar

- May have deep distal root concavity

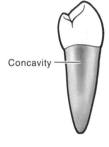

Concavity

Mesial   *Distal*

Maxillary First Premolar

- Deep linear mesial concavity
- Distal concavity is less pronounced

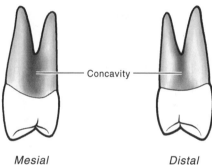

Concavity

Mesial   *Distal*

Mandibular First Molar

- Deep depression on root trunk extending from bifurcation to cervical line, depression becomes more shallow toward the cervical line

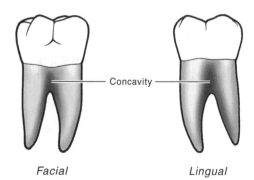

Concavity

Facial   *Lingual*

Root Morphology: Posterior Teeth *Continued*

Tooth	Root Morphology
Mandibular First Molar, • Wide, shallow root concavity on mesial root	 *Mesial* *Distal*
Maxillary First Molar • Deep depression on root trunk extending from the furcation to cervical line • Longitudinal groove extending the length of the lingual (palatal) root	 *Facial* *Lingual*
Maxillary First Molar, Proximal Views • Concavities extending from the furcation to cervical line	 *Mesial* *Distal*

Skill Evaluation #1: Area-Specific Curets, Anterior Sextants

Student: _____   Area 1 = _____

Evaluator: _____   Area 2 = _____

Date: _____   Area 3 = _____

                                 Area 4 = _____

DIRECTIONS: For each area, use **Column S** for student self-evaluation and **Column I** for instructor evaluation. For each skill evaluated, indicate the skill level as: **S** (satisfactory), **I** (improvement needed), or **U** (unsatisfactory).

CRITERIA:	Area 1		Area 2		Area 3		Area 4	
	S	I	S	I	S	I	S	I
Uses correct patient head position								
Index finger & thumb are across from one another and not touching; middle finger rests lightly on shank								
Ring finger acts as "support beam"; finger rest is on a stable tooth surface								
Handle placement correct								
Uses mirror appropriately								
Gently inserts working-end beneath gingival margin								
Maintains adaptation of toe-third of cutting edge								
Maintains correct face-to-tooth surface angulation								
Uses controlled work strokes								
Applies stroke pressure in a coronal direction only								
Uses appropriate motion activation								
Uses correct sequence								

Skill Evaluation #1: Area-Specific Curets, Anterior Sextants

Student: _____

Evaluator Comments:

_____

_____

_____

_____

_____

_____

_____

_____

_____

_____

_____

_____

_____

_____

_____

_____

Box for sketches pertaining to written comments.

Skill Evaluation #2: Area-Specific Curets, Posterior Sextants

Student: _____   Area 1 = _____

Evaluator: _____   Area 2 = _____

Date: _____   Area 3 = _____

                                     Area 4 = _____

DIRECTIONS: For each area, use **Column S** for student self-evaluation and **Column I** for instructor evaluation. For each skill evaluated, indicate the skill level as: **S** (satisfactory), **I** (improvement needed), or **U** (unsatisfactory).

CRITERIA:	Area 1 S	Area 1 I	Area 2 S	Area 2 I	Area 3 S	Area 3 I	Area 4 S	Area 4 I
Uses correct patient head position								
Index finger & thumb are across from one another and not touching; middle finger rests lightly on shank								
Ring finger acts as "support beam"; finger rest is on a stable tooth surface								
Handle placement correct								
Uses mirror appropriately								
Gently inserts working-end beneath gingival margin								
Maintains adaptation of toe-third of cutting edge								
Maintains correct face-to-tooth surface angulation								
Uses controlled work strokes								
Applies stroke pressure in a coronal direction only								
Uses appropriate motion activation								
Uses correct sequence								

Skill Evaluation #2: Area-Specific Curets, Posterior Sextants

Student: _____

Evaluator Comments:

_____

_____

_____

_____

_____

_____

_____

_____

_____

_____

_____

_____

_____

_____

_____

_____

_____

Box for sketches pertaining to written comments.

Problem Identification: Difficulties in Instrumentation

This module provides solutions for the most common instrumentation problems encountered by beginning clinicians. These problems are divided into seven categories:

Here's how to use the problem charts:

1. First select the category <u>that most closely describes the problem</u> that you are having. Turn to the problem chart for that category.

2. The "Cause" column lists possible causes of the problem. In each category, the causes are listed in order from the most likely cause to least likely cause.

3. Read the "Solution" column for suggestions on how to correct the problem.

Problem Chart 1: Can't See the Treatment Area!	
Cause	**Solution**
Clinician seated in wrong "clock position" for treatment area	Refer to Positioning Summary Sheet Right-handed-p.34; left-handed-p.42.
Patient positioned too high	Lower patient chair until the patient's mouth is below your elbow when you hold your arms against your side.
Patient head position	Mandibular arch = chin-down Maxillary arch = chin-up Aspect toward = turned slightly away Aspect away = turned toward
Not using indirect vision	A combination of direct vision and indirect vision is required in most treatment areas.
Using mirror, but still can't see	Be sure that you are using the mirror to fully retract the tongue or cheek away from the treatment area. If you can't see the treatment area in the mirror's reflecting surface, try rotating the mirror head slightly. Move mirror further away from treatment area. For mandibular lingual aspects, move mirror toward midline of the mouth. For maxillary anteriors, move mirror closer to the mandibular arch.
Finger rest too close to surface to be instrumented	Move rest slightly forward in the mouth so that your finger isn't covering up the surface to be instrumented.
Hand is blocking view	Swivel or pivot your hand and arm until you can see the treatment area.

Problem Chart 2: Can't Locate the Calculus!	
Cause	**Solution**
Middle finger not resting on shank	You will receive more tactile information if your finger is resting on the shank.
Using middle finger to hold the instrument (index finger is just "going along for the ride" rather than holding the handle)	Using the middle finger to hold the handle prevents it from detecting vibrations. The thumb and index finger should be across from one another. You should be able to lift your middle finger off of the shank and not drop the instrument.
Using "death grasp" on handle	Relax your fingers and grasp the handle as lightly as possible. Try working on a typodont without wearing gloves—if your fingers are blanched, you are holding the handle too tightly.
Not beginning strokes at the junctional epithelium	Be sure to insert the working end to the base of the sulcus or pocket before initiating an assessment stroke. If you can't tell where the base is, get an instructor to help you.
Too few strokes, not overlapping strokes	When working subgingivally, use instrumentation zones and overlapping strokes to cover the entire root surface.
Not detecting calculus at line angles on posterior teeth	Position the working-end distal to the line angle with the explorer tip aimed toward the junctional epithelium (but NOT touching the J.E.) and make short horizontal strokes "around" the line angle toward the front of the mouth.
Not detecting calculus at midlines of anterior teeth	Make small, controlled horizontal strokes at the midline on facial or lingual surfaces.

Problem Chart 3: Poor Illumination of Treatment Area!	
Cause	**Solution**
Unit light too close to mouth	Positioning the light close to the patient's mouth creates excessive shadowing and actually makes it harder to see. Light should be an arm's length above or in front of the clinician.
Patient's head positioned incorrectly for treatment area	Mandibular arch = chin-down Maxillary arch = chin-up Aspect toward = turned slightly away Aspect away = turned toward
Not using mirror for indirect illumination	Use mirror to direct light onto the treatment area.

Problem Chart 4: Can't Adapt Cutting Edge to Tooth Surface!	
Cause	**Solution**
Trying to adapt the toe- and middle-third of cutting edge	Usually only the tip-third or toe-third of the cutting edge can be adapted.
Using the wrong cutting edge for the tooth surface	Review the visual guidelines for the instrument classification.
Using the wrong instrument for the task or area of the mouth	Review uses and applications of instrument classifications.
Finger rest too far away	Establish a finger rest near to the tooth to be instrumented.
Lower shank not parallel to facial or lingual surface of posterior tooth	On posterior teeth, the lower shank should be parallel to the tooth surface, but not touching it at any point.

Problem Chart 5: Can't Maintain Adaptation!	
Cause	**Solution**
Incorrect grasp; not rolling instrument handle	Sloppy technique with grasp makes it difficult to control the instrument. As you work around the circumference of the tooth, roll the handle between your index finger and thumb to maintain adaptation.
Split grasp	Keep fingers together in the correct grasp position.
Fulcrum too close or too far away from tooth to be instrumented	Finger rest should be near (but not on) the tooth to be instrumented.
Fulcrum finger lifts off of the tooth as stroke is made	Fulcrum finger should be maintained in a straight, upright position throughout the stroke (acting as a "support beam"). Press down against the tooth with your fulcrum finger so finger can act as a "brake" to stop the stroke.
Tilting the instrument face away from the tooth surface during stroke (so lateral surface or back of working-end contacts tooth)	Maintain correct face-to-tooth surface angulation, as you use a pull stroke to move the working-end in a coronal direction. Handle position should stay parallel to the tooth surface as you make strokes (it should not tilt away from the tooth surface).
Not pivoting on finger rest	On posterior teeth, pivot at line angles to maintain adaptation. In anterior sextants, as you work toward yourself, your hand and arm should gradually pivot closer to your body.

Problem Chart 6: Uncontrolled or Weak Work Stroke!	
Cause	**Solution**
Instrument handle is supported solely by index finger and thumb	Handle should rest against the index finger or hand for support.
Split grasp—fingers not in contact	Keep fingers together in correct grasp position for control of strokes.
"Death grip" on handle	Use a firm grasp, but not a choking grasp.
Fulcrum finger lifts off of the tooth as stroke is made	Press down against the tooth with your fulcrum finger so finger can act as a "brake" to stop the stroke.
Fulcrum finger is relaxed and bent	Fulcrum finger should be straight and apply pressure against rest point on tooth (acting as a "support beam").
Stroke not stabilized; no lateral pressure with cutting edge against tooth surface	During a work stroke, the index finger and thumb should apply equal pressure against the instrument handle and the fulcrum finger applies pressure against the tooth surface.
Wrist and arm not in neutral position	Assess patient position, clinician position, and arm position.
Using a push-pull stroke	Apply lateral pressure only with the pull stroke, away from junctional epithelium.
Working too rapidly, strokes too fast	Pause briefly after each stroke. Make slow, controlled strokes.
On posterior teeth, lower shank not parallel—shank rocks on height of contour	On posterior teeth, the lower shank should be parallel to the facial or lingual surface, but not touching it at any point.

Problem Chart 7A: Missed Calculus Deposits!
Deposits Missed at Midlines of Anterior Teeth.

Cause	Solution
Not using horizontal strokes at midline of facial or lingual surface	Position the curet to the side of the midline with the toe aiming toward the junctional epithelium (but not touching the J.E.). Make a series of short controlled horizontal strokes.
Not overlapping vertical strokes at midline	Position the working-end so that strokes will overlap for surfaces toward and away.
Not using a specialized instrument when indicated	Use an area-specific curet with a miniature working-end at midlines.

Problem Chart 7B: Missed Calculus Deposits!
Deposits Missed at Line Angles of Posterior Teeth.

Cause	Solution
Not using horizontal strokes at the line angles	Position the curet distal to the line angle with the toe aiming toward the junctional epithelium (but not touching the J.E.). Make a series of short strokes around the line angle.
Not rolling handle to maintain adaptation to line angle	As you work around a line angle, it is necessary to roll the instrument handle between the index finger and thumb to maintain adaptation.

Problem Chart 7C: Missed Calculus Deposits!
Deposits Missed on Proximal Surfaces.

Cause	Solution
Not using indirect vision	Beginning clinicians often have trouble learning to use indirect vision and so try to view all surfaces directly. Use of indirect vision is vital for proximal surfaces.
Not rotating reflecting surface to view proximal surfaces	This problem is common on lingual surfaces of anterior teeth. First, angle the mirror to view the surfaces toward you, then turn the mirror to view the surfaces away from you.
Strokes not extended under contact area	Instrument at least one-half of a proximal surface from the facial and lingual aspects. Place curet between the papilla and insert it to the junctional epithelium. (Do not "trace" papilla with working-end.)
Not rolling handle to maintain adaptation	As you work around a line angle and onto the proximal surface, make small, continuous adjustments in adaptation by rolling the handle.
Working-end not "aimed" toward surface to be instrumented	For distal surfaces of posterior teeth, the toe should aim toward the back of the mouth. Don't try to "back the working-end" onto the distal surface.

Instrument Sharpening

In this module you will learn the moving-stone technique for sharpening hand-activated instruments.

Required Equipment:

- a variety of hand-activated instruments
- sharpening stone(s) and plastic test stick

Section 1: Introduction to Sharpening Concepts

Advantages of Sharp Instruments

The cutting edges of a hand-activated instrument must be sharp to achieve efficient periodontal debridement with minimal tissue trauma.

A sharp cutting edge allows:
1. **Easier calculus removal.** A sharp cutting edge "bites into" the calculus deposit, removing it in an efficient manner. A dull cutting edge will slide over the calculus deposit and may burnish it.

2. **Improved stroke control**. A dull cutting edge must be pressed with greater force against the tooth surface to achieve calculus removal. Excessive force used with a dull cutting edge increases the likelihood of losing control of the stroke. The clinician is more likely to slip or obtain an instrument stick.

3. **Reduced number of strokes.** It takes fewer strokes to remove a calculus deposit with a sharp cutting edge. Sharp instruments reduce the overall treatment time.

4. **Increased patient comfort**. A sharp instrument allows the clinician to use less force and make fewer, better-controlled instrument strokes. A sharp cutting edge, therefore, increases patient comfort.

5. **Reduced clinician fatigue**. A dull cutting edge requires greater stroke pressure and more instrumentation strokes for calculus removal. The excessive lateral pressure and extra number of strokes places unnecessary strain on the clinician's musculoskeletal system.

Understanding Working-End Design

To sharpen a hand-activated periodontal instrument correctly, you need to have a clear understanding of the following design features of the working-end: (1) the cutting edge and (2) the relationship of the lateral surface to the instrument face.

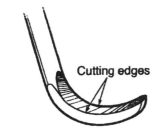

1. The union of the instrument face and a lateral surface forms the cutting edge. This illustration shows the two cutting edges of a universal curet.

    A sharp cutting edge is a **line**. It has length, but no width.

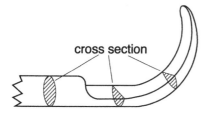

2. In order to understand the relationship of the lateral surface to the face, you must view the working-end in cross section.

    The illustration shows a universal curet.

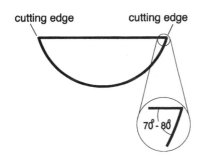

3. The lateral surfaces meet the instrument face at an internal angle of between 70° and 80°.

    This 70°- 80° angulation is found on sickles, universal curets, and area-specific curets.

The Dull Cutting Edge

The metal of the cutting edge gradually is worn away, over time, as the working-end is used against the tooth surface. The cutting edge changes from a sharp point to a <u>rounded surface</u>. A sharpening stone is used to remove the rounded edge and restore a sharp cutting edge to the instrument. The goal of sharpening is to restore an internal angle of 70°- 80° between the lateral surface and the instrument face.

A dull cutting edge. When the cutting edge is dull, the face and lateral surface meet in a wide, rounded surface. This rounded surface will slide over the calculus deposit instead of biting into it.

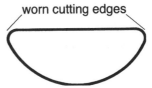

The rounded edge must be removed. The shaded area on the illustration shows the portion of the lateral surface that must be removed in order to restore a fine, sharp cutting edge.

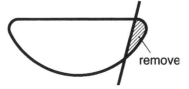

Skill Practice: Establishing the Correct Angulation

Follow the directions on this page to gain experience in establishing the correct angulation between the sharpening stone and the instrument face.

Equipment: (1) a rectangular sharpening stone and (2) the illustration on the next page.

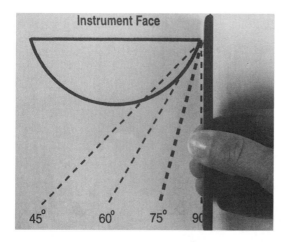

Step 1: Establish a 90° angle.

Place your sharpening stone on the dotted line labeled as a 90-degree angle. Your sharpening stone is now positioned at a 90-degree angle to the instrument face.

This position gives you a visual starting point from which to establish the correct angulation

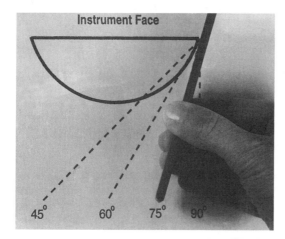

Step 2: Establish a 75° angle.

Swing the lower end of the sharpening stone toward the instrument back. Align your stone with the dotted line labeled as a 75° angle. Your sharpening stone is now at the proper angle to the face.

Practice with angles. Use this illustration to practice establishing the correct angle between the instrument face and the sharpening stone.

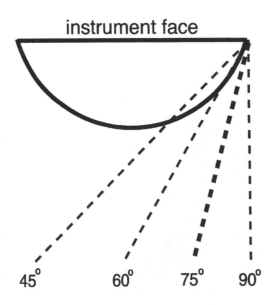

Positioning Curets and Sickles for Sharpening

The face of a sickle scaler, universal curet, or area-specific curet should be positioned parallel to the countertop for sharpening.

Universal Curets or Sickle Scalers:
With a universal curet or sickle scaler, when the face is positioned correctly, the lower shank will be perpendicular (⊥) to the countertop.

Two cutting edges are sharpened on the working-end of a sickle scaler or a universal curet.

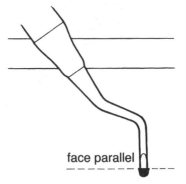

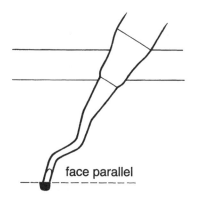

face parallel

Area-Specific Curets:
With an area-specific curet, when the face is positioned correctly, the lower shank will <u>not</u> be perpendicular to the countertop.

One cutting edge, the working cutting edge, is sharpened on each area-specific curet.

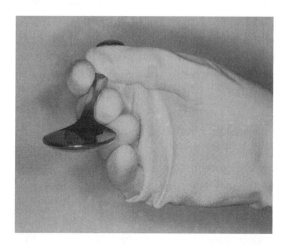

A spoonful of cough syrup. Imagine that you are holding a tablespoon filled with red, sticky cough syrup.

You must hold the spoon so that the sides of the bowl are level with each other or the cough syrup will spill!

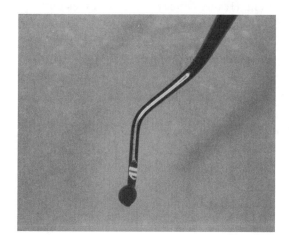

Imagine a curet face that is covered with red cough syrup. You must position the face so that it is level or the imaginary cough syrup will spill.

When to Sharpen

Frequency

Calculus removal will be easier and instruments will last longer if you <u>sharpen the instruments after each use</u>. Instruments on your instrument tray that were not used do not need to be sharpened; modern stainless steel instruments are not dulled by autoclaving. All instruments used during the appointment for debridement should be sharpened.

If you sharpen your instruments routinely after use, a few light strokes with the stone will restore a sharp cutting edge. Sharpening can be a quick, easy procedure if done in this manner. Sharpening becomes a difficult and time-consuming process when instruments are used repeatedly without sharpening. In this case, you will need to use many strokes with the stone to restore the cutting edge. Dull, neglected cutting edges require extensive re-contouring. The original design features of the working-end can be easily altered when extensive sharpening is necessary.

Precautions

Ideally, it is best to sharpen your instruments after autoclaving and then re-autoclave them prior to patient treatment. This approach eliminates the risk of disease transmission to the healthcare provider from the contaminated instruments. Unfortunately, this approach is not always practical since instruments may require sharpening during treatment. After treatment, time constraints often make it difficult to autoclave the instruments prior to sharpening.

When an instrument becomes dull during treatment, the best approach is to set the instrument aside and obtain another instrument. (If one Gracey 11/12 becomes dull, lay it aside and obtain a second Gracey 11/12). This approach is more efficient than sharpening a dull instrument at chairside. Also, this approach does not expose the clinician to the risk of an accidental instrument stick during the sharpening of the contaminated instrument.

If time constraints do not allow for the autoclaving of dull instruments prior to sharpening, the clinician should employ infection control precautions. Thick household gloves should be worn while handling contaminated instruments because they offer better protection against instrument sticks than surgical or exam gloves. Clean the instruments in an ultrasonic bath and pat dry with paper towels before sharpening. Aerosols can be generated during the sharpening of contaminated instruments, so wear a mask and eye protection while sharpening.

Section 2: Equipment

The following equipment should be assembled for sharpening:
*   A heat-sterilized rectangular sharpening stone.

*   A heat-sterilized plastic sharpening test stick. This plastic stick is used to test the sharpness of the instrument's cutting edge.

*   Protective eyewear and household gloves. If sharpening contaminated instruments, wear a mask.

Sharpening Stones

Types of Sharpening Stones			
Type	**Texture**	**Use**	**Lubrication**
Composition stone	Course	A synthetic (man-made) stone used for extensive reshaping of working-ends that have been improperly sharpened or have extremely dull, worn cutting edges.	Water
India stone	Medium	A synthetic stone used to sharpen very dull cutting edges.	Water or oil
Arkansas stone	Fine	A natural stone used for routine sharpening of instruments.	Mineral oil
Ceramic stone	Fine	A synthetic stone used for routine sharpening of instruments.	Water

Lubrication and Care of Stone

A sharpening stone may be used in a dry state or it may be lubricated. Lubricating the sharpening stone with either water or oil will help to prevent the metal shavings removed from the instrument from sticking to the surface of the stone. (These metal shavings can become embedded in the surface of the sharpening stone and reduce its effectiveness.) In addition, lubrication reduces frictional heat between the metal instrument and the stone. Stones that are used without lubrication will need to be replaced more frequently than stones used with lubricant.

A sharpening stone that can be lubricated with water is recommended for use when sharpening instruments during patient treatment. (Distilled water can be used for sharpening during treatment.) Oil is not recommended for use when sharpening during patient treatment because it cannot be effectively sterilized.

After using, wipe the surface of the stone with a wet 4-x-4 gauze square. Clean the stone in an ultrasonic cleaner or scrub the stone with a brush. (If cleaning a contaminated stone by hand, it is recommended to fill a sink with water and to scrub the stone under water to prevent aerosol production.) Dry the stone on a paper towel; place it in an autoclave bag and sterilize.

Work Area

The right work area is important in assuring an efficient and safe sharpening procedure.

- A stable work surface is essential for good sharpening technique. A countertop in the treatment room makes a good surface. A bracket table or other unstable surface is not appropriate for the sharpening procedure.
- The work area should be disinfected and covered with a barrier such as plastic wrap or an impervious-backed paper. The barrier should cover both the top and edge of the countertop.
- A good light source, such as the dental unit light directed over the working area.
- A magnifying lens is helpful for examining the working-end during sharpening.

Section 3: Sharpening Guides

Suggestion: Photocopy this page and Sharpening Guides R and L. Place the photocopied pages in plastic page protectors for longer use.

Reference Sheet: Sharpening

1. Grasp the instrument handle and rest your hand and arm on a stable work surface.

2. Position the instrument with the toe (or tip) toward you and the face parallel (=) to the countertop.

3. Grasp the lower third of the sharpening stone. Place the stone at a 90° angle to the instrument face.

4. Swing the lower end of the stone closer to the back of the working-end until the stone meets the face at about a 75-degree angle.

5. Activate a few light strokes on the heel-third of the cutting edge. Reposition the stone to sharpen the middle-third, then the toe/tip-third.

6. For curets, re-contour the toe. Turn the working-end so that you are looking at the lateral surface. Sharpen the *toe* of the instrument.

7. For curets, re-contour the back. Turn the working-end so that you are looking at the toe. Use semicircular strokes around the *back*.

8. Use a plastic test stick to test for sharpness.

9. Repeat Steps 1-8 to sharpen other cutting edge(s) on the same instrument.

Sharpening Guides R and L

Directions: Photocopy both Sharpening Guides (R and L) and place them back-to-back in a single plastic page protector.

Sharpening Guide—R

Use **Sharpening Guide–R** for:
- the right cutting edge of a universal curet or sickle scaler
- for ODD numbered Gracey curets, such as a G11 and G13

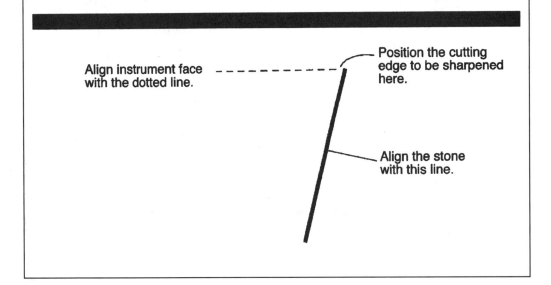

Sharpening Guide—R

Fold the page in half along the heavy black line. Place the folded page on a countertop so that the black line is aligned with the edge of the counter.

Align instrument face with the dotted line.

Position the cutting edge to be sharpened here.

Align the stone with this line.

Sharpening Guide—L

Use **Sharpening Guide–L** for:
- the left cutting edge of a universal curet or sickle scaler
- for EVEN numbered Gracey curets, such as a G12 and G14

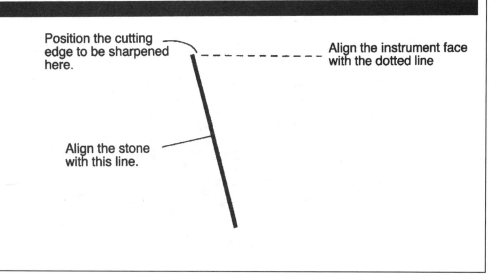

Sharpening Guide—L

Fold the page in half along the heavy black line. Place the folded page on a countertop so that the black line is aligned with the edge of the counter.

Position the cutting edge to be sharpened here.

Align the instrument face with the dotted line

Align the stone with this line.

Technique Practice With Sharpening Guide

Directions: For the purposes of this technique practice, begin by using **Sharpening Guide—R**. If using a Gracey curet, select an ODD numbered Gracey curet, such as a G11 or G13.

1. Fold **Sharpening Guide—R** along the heavy black line. Place it on the counter so that the heavy black line falls along the edge of the counter.

   Place a book on the top of the page to secure it to the counter or tape the page to the counter.

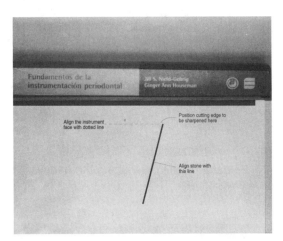

2. Hold the <u>instrument handle</u> in your <u>left hand</u>.

   Grasp the <u>stone</u> in your <u>right hand</u>.

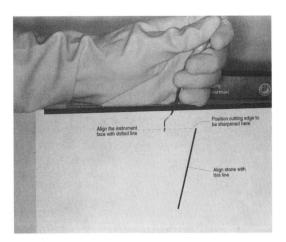

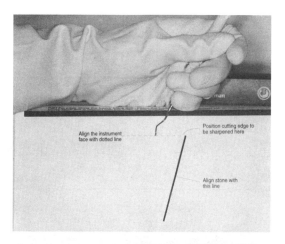

3. Align the instrument face with the fine dotted line.

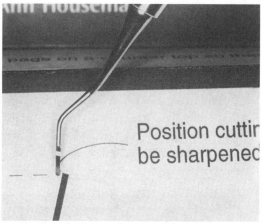

4. Keeping the face aligned with the dotted line, slide your left hand over until the cutting edge to be sharpened is positioned <u>at the far right-hand side</u> of the dotted line.

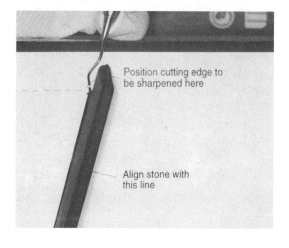

5. Align the sharpening stone with the vertical black line. This is the correct angulation for sharpening.

6. Use **Sharpening Guide—L** to sharpen the other cutting edge of a universal curet and for the working cutting edge of EVEN numbered Gracey curets.

Section 4: Step-by-Step Technique

Directions: For the purposes of this technique practice, begin by sharpening either a universal curet or a Gracey curet.

If using a Gracey curet, select an ODD numbered Gracey curet, such as a G11 or G13.

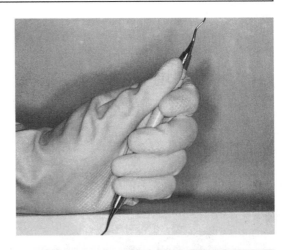

1. **Grasp the instrument.** Grasp the instrument handle in the palm of your <u>left hand</u>. Rest your hand and arm on the countertop. Stabilize the upper shank with your thumb.

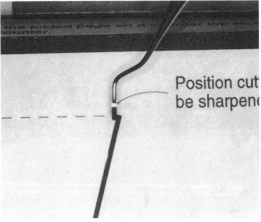

2. **Position the instrument face.** Position the working-end so that the face is parallel (=) to the countertop. (Imagine the face is covered with red cough syrup!)

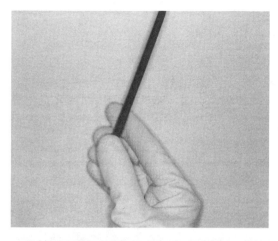

3. **Grasp the sharpening stone** in your <u>right hand</u>.

   Hold the stone on the edges so that your fingers do not get in the way when sharpening. Confine your grasp to the lower third of the stone.

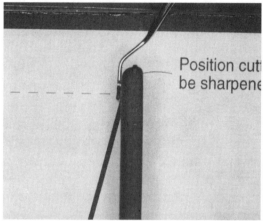

4. **Position the stone** at a 90° angle to the instrument face. From this position, you only need to swing the lower portion of the stone slightly closer to the back of the instrument in order to establish the correct angle for sharpening.

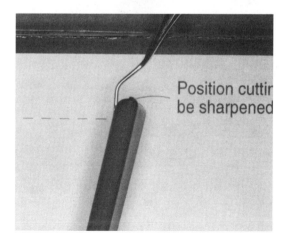

5. **Establish a 75° angle** to the face by swinging the lower part of the stone closer to the lateral surface and back of the instrument. If the stone is in proper position, the lower part of the stone will <u>tilt away from the palm of your hand</u>.

Technique Strategy: Sharpen the Cutting Edge in Sections

Divide the cutting into 3 imaginary sections for sharpening.

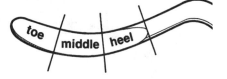

---

6. **Adapt the stone to the heel-third of the working-end.** The photograph shows a bird's-eye-view looking down at the instrument face.

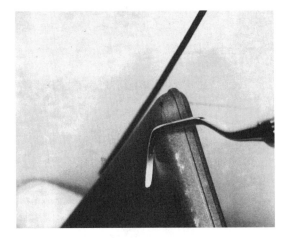

7. **Activate Sharpening strokes.** Move the sharpening stone up and down in short, rhythmic strokes to remove metal from the lateral surface.

   Finish each series of strokes in a down stroke to avoid leaving metal burs on the cutting edge.

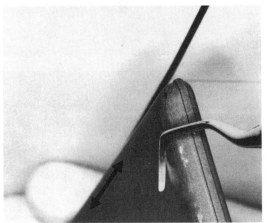

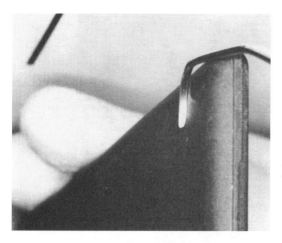

8. **Sharpen the middle-third of the cutting edge.** When the heel section is sharp, reposition the stone so that it is in contact with the middle-third of the cutting edge. Sharpen this section of the cutting edge, ending with a down stroke.

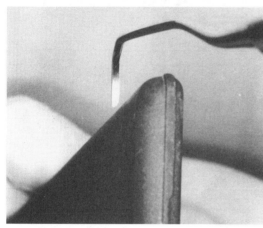

9. **Sharpen the toe-third of the cutting edge.** Reposition the stone so that it is in contact with the toe-third (or tip-third) of the cutting edge. Sharpen this section of the cutting edge.

10. If sharpening a curet, read the "Technique Strategy" below and proceed to Step 11. If sharpening a sickle scaler, skip to Step 13.

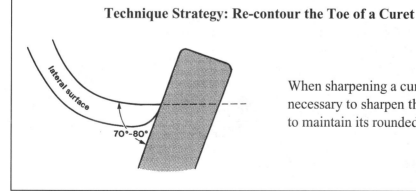

Technique Strategy: Re-contour the Toe of a Curet

When sharpening a curet, it is necessary to sharpen the toe in order to maintain its rounded contour.

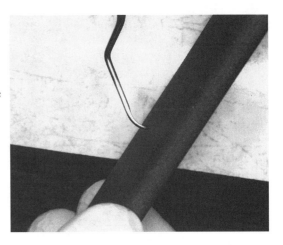

11. To re-contour the curet toe, turn the working-end so that you are looking at the lateral surface of the cutting edge. Be careful to keep the face parallel (=) to the countertop. Move the stone in up and down strokes as you work your way around the toe.

Technique Strategy: Re-contour the Back of a Curet

Re-contour the back of a curet to maintain the rounded surface.

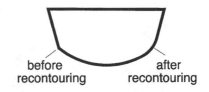

before recontouring   after recontouring

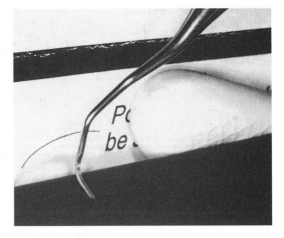

12. To re-contour the back, turn the working-end so that you are looking at the toe. Use semicircular strokes around the back of the curet.

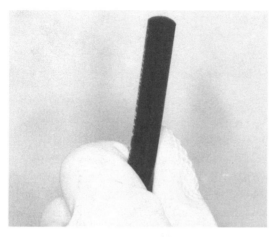

13. **Test for sharpness.** Obtain a plastic test stick. Hold the stick at waist level in your <u>non-dominant</u> hand.

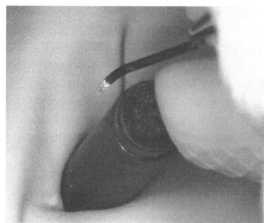

14. **Establish finger rest.** Hold the test stick so that you are looking down at the very top of the stick.

    Establish a finger rest with the ring finger of your dominant hand on the top of the stick. (The photograph shows a right-handed clinician.)

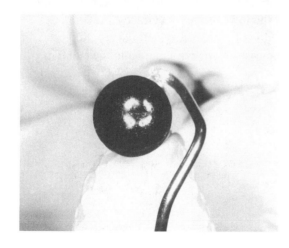

15. **Adapt the cutting edge.** Position the stick so that you are looking down on the top. Adapt the cutting edge at a 70°-to-80° angle to the stick. The cutting edge must be adapted in the same manner as on a tooth surface.

16. **Test for sharpness.** If the cutting edge is sharp, it will grasp the test stick. A dull edge will slide over the surface of the test stick.

    Note that it is possible for one section of the cutting edge to be sharp while other sections are dull.

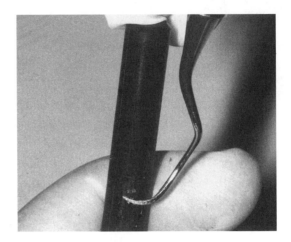

17. **Sharpen the other cutting edge(s) on the instrument.**
    If sharpening a sickle scaler or universal curet:
    - Grasp the instrument handle in your right hand; hold the stone with your left hand.
    - Repeat Steps 1 through 16 to sharpen the second *cutting edge* on the same working-end.
    - When finished, sharpen both cutting edges on the other end of a double-ended instrument.

    If sharpening a double-ended area-specific curet:
    - Flip the instrument over and position the opposite working-end for sharpening. For example, if you just sharpened the lower edge of a Gracey 11, flip the instrument and position the lower edge of the Gracey 12 for sharpening.
    - Hold the EVEN numbered Gracey curet in your right hand and the stone in your left.
    - Follow Steps 1 through 16.

Skill Evaluation: Sharpening

Student: _____   Instrument 1 = _____

Evaluator: _____   Instrument 2 = _____

Date: _____   Instrument 3 = _____

DIRECTIONS: For each instrument, use **Column S** for student self-evaluation and **Column I** for instructor evaluation. For each instrument sharpened, indicate the skill level as: **S** (satisfactory), **I** (improvement needed), or **U** (unsatisfactory).

CRITERIA:	Area 1		Area 2		Area 3	
	S	I	S	I	S	I
Assembles sharpening and personal protective equipment						
Describes the working-end design characteristics prior to initiating sharpening procedure						
If desired, lubricates stone						
Stabilizes instrument with the face parallel to countertop						
Establishes a 70-to-80 degree angle between the stone and instrument face						
Uses rhythmic up and down strokes						
Finishes with a downward stroke						
Preserves original design characteristics of the working-end						
Evaluates sharpness using a plastic test stick						
States the advantages of a sharp cutting edge						
Describes infection control procedures for sharpening during and after patient treatment						
Describes care of sharpening stone						

Skill Evaluation: Sharpening

Student: _____

Evaluator Comments:

_____

_____

_____

_____

_____

_____

_____

_____

_____

_____

_____

_____

_____

_____

_____

_____

Box for sketches pertaining to written comments.

20
MODULE

Instrumentation Strategies

The first section of this module introduces appointment planning for calculus removal. The second part discusses instrument sequencing for calculus detection and removal.

Key Terms:

Full-mouth debridement

Multiple appointments

Gross scaling (prescaling)

Circuit scaling

Incomplete instrumentation

Section 1: The Calculus Removal Game Plan

Full-Mouth Debridement

Recent research findings suggest that the best response to nonsurgical periodontal therapy is obtained when periodontal debridement is completed in a single appointment or in two appointments within a 24 hour period. [1-5] In these research studies, full-mouth debridement was combined with the use of topical antiseptic therapy (full-mouth disinfection). Traditionally, debridement of periodontal patients has been accomplished a quadrant at-a-time over a period of 2 to 4 weeks. Since periodontal disease is an infection, the full-mouth approach to periodontal debridement is based on the assumption that the remaining untreated areas of the mouth can reinfect the treated areas. Full-mouth debridement is best accomplished by a clinician (dental hygienist or periodontist) working with an assistant.

Multiple Appointments for the Student Clinician

Full-mouth debridement of difficult patient cases is not a realistic goal for beginning student clinicians. For this reason, the student clinician must decide how many teeth can be successfully instrumented at each appointment.

The Gross Scaling Approach to Multiple Appointments (Not Recommended)

When multiple appointments are needed for calculus removal, one strategy involves devoting the first appointment to "gross scaling" followed by one or more appointments for "fine scaling". **Gross scaling** (or **prescaling**) is done throughout the entire mouth for the purpose of removing medium- or large-sized calculus deposits located supragingivally and just beneath the gingival margin. In the following days or weeks, fine scaling appointments are used to remove subgingival deposits. Usually the entire mouth is treated at each appointment, "whittling away" the calculus bit-by-bit until all deposits are finally removed. This approach of instrumenting the entire mouth at each appointment is known as **circuit scaling** (because the clinician goes around and around the mouth at appointment after appointment).

The gross scaling approach to multiple appointments is <u>NOT recommended</u> because undesirable consequences can result from incomplete calculus removal. Gross scaling removes bacterial plaque and dental calculus near the gingival margin allowing the marginal tissues to shrink and tighten around the tooth. In addition, these marginal tissues may exhibit improved tissue color and contour that may be mistaken by the patient as the complete return to a healthy state.

Incomplete calculus removal (subgingival deposits not removed) combined with healing at the gingival margin presents several potential problems:

1. **Proliferation of Microorganisms.** Gross scaling leaves behind partially removed deposits that are rough, irregular, and covered with bacterial plaque. As the marginal tissue shrinks, it closes off the entrance to the pocket, providing a protected environment within the pocket in which the microorganisms continue to multiply.

2. **Abscess Formation.** When deep pockets are present, incomplete calculus removal allows the gingival margin to tighten around the tooth, like the drawstring of a pouch. This prevents drainage of bacterial toxins and other waste products from the pocket. This situation can result in the development of a periodontal abscess. Certain patients are particularly prone to abscess formation:
   a. Medically compromised individuals, such as immunosuppressed or patients with uncontrolled diabetes, are especially prone to infection.
   b. Patients with deep periodontal pockets, especially infrabony pockets or pockets with furcation involvement.

3. **Difficult Instrumentation.** Instrument insertion is often more difficult at those appointments following the gross scale appointment because the gingival margin is more closely adapted to the tooth surface.

4. **Decreased Patient Motivation for Treatment.** Many patients are motivated to seek treatment for esthetic (appearance) reasons. Removal of the visible supragingival deposits combined with the improved appearance of the gingival tissues may influence the patient to forego further treatment. It is hard for patients to recognize that "what they can't see can hurt them".

5. **Patient Frustration.** When the patient undergoes multiple appointments at which the entire mouth is instrumented, he begins to feel that nothing is being accomplished by the treatment. All he knows is that the clinician goes around and around his mouth at each appointment, seemly without end. ("I thought you cleaned all of my teeth at the LAST appointment!")

Sextant/ Quadrant Approach to Multiple Appointments (Recommended)

This approach to multiple appointments is based on the concept of complete instrumentation of the areas treated at each appointment. When calculus removal is begun on a tooth, it undergoes complete instrumentation at that time (removal of large deposits all the way through root surface debridement of *treated* teeth is completed at one appointment). The clinician undertakes to treat only as many teeth, sextants, or quadrants as he or she can thoroughly debride in an appointment. For example, the clinician may complete a single sextant (facial and lingual aspects) on a patient with advanced periodontitis or complete two quadrants (half the mouth) on a patient with gingivitis. The sextant/quadrant approach to multiple appointments is the *recommended* approach for calculus removal by a student clinician.

Dividing Up the Work

When multiple appointments are necessary, the student clinician must decide how to divide up the work. The following approaches are recommended:

1. **Complete one sextant or quadrant.** With more involved cases, it is often possible only to complete one sextant or quadrant at an appointment. The clinician can begin by treating a posterior sextant. Treatment can end here for the appointment, or if time permits, the adjacent anterior teeth are completed to the midline of the arch (resulting in completion of the quadrant).
2. **Complete two quadrants on the same side of the mouth.** When two quadrants are completed at one appointment, treatment of a maxillary and mandibular quadrant on the same side of the mouth is recommended (versus treating the entire maxillary arch or the entire mandibular arch). Doing one side of the mouth is preferred for several reasons. First, this approach gives the patient an untreated side on which to chew comfortably. This option usually divides the work more evenly for the clinician since the maxillary arch is more difficult for most clinicians. When local anesthesia is indicated for two quadrants, it is recommended that a maxillary and mandibular quadrant on the same side of the mouth be selected.
3. **Divide posterior and anterior teeth within a quadrant.** Different instruments are often required for anterior and posterior teeth (e.g., anterior and posterior sickles; area-specific curets). When instrumenting a quadrant, it is more efficient to complete instrumentation on the posterior teeth before progressing to the anterior teeth in the quadrant.

Sequence for Instrument Use

Instrument selection is determined by the type and location of the calculus deposits. First, periodontal probes (calibrated and furcation) and an explorer are used to assess the mouth. Periodontal probes are used to determine the extent, location, and characteristics of clinical attachment loss. An explorer is used to determine calculus size (small, medium, or large deposits), distribution (localized or generalized) and location (supragingival or within deep pockets or furcations). Supragingival calculus deposits <u>in the treatment area</u> are removed first with an appropriate instrument (e.g., sickle scaler, curet). Subgingival deposits are removed next with an appropriate curet. Root surface debridement work strokes with a curet are used to remove small deposits and for root surface debridement. During instrumentation, a curet should be used for calculus detection to minimize switching back and forth between the explorer and curet. When all deposits detected with the curet have been removed, the treatment area is assessed with an explorer for definitive detection of any remaining deposits.

Sample Calculus Removal Game Plan

A case example is presented here to help you understand how to formulate a calculus removal game plan that is appropriate for a student clinician.

Case Example:

The illustration is an example of the conditions throughout the entire mouth. When you assess the mouth you find the following presenting conditions:

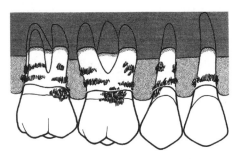

- generalized, large-sized supragingival and subgingival calculus deposits
- generalized 5 to 6 mm clinical loss of attachment
- bacterial plaque on 90% of tooth surfaces

Calculus Removal Plan	
1. Number of appointments planned for calculus removal: 4	
2. Areas to be treated at each appointment appointment, listed in order of use	3. Instrument(s) selected for each
Appt. #1: Mandibular right quadrant	anterior and posterior sickle scalers universal curet area-specific curets
Appt. 2: Maxillary right quadrant	anterior and posterior sickle scalers universal curet area-specific curets
Appt. 3: Mandibular left quadrant	anterior and posterior sickle scalers universal curet area-specific curets
Appt. 4: Maxillary left quadrant	anterior and posterior sickle scalers universal curet area-specific curets

Section 2: Skill Building Activities

Instrument Set for Skill Building Activity 1 and 2

For purposes of these activities, assume that your instrument set contains the selection of hand-activated instruments shown below.

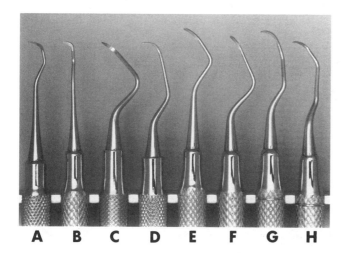

A—anterior sickle
B—posterior sickle
C—posterior sickle
D—Gracey 3/4
E—universal curet
F—universal curet
G—Gracey 11/12
H—Gracey 13/14

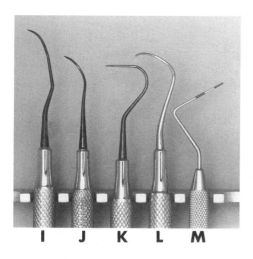

I—11/12-type explorer
J—Pigtail explorer
K—Shepherd Hook explorer
L—furcation probe
M—calibrated probe

Activity #1: Instrument Selection

This activity is designed to provide practice in instrument selection. When selecting an instrument, the clinician should consider factors such as access to the tooth surface and the size or tenacity of the calculus deposits.

Directions: Using the set of instruments pictured on page 437, select the best instrument for each condition or task described below.

1. Which instrument would be the best choice for removing medium-sized <u>supragingival</u> deposits from the mandibular anterior teeth? _____

2. Which instrument would be best for removing large-sized deposits from posterior teeth? _____

3. Which instrument would you select to determine the presence of loss of attachment? _____

4. Which instrument would you select to detect furcation involvement? _____

5. Would universal curet E or F work better for removing a deposit located 4 mm below the CEJ on a mandibular molar? _____

6. Which instrument would you select to remove a spicule of calculus located within a deep periodontal pocket found on the distal surface of a molar? _____

7. Which instrument would you select to remove a spicule of calculus located within a deep periodontal pocket found on an anterior tooth? _____

8. Which instrument should you use to detect dental caries? _____

9. Would you use explorer I or J to detect calculus deposits located within a deep periodontal pocket? _____

(See page 441 for the suggested answers.)

Activity #2: Plan for Calculus Removal

Directions: (1) Develop a calculus removal game plan. (2)Using the instrument set pictured on page 437, develop a sequence for instrument use that would be appropriate for a student clinician. Indicate the number of anticipated appointments for calculus removal, which area or areas will be treated at each appointment, and the instrument selection for each appointment.

Patient Case
When you assess the mouth you find the following:
- heavy <u>subgingival</u> calculus rings encircling every tooth in the mouth
- 4- to 6-mm clinical attachment levels throughout the mouth

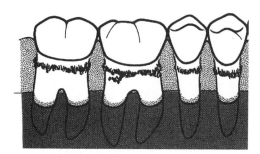

This sextant is an example of the calculus deposits *found on the entire dentition*.

Use the form on page 440 to record your plan. Refer to page 436 for an example of a completed form.

My Calculus Removal Plan	
1. Number of appointments planned for calculus removal: _____	
2. Areas to be treated at each appointment	3. Instrument(s) selected for each appointment, listed in order of use
Appt. 1:	
Appt. 2 (if needed):	
Appt. 3 (if needed):	
Appt. 4 (if needed):	
Appt. 5 (if needed):	
Appt. 6 (if needed):	

(Turn to page 441 for suggested calculus removal plans for this case.)

Solutions for Skill Building Activities

Activity #1: Instrument Selection

1-A	6-H
2-B or C	7-D
3-M	8-K
4-L	9-I
5-F	

Activity #2: Plan for Calculus Removal

A suggested calculus removal plan is given below for the patient case. If your answer doesn't exactly match this plan, discuss your plan with an instructor. Your plan may work equally well as the answer given here.

Four to six appointments would be planned for calculus removal on this case—planning either for one quadrant or one sextant per appointment, depending on the experience of the student clinician.

Instrument selection: Begin debridement with a sickle scaler to remove heavy supragingival deposits in the treatment area. Next use a universal curet to remove heavy and medium-sized subgingival deposits, then use area-specific curets to remove light calculus deposits and for root surface debridement.

Section 3: References

1. Bray, K.K. and Wilder, R.S., *Full-mouth disinfection: A new approach to nonsurgical periodontal therapy.* Access, 1999. **13**(8): p. 57-61.
2. Mongardini, C., et al., *One stage full- versus partial-mouth disinfection in the treatment of chronic adult or generalized early onset periodontitis.* J Periodontol, 1999. **70**: p. 632-645.
3. Quirynen, M., et al., *The effect of a 1-stage full mouth disinfection on oral malodor and microbial colonization of the tongue in periodontitis patients. A pilot study.* J Periodontol, 1998. **69**: p. 374-382.
4. Quirynen, M., et al., *Full- vs. partial-mouth disinfection in the treatment of periodontal infections: Short-term clinical and microbial observations.* J Dental Research: 1995. **74**: p. 1459-1467.
5. Vanderkerckhove, B.N.A., et al., *Full- vs. partial-mouth disinfection in the treatment of periodontal infections. Long-term clinical observations in a pilot study.* J Periodontol, 1996. **67**: p. 1251-1259.

Basic Concepts of Ultrasonic Instrumentation

This module presents the basic principles of ultrasonic instrumentation. Module 22 contains instructions for the use of magnetostrictive and piezoelectric ultrasonic equipment.

Key Terms:

Mechanized instrument
Ultrasonic unit
Standard size instrument tip
Precision-thin instrument tip
Deplaquing
Cavitation
Acoustic turbulence
Fluid lavage
Iatrogenic damage to periodontium

Biofilms
Bacteremia
Aerosols
Surfaces of instrument tip
Power setting
Clinical power
Active tip area
Fluid adjustment

Section 1: Introduction to Ultrasonic Instruments

Equipment

Types of Ultrasonic Units

Mechanized instruments use a water-cooled instrument tip, vibrating at a high-frequency, to remove supragingival and subgingival calculus deposits from the teeth and bacterial plaque from periodontal pockets. The two categories of mechanized instruments are ultrasonic units and sonic handpieces. Ultrasonic units are comprised of an electric generator, a handpiece, and interchangeable instrument tips. Sonic handpieces consist of a handpiece that attaches to the dental unit's compressed air line and interchangeable instrument tips. This chapter will discuss the basic concepts of ultrasonic instrumentation. Sonic instruments are covered in Module 23.

<u>Ultrasonic devices</u> <u>work by converting electrical current to mechanical energy in</u> <u>the form of high-frequency vibrations of the instrument tip</u>. Ultrasonic devices operate at frequencies above the audible range. In dentistry, this includes systems in the 18,000 to 50,000 cycles per second (18 to 50 kHz) range. The two types of ultrasonic units are the **magnetostrictive** (mag'-net-oh) ultrasonic units and **piezoelectric** (pie-e'-zoe) ultrasonic units.

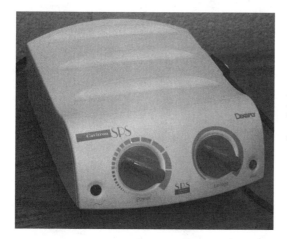

Magnetostrictive Ultrasonic Unit. This Dentsply Cavitron is an example of a magnetostrictive ultrasonic unit.

A magnetostrictive insert tip.
Interchangeable insert tips are
inserted into a handpiece that
connects to the magnetostrictive unit.

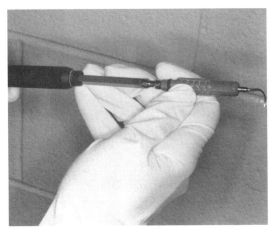

Piezoelectric Ultrasonic Unit.
This EMS unit is an example of
piezoelectric ultrasonic instrument.

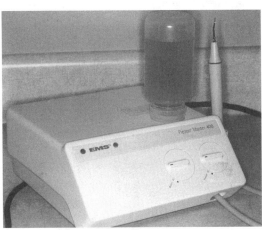

**A piezoelectric handpiece with
instrument tip.** Interchangeable
instrument tips screw onto the
handpiece that attaches to the
piezoelectric unit.

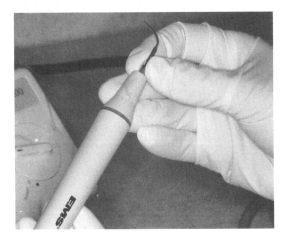

Fluid Delivery

Ultrasonic instrument tips must be cooled by fluid to prevent overheating of the vibrating instrument tip. Fluid constantly flows through the ultrasonic handpiece and exits near the point of the instrument tip. Most commonly, the ultrasonic unit is connected by a hose to a water outlet on the dental unit. In this case, water is the fluid used to cool the instrument tip.

Some ultrasonic units have independent reservoirs that can be used to deliver distilled water or other fluid solutions to the instrument tip. The independent fluid reservoir allows the clinician to select the fluid solution appropriate for the patient's periodontal health status and the fluid temperature that is most comfortable for the patient. Solutions commonly used for irrigation include distilled water, sterile saline, stannous fluoride, and chemotherapeutic agents (antimicrobials), such as chlorhexidine. The use of chemotherapeutic agents with ultrasonic instruments has been shown to enhance pocket depth reduction beyond that achieved by hand instrumentation or ultrasonic instrumentation with water.[1-3]

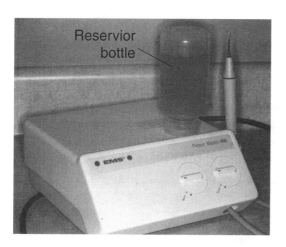

The EMS Master 400 is an example of a piezoelectric ultrasonic unit with an independent reservoir.

Indications for Use

Introduced in the late 1950s, the first ultrasonic instruments had working-ends that were large in size and limited in adaptation. Throughout the 1960s, 70s, and early 80s, ultrasonic and sonic scalers were used primarily for removing heavy *supra*gingival calculus deposits, followed by hand-activated instruments for subgingival instrumentation. In the late 1980s, precision-thin working-ends, significantly smaller than the standard Gracey curet, were developed. Modern ultrasonic instruments are as effective as hand instruments in removing bacterial plaque, plaque retentive supra- and subgingival calculus deposits, and bacterial endotoxins. In addition, these instruments efficiently remove extrinsic stains and orthodontic cement. The 1996 World Workshop in Periodontics review of nonsurgical periodontal instrumentation states that the best instrumentation results are probably achieved by the combined use of ultrasonic and hand-activated instrumentation.

Ultrasonic instrumentation has been shown to be as effective as hand instruments in subgingival calculus removal [4-6], removal of attached and unattached subgingival bacterial plaque [7-10], removal of toxins from root surfaces [11], and in reduction and maintenance of pocket depths.[8, 9, 12] Ultrasonic instruments are especially effective in deplaquing. **Deplaquing** is the disruption or removal of subgingival bacterial plaque and its byproducts from root surfaces and the pocket space. Bacterial plaque has been shown to thrive in the pocket space as well as on the root surface.[13, 14] Ultrasonic instrumentation is uniquely effective in deplaquing the subgingival pocket environment.

Advantages of Ultrasonic Instrumentation

As recently as 10 years ago, the Gracey curet was considered to be the primary instrument for use within a periodontal pocket; today, it is the precision-thin ultrasonic tip. Research investigations indicate not only that ultrasonic instrumentation is as effective as hand instrumentation, but that ultrasonic instrumentation has significant advantages over hand instrumentation in the treatment and maintenance of periodontal pockets. These advantages are the (1) mechanisms of action, (2) instrument tip design, and (3) instrumentation technique.

Mechanisms of Action

A hand-activated instrument has only *one* mechanism of action in the treatment of periodontal disease, that is the mechanical removal of dental calculus and bacterial plaque. Ultrasonic instrumentation has several mechanisms of action including cavitation, acoustic turbulence, fluid lavage, and mechanical action. A hand instrument removes only what it touches. Ultrasonic instruments have the ability to disrupt and destroy bacteria from a distance. Unlike hand instruments, the ultrasonic instrument does not have to come in direct contact with dental calculus or bacterial plaque. Ultrasonic mechanisms of action produce the following disease-fighting effects:

1. **The ability to flush debris, bacteria, and unattached plaque from the periodontal pocket.** A constant stream of fluid runs through the ultrasonic handpiece and exits near the point of the ultrasonic tip. This fluid stream within the periodontal pocket is termed the <u>fluid lavage</u>. The fluid lavage produces a <u>flushing action</u> that washes debris, bacteria, and unattached plaque from the periodontal pocket. The flushing action also provides better vision during instrumentation by removing blood from the treatment site. The fluid lavage has been shown to infiltrate the pocket to a depth that is equal to the depth reached by the ultrasonic tip.[1]

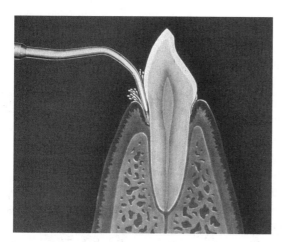

Infiltration of the fluid has been shown to be equal to the depth reached by the ultrasonic tip.
(Illustration courtesy of DENTSPLY Preventive Care.)

2. **The ability to disrupt and destroy bacteria from a distance**. The continuous stream of fluid flowing over the ultrasonic tip creates cavitation and acoustic turbulence within the periodontal pocket. Just the act of holding an activated ultrasonic tip in the periodontal pocket is destructive to the bacteria. This ability to "destroy from a distance" might be likened to an opera singer's ability to break a glass by singing a certain note.

    As the fluid flow strikes the vibrating ultrasonic tip it creates a spray comprised of millions of tiny bubbles. <u>Cavitation</u> (kav"ah-tay'-shun) results when these tiny bubbles collapse, releasing energy that destroys bacteria by tearing the bacterial cell walls and assists in the removal of plaque and endotoxins from the root surface.[15-17]

    <u>Acoustic turbulence</u> (ah-koos'-tic), also called <u>acoustic microstreaming</u>, is the pressure produced within the confined space of a periodontal pocket by the continuous stream of fluid flowing over the vibrating instrument tip. The vibrating

tip acts to churn the fluid within the confined space of the pocket. Acoustic turbulence has an antimicrobial effect within the environment of the pocket, can disrupt bacterial plaque, and destroy subgingival pathogens, especially gram-negative bacteria.[18, 19]

3. **The ability to mechanically remove dental calculus and bacterial plaque.** Just as with hand-activated instrumentation, ultrasonic instrumentation has a mechanical action. The mechanical action of the vibrating instrument tip removes supra- and subgingival calculus deposits as effectively as hand instrumentation.[6] In fact, several research studies have shown that precision-thin ultrasonic tips produce better calculus removal [5] and provide better access within periodontal pockets [20] and Class II and III furcations.[8, 21-23]

Instrument Tip Design

Hand instruments are challenging to use in deep periodontal pockets because of the size of the working-ends and the exactness with which the working-end must be adapted and angulated. Some ultrasonic tips are smaller in size than the working-end of a curet. Ultrasonic tips do not require precise adaptation or angulation to be effective. The instrument tip design of an ultrasonic tip has the following advantages over the design of a hand-activated instrument:

1. **A significantly smaller size than the working-end of a curet.** A precision-thin tip is an ultrasonic tip that is thin in diameter, significantly smaller in size than the working-end of a curet, and approximately 40% thinner than a standard size ultrasonic instrument tip. Standard Gracey curets are too wide to enter the furcation area of over 50% of all maxillary and mandibular molars.[21] The average facial furcation entrance of maxillary and mandibular first molars is from 0.63 to 1.04 mm in width.[25] The width of a new Gracey curet ranges from 0.76 to 1 mm while the diameter of a precision-thin ultrasonic tip is 0.3 to 0.6 millimeter.[26] Precision-thin tips have been shown to reach 1 mm deeper than hand instruments [27] and to reach the base of the pocket in 86% of 3-to-9 mm pockets.[24]

2. **A 365-degree circle of ultrasonic activity.** Only the cutting edge of a hand instrument is capable of calculus removal. Energy is generated by the lateral surfaces, back, face, and point of an ultrasonic tip creating a 360-degree circle of activity around the ultrasonic tip. In other words, the ultrasonic tip is effective no matter which surface of the tip is in contact with the calculus deposit. This allows the clinician to debride the tooth with the surface of the instrument tip that adapts most easily to the area.[28] Ultrasonic instrument tips do not need a sharp cutting edge to remove calculus deposits. In addition, hand-activated curets must be

positioned beneath (apical to) the calculus deposit before initiating a work stroke; this position causes considerable distention (stretching) of pocket wall away from the tooth surface. The thin ultrasonic tip can be positioned at the coronal (uppermost) edge of the deposit to chip away at the deposit from above. Positioning of the thin insert with less tissue distention increases patient comfort and results in less tissue trauma.

3.   **A handpiece that is large in diameter.** The pinch pressure used to grasp the instrument handle is one of the most harmful elements to the clinician's fingers and hands. Smaller diameter handles require a greater pinch pressure to grasp the instrument.[29] Ultrasonic handpieces are larger in diameter than hand instruments and therefore, require less pinch pressure to hold.

Instrumentation Technique

Ultrasonic instrumentation has the following advantages over hand instrumentation:

1.   **Minimal stroke pressure.** Hand instruments require the clinician exert moderate to firm lateral pressure against the tooth surface for calculus removal. Ultrasonic instruments are used with light stroke pressure and a relaxed grasp.

2.   **Shorter instrumentation time.** Less time is required for calculus removal using ultrasonic instrumentation than with hand instrumentation.[30, 42] Shorter instrumentation time combined with a more relaxed grasp and less stroke pressure make ultrasonic instrumentation less tiring and reduces the risk of musculoskeletal injury for the clinician.

3.   **Less iatrogenic damage to periodontium.** Iatrogenic damage is injury to the periodontium that occurs as a result of periodontal instrumentation, such as tissue trauma or loss of cementum.
   * Gentler to the tissues. Ultrasonic instruments have no cutting edges to cut or tear the tissue and can be inserted in deep pockets with less tissue distention. Less tissue trauma results in faster healing rates for sites treated with ultrasonic instruments.[31]
   * Minimal cementum removal. Conservation of cementum is advantageous to periodontal health.[34, 35] A precision-thin tip removes less cementum than a curet and therefore, provides a more conservative approach to subgingival debridement.[32] Ritz, et al. found that only a thin layer (11.6 microns) of cementum was removed by an ultrasonic scaler compared to much greater losses of 108.9 microns with a curet.[33]

Summary Sheet: Hand Versus Ultrasonic Instrumentation

Ultrasonic Instrumentation	Hand Instrumentation
1. Several mechanisms of action: cavitation, acoustic turbulence, fluid lavage, and mechanical action	1. Only one mechanism of action: mechanical action
2. Ability to disrupt and destroy bacteria from a distance	2. Can remove only what it touches
3. Flushing action removes debris and bacteria from pocket	3. Some debris remains in pocket to cause irrigation to tissue
4. Small tip size (0.3-0.6 mm)	4. Larger in size (0.76-1.0 mm)
5. Tip has 360° circle of activity and is effective no matter which surface is in contact with a deposit	5. Only a correctly adapted cutting edge is capable of calculus removal
6. Light lateral pressure and relaxed grasp is used for calculus removal	6. Moderate to firm lateral pressure is needed for calculus removal
7. Less time needed for calculus removal	7. More time needed for calculus removal
8. Easily inserted in pocket with minimal distention (stretching) of pocket wall away from the tooth	8. Must be positioned apical to deposit resulting in considerable distention of pocket wall
9. Less tissue trauma and faster healing rate	9. More tissue trauma and slower healing rate
10. Less cementum removal	10. More cementum removal
11. No sharpening needed	11. Frequent sharpening needed

Section 2: Treatment Considerations

Contraindications for Use

With all of the benefits of mechanized instruments, it is important to remember that these instruments are not recommended for use with all patients.

Contraindications for Mechanized Instrumentation

1. **Communicable disease.** Individuals with communicable diseases that can be disseminated by aerosols (e.g., tuberculosis, respiratory infections).

2. **High susceptibility to infection.** Individuals with a high susceptibility to opportunistic infection that can be transmitted by contaminated dental-unit water or aerosols, such as, uncontrolled diabetics, debilitated individuals with chronic medical conditions, or immuno-suppressed individuals.

3. **Respiratory risk.** Individuals with respiratory disease or difficulty in breathing (e.g., history of emphysema, cystic fibrosis, asthma). This patient would have a high infection risk if he or she were to aspirate septic material or microorganisms from plaque and periodontal pocket into the lungs.

4. **Unshielded pacemaker.** Magnetostrictive instruments may effect certain styles of cardiac pacemakers. <u>Check with cardiologist</u>. Piezoelectric instruments do *not* interfere with pacemaker functioning.

5. **Difficulty in swallowing or prone to gagging.** Individuals with multiple sclerosis, amyotrophic lateral sclerosis, muscular dystrophy, or paralysis may experience difficulty in swallowing or be prone to gagging.

6. **Age.** Primary and newly erupted teeth of young children have large pulp chambers that are more susceptible to damage from the vibrations and heat produced by ultrasonic instrumentation.

7. **Oral conditions.** Avoid contact of instrument tip with porcelain crowns, composite resin restorations, demineralized enamel surfaces, or exposed dentinal surfaces. Not for use with titanium implants, unless the ultrasonic instrument is covered with a specially designed plastic sleeve.

Biofilm Contamination in Waterlines

Scientific investigations have shown that dental unit waterlines may become significantly contaminated with microorganisms including Staphylococcus, Legionella, Pseudomonas, and Moraxella.[36-38] This contaminated water is delivered to mechanized instruments, dental handpieces, and air/water syringes. Although water from a municipal water source is safe for drinking, the presence of even small numbers of organisms can present problems for dental unit water quality. Potable drinking water is defined as less than 500 bacterial colony-forming units per milliliter (CFU/ml). Water recovered from dental units connected to municipal water supplies may contain millions of bacterial colony forming units per milliliter.

Biofilms are microbial accumulations that adhere to the interior surfaces of waterline tubing. These biofilms have been shown to be the primary source of contaminated water delivered by dental units. Stagnant water at room temperature is an ideal culture medium for many microorganisms. Dental tubing presents a favorable environment for bacterial colonization because fluid flow is practically stagnant near the tubing walls. Stagnant fluid flow allows floating bacteria to form organized intricate colonies on the tubing walls. These bacterial colonies are embedded in a polysaccharide slime layer that protects the bacteria from physical or chemical destruction. Parts of the biofilm frequently disengage from the tubing walls and can be carried into the patient's mouth. Organisms in the structure of a biofilm are highly resistant to chemical germicides and therefore, act as a source for the continuous recontamination of dental unit water. Improving the quality of dental water is a growing concern for dental healthcare providers striving to maintain high quality patient care.

Patients at risk of infection linked to dental treatment include the elderly, individuals with chronic medical conditions, diabetics, smokers, alcoholics, immuno-suppressed (i.e., organ-transplant or cancer patients), and HIV-positive individuals. Patients and clinicians temporarily compromised by infections and stresses also may be at risk of infection. The medical risk from the microbial contamination of dental water is most significant to immuno-suppressed individuals.

Options to control contamination of ultrasonic handpiece tubing include a combination of:

1. **Self-contained reservoir.** Use an ultrasonic unit with a self-contained reservoir bottle that requires no waterline hook-up. The reservoir can be used to deliver distilled water or antimicrobial to ultrasonic instrument tip.
2. **Point-of-use filter.** Install a filter in the ultrasonic waterline to physically reduce the numbers of microorganisms in the water flowing over the instrument tip. These filters are easily installed in existing dental unit waterlines.

3. **Flush the ultrasonic handpiece tubing**. Flush the ultrasonic handpiece tubing at the beginning of each day by stepping on the foot pedal to allow water to flow through the handpiece for at least 2 minutes. Flushing clears stagnant water from the tubing.

Prevention of Bacteremias

Bacteremia is the presence of bacteria in the bloodstream. Bacteria from the oral cavity are introduced into the bloodstream during hand and ultrasonic instrumentation.[39] Bacteremias of oral origin present a risk of **bacterial endocarditis** (bacterial infection of the lining of the heart chambers and heart valves) for some individuals, such as those with a history of certain heart conditions and total joint replacement. For patients who are at risk of developing bacterial endocarditis, the American Heart Association recommends the use of antibiotic premedication, pre-procedural rinses, and subgingival irrigation. Pre-procedural rinsing and subgingival irrigation with an antimicrobial solution has been shown to significantly reduce the level of blood borne microorganisms resulting from nonsurgical dental procedures, including instrumentation with ultrasonic instruments.

Pre-procedural rinsing with either chlorhexidine or an antiseptic mouthrinse, such as Listerine Antiseptic, for 20 to 30 seconds prior to treatment is recommended for all patients. This procedure is recommended to reduce the number of bacteria introduced into the patient's blood stream and for control of aerosols into the surrounding environment.

Pre-procedural subgingival irrigation of the treatment area with either chlorhexidine or an antiseptic mouthrinse, such as Listerine Antiseptic, is recommended for patients with gingivitis or periodontitis. The antimicrobial solution may be delivered with an irrigating syringe, a subgingival irrigation delivery device (such as a Teledyne Perio Pik), or an ultrasonic unit with a fluid reservoir.

Aerosol Production

Mechanized instruments have been shown to generate high levels of aerosols. Dental **aerosols** are airborne particles dispersed into the surrounding environment by dental equipment such as high-speed handpieces and ultrasonic instruments. Particles found in dental aerosols include oral microorganisms, blood, saliva, and oral debris. Microorganisms in the dental aerosols have been shown to survive for up to 24 hours.

The use of surface disinfection and barriers are particularly important when using an ultrasonic instrument. Independent water reservoirs or point-of-use filters and pre-procedural rinsing by the patient are recommended to reduce the number of airborne microorganisms in aerosols. Laminar airflow systems that filter microorganisms from the air can significantly reduce the number of airborne organisms in the dental environment.

Fluid control measures reduce aerosol production, improve visibility of the treatment area and increases patient comfort. A disposable high-volume evacuation tip or a saliva ejector is recommended for fluid control. The PERIOgiene is a high volume suction device that attaches directly to the Cavitron ultrasonic handpiece. This device reduces aerosol production by 93% and fluid buildup in the patient's mouth by 76%.[40]

Universal Precautions

As with any dental procedure, universal precautions must be used during ultrasonic instrumentation. The clinician should wear a gown with a high neck and long sleeves, hair-covering, high bacterial filtration efficiency (HBFE) mask, protective eyewear, face shield, and gloves. The mask should be changed every 20 minutes, as a damp mask will not provide adequate protection. Personal protective gear for the patient should include a plastic drape, towel or bib, and protective eyewear. The patient may prefer to cover his or her nose with a flat-style mask to limit inhalation of aerosols.

Magnetic Fields

Recently, some dental healthcare workers have expressed concern regarding occupational exposure to weak time-varying magnetic fields. Magnetostrictive ultrasonic units, amalgamators, composite light curing units, x-ray view boxes, and dental unit chair lights all produce weak magnetic fields. To date, there is no scientific evidence of any adverse health effect occurring as a result of exposure to weak magnetic fields.[41]

Section 3: Ultrasonic Instrument Tip

Tip Selection

Modern ultrasonic instrument tips range in size from large, broad tips (standard size) to thin, slender tips (precision-thin). Each manufacturing company produces unique instrument tips for their ultrasonic units. The variety of instrument tip designs varies from company to company and a full range of tip sizes is not available from all manufacturers. In addition, instrument tips from one manufacturer do not necessarily fit another company's ultrasonic unit.

Ultrasonic tips should be selected in a similar manner to hand instruments. Standard instrument tips with large, broad working-ends are designed to remove heavy supragingival calculus deposits. Standard instrument tips with medium-sized working-ends are used to remove moderate supragingival deposits and subgingival calculus deposits if tissue distention permits easy insertion of the tip. Precision-thin tips provide the best access to deep pockets and furcation areas and are used to remove light subgingival deposits.

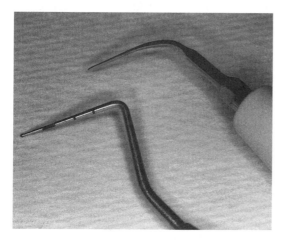

Precision-thin ultrasonic tips are similar in diameter to periodontal probes.

The range of instrument tips available for a particular unit should be a major determining factor when selecting an ultrasonic unit for purchase. A few examples of instrument tip designs are shown on the next two pages.

Instrument Tip Designs

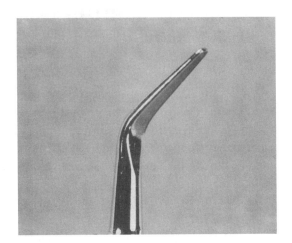

This broad <u>standard size</u> instrument tip is commonly referred to as a "beavertail" tip. It is an example of a tip designed to remove heavy <u>supra</u>gingival calculus, especially from the lingual aspect of anterior teeth.

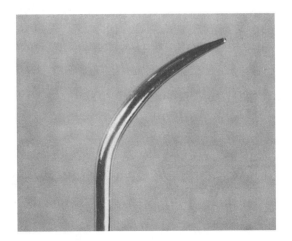

This <u>standard size</u> instrument tip is commonly referred to as a "universal tip". It is used to remove medium-sized calculus deposits and may be used subgingivally if tissue distention allows easy insertion of the tip. It has universal application (instrumentation of anterior and posterior teeth).

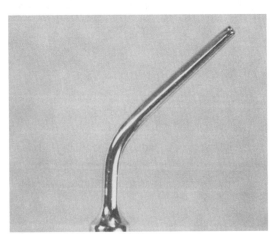

This <u>standard size</u> tip is commonly referred to as the "probe tip". It is used to remove moderate and light subgingival calculus deposits. It has universal application (instrumentation of anterior and posterior teeth).

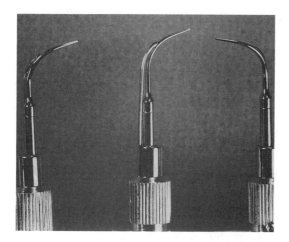

These <u>precision-thin</u> inserts come in a left style, straight style, and right style. These instruments are used for light calculus removal and deplaquing. The right and left tips facilitate access and adaptation to root concavities, proximal surfaces, and furcation areas.

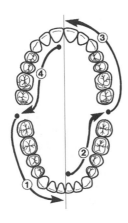

The **right** tip adapts to the following areas:

1-mand. right quadrant, facial aspect
2-mand. left quadrant, lingual aspect
3.-max. left quadrant, facial aspect
4-max. right quadrant, lingual aspect

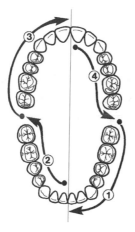

The **left** tip adapts to the following areas:

1-mand. left quadrant, facial aspect
2-mand. right quadrant, lingual aspect
3-max. right quadrant, facial aspect
4-max. left quadrant, lingual aspect

Energy Dispersion of Tip Surfaces

Ultrasonic instrument tips are active on all surfaces. The point of the tip generates the most energy. The face (concave surface) is the second most powerful surface, followed by the back (convex surface). The lateral surfaces (sides) of the tip generate the least amount of energy. Understanding the levels of energy generated by the different tip surfaces is important in determining which surface should be adapted to the tooth surface or calculus deposit. By adapting the appropriate tip surface, the clinician can control energy dispersion and patient sensitivity (e.g.: higher energy for heavy deposits; lower energy for sensitive areas.)

Clinicians should follow manufacturer's recommendations for tip-surface adaptation. The face and point of the tip are not used against the tooth surface; the high amount of energy generated by these surfaces would result in damage to the tooth surface. The point of the tip can be adapted to calculus deposits, but should never be adapted directly to the tooth surface. With magnetostrictive instrument tips, the lateral surfaces and back of the working-end can be adapted to the tooth surface. Adaptation of the lateral surfaces of the instrument tip is recommended when using piezoelectric instruments.

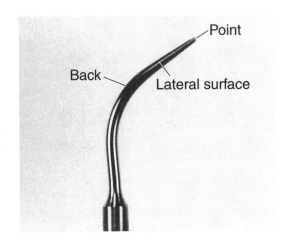

Energy generated by tip surfaces. The point generates the most energy. The face is the second most powerful surface, followed by the back. The lateral surfaces generate the least amount of energy.

Tip Frequency

Ultrasonic sound waves do not remove calculus deposits. It is the vibration, or movement, of the ultrasonic tip that is responsible for calculus removal. The number of times per second that the instrument tip moves back and forth during one cycle is called the **frequency**.

As the tip vibrates back and forth at 18,000 or more strokes per second, it chips away at the calculus deposit. The portion of the instrument tip that is capable of doing work is called the **active tip area**. The active tip area ranges from 2 to 4 millimeters in length depending on the tip frequency and type of unit. This means that the power to do work is concentrated in the last 2 to 4 mm of the length of the tip (on all sides).

Some ultrasonic units (**manual tune units**) allow the clinician to adjust the tip frequency by turning a knob on the unit. On **automatically tuned units**, the tip frequency is controlled automatically by the unit.

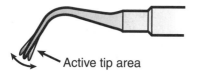

Active tip area

The power for calculus removal is concentrated in the **active tip area** (the last 2-4 mm of the tip).

Power Settings

Power is the energy in the handpiece that is used to generate the movement of the instrument tip. Higher power settings result in greater longitudinal oscillation (distance) traveled by the instrument tip. The higher the power, the longer the stroke, and the more forcefully the instrument tip strikes the surface of the tooth or calculus deposit. For this reason, higher power settings are more uncomfortable for the patient and more likely to damage the tooth surface.

The **stroke** is the maximum distance the instrument tip moves during one cycle. On ultrasonic units, the stroke is adjusted by turning the power knob on the ultrasonic unit. The power levels may be designated as ranges of "high, medium, and low" or "1, 2, 3" depending on the unit. Use of the low power setting is recommended for calculus removal and deplaquing. For tenacious calculus deposits, the medium power setting can be used with the standard size instrument tips (not with precision-thin tips). Research investigations found no difference in the effectiveness of ultrasonic instruments when operated at high power levels or medium power levels.[42] Therefore, use of power levels above the medium (middle) setting is not recommended.

Clinical Power

The resistance on an instrument tip when placed against the calculus deposit is known as the **load** (the tip must overcome the load in order to remove calculus). **Clinical power** is the ability to remove calculus deposits under load. The surface of the instrument tip in contact with the tooth, tip frequency, and power setting are the major variables that determine clinical power. Several other factors influence the force produced by the instrument tip[43]:

1. **Lateral pressure**. Moderate or firm lateral pressure applied with the instrument tip against the surface of the calculus deposit or tooth decreases or stops the vibrating tip. The tip functions most effectively with light lateral pressure against the tooth or calculus surface.
2. **Exposure time.** The longer the tip is in contact with the tooth, the greater amount of energy delivered to the tooth. The tip should be kept in constant motion to avoid damage to the tooth surface or pulp; never hold the instrument tip still in one spot.
3. **Angle of adaptation.** The highest energy is emitted from the tip when it is adapted at a 90° angle to the tooth surface. An angulation between 0° and 15° is recommended.
4. **Sharpness of the tip.** Sharpened ultrasonic tips emit high energy levels; therefore, tips should be round or blunt with no sharpened edges.

Fluid Adjustment

The ultrasonic unit converts electrical energy into high frequency sound waves in the form of rapid vibrations. These high frequency sound waves produce heat; if not cooled the instrument tip overheats. Fluid spray flowing over the instrument tip is used as a coolant. Too little fluid flow to the instrument tip can result in heat damage to the dental pulp. The most common mistake made by beginning clinicians is using too little fluid. A warm handpiece is a sign of inadequate fluid. The fluid flow should be adjusted until a fine mist or a mist with fluid droplets is observed around the instrument tip.

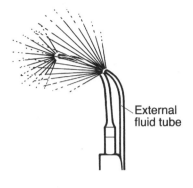

This ultrasonic instrument tip has an <u>external</u> flow tube to carry fluid to the instrument tip. Adjust the fluid flow so that it breaks into a fine mist near the end of the external flow tube.

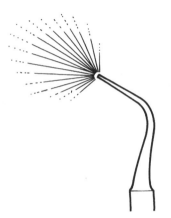

This ultrasonic instrument tip has an <u>internal</u> fluid flow system. The fluid flows directly through the instrument tip and breaks into a fine mist at the very end of the tip.

Tip Wear and Replacement

It is important to monitor the condition of ultrasonic instrument tips. Over time, the instrument tip is worn down with use. As the instrument tip wears effectiveness decreases. A rule of thumb is that 1 mm of wear results in approximately 25% loss of efficiency. Approximately 50% loss of efficiency occurs at 2 mm of wear and the tip should be discarded at this point. Some instrument manufacturers provide wear guides for their instrument tips. A tip should be replaced s soon as it shows signs of wear or damage since use of heavily worn tips can result in damage to the tooth surface. Also, check the metal stacks on magnetostrictive insert tip; if the magnetostrictive insert tip does not slide freely into the handpiece, the tip will not function effectively.

Section 4: Tip Adaptation

The technique used for adaptation of an ultrasonic instrument is very different from that used with hand-activated instruments. A curet must be adapted at the proper angulation and positioned apical to (underneath) the calculus deposit. Calculus removal with a curet is accomplished beginning at the base of the pocket, working "upward" toward the CEJ. Ultrasonic instruments are active 360° around the instrument tip; the tip is effective no matter which surface of the instrument tip is in contact with the calculus deposit. Calculus removal with an ultrasonic instrument is accomplished from coronal to (above) the calculus deposit, working "downward" toward the junctional epithelium. The instrumentation technique used depends on whether you are adapting the instrument tip to a tooth surface or against a calculus deposit:

Against the tooth surface. Position the instrument tip in a manner similar to that of a calibrated periodontal probe, with the point directed toward the junctional epithelium and the length of the tip at a 0° to 15° angle to the tooth surface. Remember that the last 2 to 4 mm of the length of the tip are the most active portion of the tip. In most cases, the lateral surface of the instrument tip is used against the tooth surface. With a magnetostrictive instrument, the instrument back also may be applied to the tooth surface for removal of a tenacious calculus deposit. The point of the tip should never be applied directly to the tooth at a 90° angle; this angulation can gouge cementum and dentin surfaces.

Against calculus deposits. With the instrument tip in a similar position to a periodontal probe, the point is placed directly against the uppermost edge of the calculus deposit. You might think of the instrument tip as being somewhat like a miniature jackhammer used to chip away at the deposit. When removing a large interproximal calculus deposit from either the facial or lingual aspect, the point of the instrument tip may be applied directly against the "front or back" of the calculus deposit.

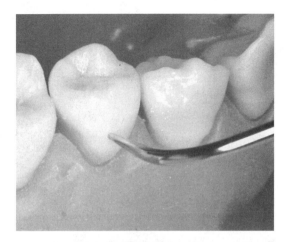

Incorrect adaptation. Never adapt the point of the instrument tip at a 90-degree angle to the tooth surface.

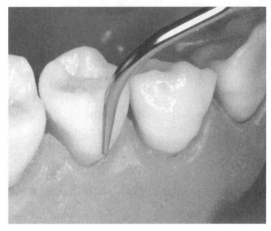

Correct adaptation. Adapt the instrument tip in a similar manner to a periodontal probe, with the point directed toward the junctional epithelium and the lateral surface at a 0° to 15° angle to the tooth surface.

Use of Lateral Surfaces of Instrument Tip

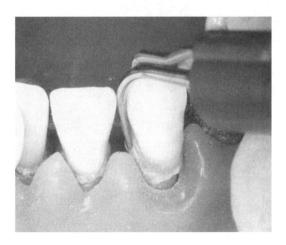

Correct adaptation of a lateral surface of the instrument tip to the proximal surface of an anterior tooth.

Correct adaptation of a lateral surface of the instrument tip (horizontal position) to the proximal surface of an anterior tooth.

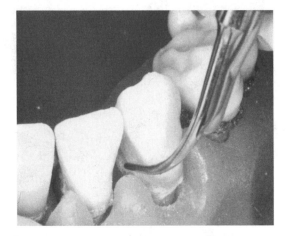

Incorrect adaptation. A traditional intraoral finger rest can make it difficult to adapt the lateral surface of the instrument tip to the lingual surface of a mandibular anterior tooth. Shown is the incorrect adaptation of the point of the instrument tip to the tooth surface.

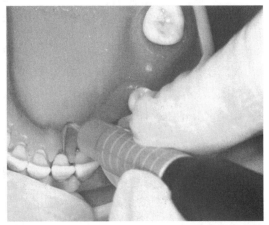

Correct adaptation. Rotating the instrument handpiece to the side of the mouth and establishing a finger rest several teeth away makes it easier to correctly adapt a lateral surface of the instrument tip to the lingual surface of a mandibular anterior tooth.

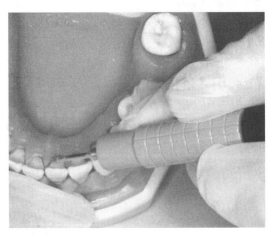

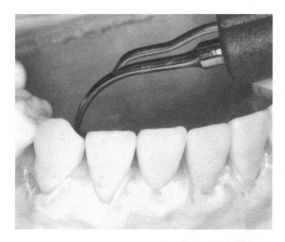

Correct adaptation of a lateral surface of the instrument tip to the lingual surface of the mandibular right canine. Note that the instrument handle is rotated to the side of the patient's mouth.

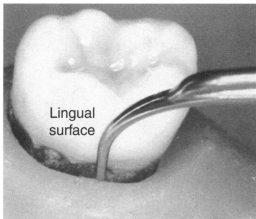

Correct adaptation of a lateral surface of the instrument tip to the lingual surface of a molar.

Use of Back of Instrument Tip

The back of the instrument tip can be used with some ultrasonic instruments. Usually use of the back of the instrument tip is only recommended for <u>magnetostrictive</u> ultrasonic instruments. Tip design specifications vary from manufacturer to manufacturer (follow manufacturer's recommendations).

Adaptation of the back of the instrument tip to the mesial surface of the mandibular left canine (from the lingual aspect).

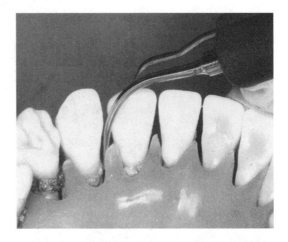

Establishing a finger rest on the opposite side of the arch from the treatment area allows adaptation of the back of the instrument tip to the lingual surface of a mandibular molar.

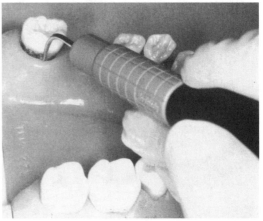

Adaptation of the back of the instrument tip to the mesial surface of a mandibular right first molar.

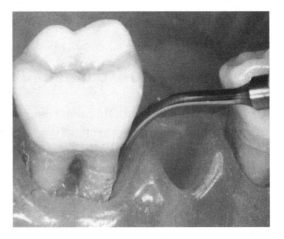

Access to Palatal Root of Maxillary Molars

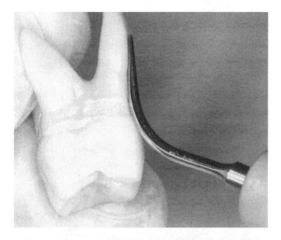

The palatal root of a maxillary molar flares in a lingual direction. For this reason, the best adaptation to the lingual surface of the palatal root is obtained with the back of the instrument tip.

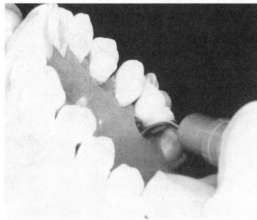

Establishing a finger rest on the opposite side of the arch from the treatment area allows the clinician to adapt the back of the instrument tip to the palatal root of this maxillary molar.

Access to Furcation Areas

Curved precision-thin tips work best for instrumentation of furcation areas. The easiest way to locate the furcation area is to *deactivate* the ultrasonic instrument tip (remove foot from foot pedal). Use the inactivated instrument tip to locate the furcation. Position the instrument tip in the furcation and activate the tip to instrument the furcation area.

Adaptation of an ultrasonic instrument with a ball-tip in the crotch area of a furcation.

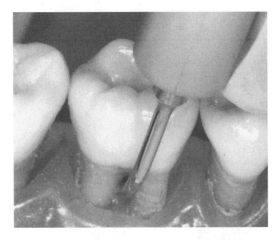

Adaptation of the back of the instrument tip to the mesial surface of the <u>distal root</u> on a mandibular first molar.

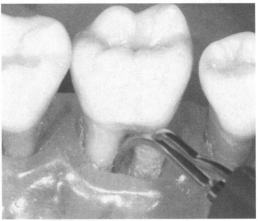

Adaptation of a lateral surface of the instrument tip to the distal surface of the <u>mesial root</u> on a mandibular first molar.

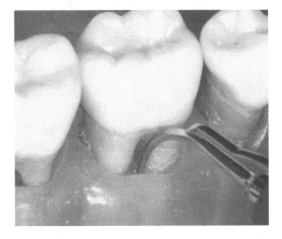

Section 5: Instrumentation Strokes

Stroke Motion

With ultrasonic instruments, the calculus removal work stroke is made with either a **tapping** motion against a calculus deposit or with a **sweeping**, eraser-like motion to deplaque the root surface. With both stroke motions <u>light pressure</u> is used, as firm pressure diminishes the effectiveness of the instrument.

An <u>inactivated</u> instrument tip (no pressure on the foot pedal) may be used to assess (explore) the subgingival tooth surfaces in a similar manner to the way in which a curet is used to assess the tooth during calculus removal.

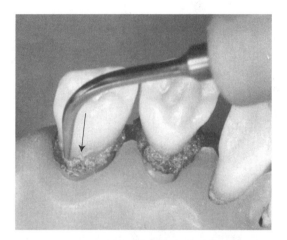

Tapping Motion: For calculus removal, the point of the instrument tip is positioned at the uppermost edge of the deposit. The instrument tip is directed against the deposit in a light tapping motion. Only gentle tapping pressure is used, as firm pressure will reduce the effectiveness of the instrument.

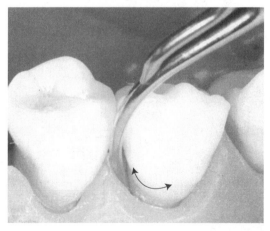

Sweeping Motion: For deplaquing, the instrument tip is used in an eraser-like motion. Overlapping strokes with the instrument tip should cover every square millimeter of the root surface. Imagine that you are using the side of a crayon (rather than the point) to color the entire root surface.

Stroke Direction

Keep the instrument tip moving at all times, using overlapping vertical, oblique, and horizontal strokes. The stroke pattern should be long and flowing with overlapping strokes covering every square millimeter of the root surface.

Vertical or oblique strokes can be used in a sweeping motion to deplaque the root surface.

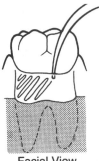
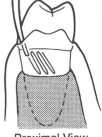

Facial View   Proximal View

Deplaquing also can be accomplished by using horizontal strokes in a sweeping motion.

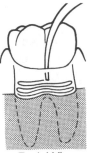

Facial View

Vertical or oblique strokes can be used with a tapping motion for calculus removal. Horizontal strokes can be used with a tapping motion against a large interproximal calculus deposit.

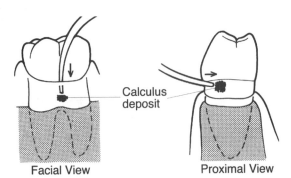

Calculus deposit

Facial View   Proximal View

Sequence for Calculus Removal

Work in a coronal-to-apical sequence, removing the coronal-most deposits first. Position the tip at the coronal (uppermost) edge of the deposit to chip away at the deposit from above (start at CEJ and move toward junctional epithelium). This differs from instrumentation with hand-activated instruments where calculus deposits are removed in an apical-to-coronal sequence (beginning at junctional epithelium and working toward CEJ).

Stubborn Calculus Deposits

A misconception of clinicians who are new to ultrasonic instrumentation is that the instrument will remove calculus with a quick pass over the deposit. The most common cause of a failure to remove calculus is not spending enough time instrumenting the area. Touch the instrument tip to the calculus and lightly tap, tap, tap away at the deposit. The deposit will not simply melt away, rather tiny pieces of the deposit will break-up as you tap, tap, tap. Sometimes very tenacious calculus deposits cannot be removed even though you are using a correct tapping technique with the instrument point and allowing enough time for calculus removal.

1. Evaluate your tip selection. Use standard sized tips for *supra*gingival deposits. Straight precision-tips work best in deep pockets on facial and lingual aspects. Curved precision-tips work best on the midlines of proximal surfaces and furcation areas.
2. Approach the deposits from different angles (attack it from a variety of directions). Approach interproximal deposits from both the facial and lingual aspects.
3. Resist the urge to use more lateral pressure, as increased stroke pressure will only diminish the effectiveness of the instrument stroke.
4. If you have a manual tune ultrasonic unit, increase the frequency.
5. If you have an automatically tuned unit or if you still cannot remove the deposit using a higher frequency, it will be necessary to increase the power setting from the low to a medium (middle) setting. Do not use the high power setting. Research has shown that a high power setting is no more effective than the medium setting at removing calculus.[42]

Section 6: Instrumentation Technique

Fundamental Skills

Fundamental instrumentation technique for ultrasonic instrumentation differs slightly from that used in hand-activated instrumentation.

1. **Grasp.** Always use a light, relaxed grasp, even for calculus removal strokes. Let the instrument do the work for you.
2. **Finger Rest.** Either an intra- or extra-oral finger rest may be used. Since the instrument does the work of mechanical calculus removal, an intraoral fulcrum is not needed to concentrate the force of the stroke. In many cases, an advanced fulcruming technique is advantageous in obtaining access to deep periodontal pockets. Advanced fulcruming techniques are explained in Module 25.
3. **Lateral Pressure.** Use light stroke pressure and allow the ultrasonic instrument to do all the work.
4. **Motion Activation.** Digital (finger) activation is recommended since the instrument is doing the work of calculus removal. Digital activation is excellent for applying the light stroke pressure needed for mechanized instrumentation.

Fluid Control and Containment

Good fluid control is achieved with the use of proper patient positioning. Position the patient in the normal supine position and work with his or her head turned to the side. The patient's head should be positioned to the side so that the fluid generated by the ultrasonic tip will pool in the corner of the mouth where it can be suctioned or evacuated. Ask the patient to turn toward you for anterior sextants and aspects toward the clinician. Ask the patient to turn slightly away from you for aspects away from the clinician.

A high-volume suction tip or a saliva ejector should be used for fluid control. A high-volume suction tip is recommended when working with an assistant or, in some instances, the clinician can hold the suction tip in the nondominant hand instead of a mirror. It may be helpful to cut the suction tip in half for easier handling when working without an assistant. Another alternative when working alone is to ask the patient to hold a saliva ejector. Position the suction tip or saliva ejector on the corner of the mouth where fluid will pool. Deactivate the ultrasonic tip occasionally to keep excessive amounts of fluid from pooling in the corner of the mouth.

It can be very frustrating to the patient to have his or her face and hair sprayed with the fluid from the instrument tip. Good fluid containment can be achieved through use of the patient's lips and cheeks as fluid-deflecting barriers. Learn to use the patient's lips and cheeks to deflect fluid back into the mouth. When working on the mandibular anterior teeth, for example, pull the patient's lip up and out away from the teeth to act as a barrier to deflect fluid back into the mouth and as a "cup" to hold the fluid. Use a similar technique for the posterior teeth, holding the cheek away from the teeth to catch the fluid.

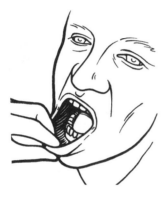

Fluid control in anterior sextants. Lower and upper lips can be cupped to contain the fluid spray.

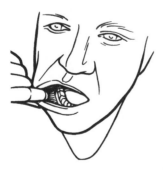

Fluid control in posterior treatment areas. Hold the cheek between the index finger and thumb and pull out and up, or down, to form a cup.

Summary Sheet: Principles of Ultrasonic Instrumentation

Basic Skills of Ultrasonic Instrumentation	
Power Setting	Use low power setting. For tenacious calculus, medium power setting can be used with standard instrument tips. Do not use high power setting, it is no more effective than the medium power setting.
Fluid Adjustment	Adjust fluid until a fine mist or a mist with fluid droplets is observed around the instrument tip.
Grasp	Maintain a light, relaxed grasp.
Finger Rest	Use intraoral or extraoral rest.
Tip Adaptation	Against the tooth surface: Position the tip similar to a probe with the point directed toward the junctional epithelium and the length of the tip at a 0° to 15° angle to the tooth surface. Against calculus deposit: Apply the point of the instrument tip against the uppermost edge of the deposit (or the "front or back" of a heavy interproximal calculus deposit.)
Motion Activation	Digital (finger) activation is excellent for applying the very light stroke pressure needed for ultrasonic instrumentation.
Sequence for Calculus Removal	Position the tip at the coronal (uppermost) edge of the deposit to chip away at the deposit from above.
Stroke Pressure	Use light stroke pressure. Moderate or firm pressure decreases the effectiveness of the instrument tip.
Stroke Motion	Calculus removal: Light tapping motion. Deplaquing: Sweeping-eraser-like motion.
Stroke Technique	Keep the instrument tip moving at all times. Cover every mm of the root surface with over-lapping, brush-like strokes.

Section 7: References

1. Nosal, G., et al., *The penetration of lavage solution into the periodontal pocket during ultrasonic instrumentation.* J Periodontol, 1991. **62**(9): p. 554-7.

2. Rams, T.E., and J. Slots, *Antibiotics in periodontal therapy: an update.* Compendium, 1992. **13**(12): p. 1130, 1132, 1134 passim.

3. Drisko, C.H., *Root instrumentation. Power-driven versus manual scalers, which one?* Dent Clin North Am, 1998. **42**(2): p. 229-44.

4. Copulos, T.A., et al., *Comparative analysis between a modified ultrasonic tip and hand instruments on clinical parameters of periodontal disease.* J Periodontol, 1993. **64**(8): p. 694-700.

5. Drisko, C.L., *Scaling and root planing without overinstrumentation: hand versus power-driven scalers.* Curr Opin Periodontol, 1993: p. 78-88.

6. Kepic, T.J., T.J. O'Leary, and A.H. Kafrawy, *Total calculus removal: an attainable objective? [see comments].* J Periodontol, 1990. **61**(1): p. 16-20.

7. Breininger, D.R., T.J. O'Leary, and R.V. Blumenshine, *Comparative effectiveness of ultrasonic and hand scaling for the removal of subgingival plaque and calculus.* J Periodontol, 1987. **58**(1): p. 9-18.

8. Leon, L.E., and R.I. Vogel, *A comparison of the effectiveness of hand scaling and ultrasonic debridement in furcations as evaluated by differential dark-field microscopy.* J Periodontol, 1987. **58**(2): p. 86-94.

9. Oosterwaal, P.J., et al., *The effect of subgingival debridement with hand and ultrasonic instruments on the subgingival microflora.* J Clin Periodontol, 1987. **14**(9): p. 528-33.

10. Thornton, S., and J. Garnick, *Comparison of ultrasonic to hand instruments in the removal of subgingival plaque.* J Periodontol, 1982. **53**(1): p. 35-7.

11. Checchi, L., and G.A. Pelliccioni, *Hand versus ultrasonic instrumentation in the removal of endotoxins from root surfaces in vitro.* J Periodontol, 1988. **59**(6): p. 398-402.

12. Badersten, A., R. Nilveus, and J. Egelberg, *Effect of nonsurgical periodontal therapy. I. Moderately advanced periodontitis.* J Clin Periodontol, 1981. **8**(1): p. 57-72.

13. Fine, D.H., et al., *Studies in plaque pathogenicity. II. A technique for the specific detection of endotoxin in plaque samples using the limulus lysate assay.* J Periodontal Res, 1978. **13**(2): p. 127-33.

14. Fine, D.H., et al., *Studies in plaque pathogenicity. I. Plaque collection and limulus lysate screening of adherent and loosely adherent plaque.* J Periodontal Res, 1978. **13**(1): p. 17-23.

15. Walmsley, A.D., W.R. Laird, and A.R. Williams, *A model system to demonstrate the role of cavitational activity in ultrasonic scaling.* J Dent Res, 1984. **63**(9): p. 1162-5.

16. Walmsley, A.D., et al., *Effects of cavitational activity on the root surface of teeth during ultrasonic scaling.* J Clin Periodontol, 1990. **17**(5): p. 306-12.

17. Baehni, P., et al., *Effects of ultrasonic and sonic scalers on dental plaque microflora in vitro and in vivo.* J Clin Periodontol, 1992. **19**(7): p. 455-9.

18. Olsen, I., and S.S. Socransky, *Ultrasonic dispersion of pure cultures of plaque bacteria and plaque.* Scand J Dent Res, 1981. **89**(4): p. 307-12.

19. Walmsley, A.D., T.F. Walsh, and W.R. Laird, *Ultrasonic instruments in dentistry: 1. The ultrasonic scaler.* Dent Update, 1988. **15**(8): p. 321-3, 325-6.

20. Walmsley, A.D., W.R. Laird, and P.J. Lumley, *Ultrasound in dentistry. Part 2—Periodontology and endodontics.* J Dent, 1992. **20**(1): p. 11-7.

21. Bower, R.C., *Furcation morphology relative to periodontal treatment. Furcation entrance architecture.* J Periodontol, 1979. **50**(1): p. 23-7.

22. Bower, R.C., *Furcation morphology relative to periodontal treatment. Furcation root surface anatomy.* J Periodontol, 1979. **50**(7): p. 366-74.

23. Bader, H., *Scaling and rootplaning: evolution or revolution?* Dent Today, 1991. **10**(9): p. 54, 56-7.

24. Shiloah, J., and L.A. Hovious, *The role of subgingival irrigations in the treatment of periodontitis [see comments].* J Periodontol, 1993. **64**(9): p. 835-43.

25. Hou, G.L., et al., *The topography of the furcation entrance in Chinese molars. Furcation entrance dimensions.* J Clin Periodontol, 1994. **21**(7): p. 451-6.

26. Holbrook, W.P., et al., *Bacteriological investigation of the aerosol from ultrasonic scalers.* Br Dent J, 1978. **144**(8): p. 245-7.

27. Young, N.A., *Periodontal debridement: re-examining non-surgical instrumentation. Part I: A new perspective on the objectives of instrumentation.* Semin Dent Hyg, 1994. **4**(4): p. 1-7.

28. Carroll, D.P., *Taking extreme care when retrieving broken tips.* Rdh, 1993. **13**(3): p. 38.

29. Radwin, R.G., et al., *External finger forces in submaximal five-finger static pinch prehension.* Ergonomics, 1992. **35**(3): p. 275-88.

30. Dragoo, M.R., *A clinical evaluation of hand and ultrasonic instruments on subgingival debridement. 1. With unmodified and modified ultrasonic inserts.* Int J Periodontics Restorative Dent, 1992. **12**(4): p. 310-23.

31. Bhaskar, S.N., M.F. Grower, and D.E. Cutright, *Gingival healing after hand and ultrasonic scaling—biochemical and histologic analysis.* J Periodontol, 1972. **43**(1): p. 31-4.

32. Cross-Poline, G.N., D.J. Stach, and S.M. Newman, *Effects of curet and ultrasonics on root surfaces.* Am J Dent, 1995. **8**(3): p. 131-3.

33. Ritz, L., A.F. Hefti, and K.H. Rateitschak, *An in vitro investigation on the loss of root substance in scaling with various instruments.* J Clin Periodontol, 1991. **18**(9): p. 643-7.

34. Moore, J., M. Wilson, and J.B. Kieser, *The distribution of bacterial lipopolysaccharide (endotoxin) in relation to periodontally involved root surfaces.* J Clin Periodontol, 1986. **13**(8): p. 748-51.

35. Smart, G.J., et al., *The assessment of ultrasonic root surface debridement by determination of residual endotoxin levels.* J Clin Periodontol, 1990. **17**(3): p. 174-8.

36. Atlas, R.M., J.F. Williams, and M.K. Huntington, *Legionella contamination of dental-unit waters.* Appl Environ Microbiol, 1995. **61**(4): p. 1208-13.

37. Dalen, P., and B. Gran, *Studying side effects of dental amalgam [letter] [In Process Citation].* Scand J Prim Health Care, 1999. **17**(2): p. 127-8.

38. Williams, J.F., et al., *Microbial contamination of dental unit waterlines: prevalence, intensity and microbiological characteristics.* J Am Dent Assoc, 1993. **124**(10): p. 59-65.

39. Lofthus, J.E., et al., *Bacteremia following subgingival irrigation and scaling and root planing.* J Periodontol, 1991. **62**(10): p. 602-7.

40. Harrel, S.K., J.B. Barnes, and F. Rivera-Hidalgo, *Reduction of aerosols produced by ultrasonic scalers.* J Periodontol, 1996. **67**(1): p. 28-32.

41. Bohay, R.N., et al., *A survey of magnetic fields in the dental operatory.* J Can Dent Assoc, 1994. **60**(9): p. 835-40.

42. Chapple, I.L., et al., *Effect of instrument power setting during ultrasonic scaling upon treatment outcome.* J Periodontol, 1995. **66**(9): p. 756-60.

43. Clark, S.M., *The ultrasonic dental unit: a guide for the clinical application of ultrasonics in dentistry and in dental hygiene.* J Periodontol, 1969. **40**(11): p. 621-9.

Ultrasonic Equipment

This module contains step-by-step instructions for the use of magnetostrictive ultrasonic equipment. <u>You should complete Module 21 and be thoroughly familiar with the concepts of ultrasonic instrumentation before attempting this module.</u>

Required Equipment:

- ultrasonic device(s) and instrument tips
- dental mirror
- personal protective equipment for clinician and patient
- antimicrobial solution for patient
- high-volume suction tip or saliva ejector

Section 1: Magnetostrictive Ultrasonic Devices

There are many brands of magnetostrictive ultrasonic units on the market; fortunately, most are operated in a similar manner.

Brand Name Examples of Magnetostrictive Equipment

Adec (Cavitron)
Dentsply Cavitron—all models
Engler Ultrason 990
Le Clean Machine
Maliga Microson 102
Parkell—all models

Periogiene Odontoson
Sonatron
Sonus V
South East Instruments Autoscaler
Tony Riso Co. Multifunction 2530
USI ultrasonic units

Components of Magnetostrictive Ultrasonic Devices

Portable unit. Magnetostrictive ultrasonic devices are housed in a portable unit that contains an electronic generator and a water control system. There usually are three "cables" attached to the portable unit: (1) a hose used to connect the unit to a water supply, (2) a cable attached to a foot pedal, and (3) tubing to which the handpiece attaches. The ultrasonic device also has a power cord that is plugged into an electrical outlet.

Foot Pedal. A foot pedal is used to activate power and fluid flow to the instrument tip in most ultrasonic units. One exception is the Odontoson unit, which has finger-switch that activates power and water to the tip.

Handpiece. The handpiece is a "tube-shaped" device into which the ultrasonic instrument inserts are placed. Some ultrasonic units have handpieces that can be removed from the tubing for sterilization, others have permanently attached handpieces that must be surface disinfected. For purposes of infection control, units with detachable handpieces are preferred.

Instrument Inserts. Most units use removable instrument inserts that fit into the handpiece. Some systems (Engler 990 and Sonus V) use screw-on tips. The electric generator produces in an alternating, low voltage electric current in the handpiece.

This current produces a magnetic field in the handpiece that causes the insert to expand and contract along its length and in turn, causes the insert tip to vibrate.

Magnetostrictive instrument inserts are available in two kilohertz options: 25 kHz and 30 kHz. A **kilohertz (kHz)** is equal to 1000 cycles per second. The working-end of a 25 kHz insert moves at 25,000 cycles per second, while the working-end of a 30 kHz insert moves at 30,000 cycles per second. The 25 kHz insert has a longer working-end stroke length than that of a 30 kHz instrument. The 30 kHz instrument inserts produce lower noise levels and have a shorter handpiece length than that of the 25 kHz inserts. The shorter 30 kHz inserts fit into a handpiece that is shorter in length and lighter in weight.

Fluid. Water or another fluid is directed onto the working-end through a metal flow tube or internal channel through the working-end. The fluid flow that is required to cool the magnetostrictive handpiece is warmed slightly to provide a fluid temperature that will be comfortable for most patients.

Tip Vibration Frequency. The tip vibration frequency of the working-end of a magnetostrictive instrument ranges from 18,000 to 42,000 cycles per second (18-42 kHz).

Tip Motion. All surfaces of the insert tip are active; this means the *face, back and both lateral sides* of the working-end are active. The active tip area is about 4.2 millimeters for both the 25 kHz and 30 kHz inserts. The active tip area of a magnetostrictive insert typically vibrates in a controlled elliptical pattern.

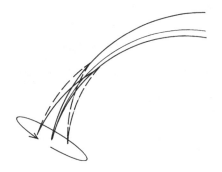

The active tip area of magnetostrictive instrument tip vibrates in an elliptical pattern.

Step-by-Step Technique: Magnetostrictive

Example: DENTSPLY Cavitron ultrasonic magnetostrictive device
[Reference—DENTSPLY Cavitron: *Instructional Manual DENTSPLY/Cavitron Dental Prophylaxis Unit.*
York, PA. DENTSPLY Preventive Care.]

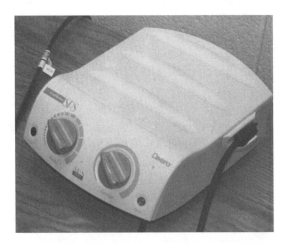

1. Place the ultrasonic power unit on a counter or cart so that you have easy access to the device at the dental chair.

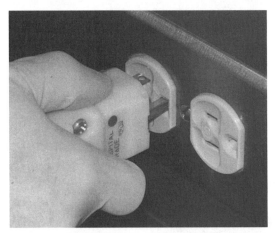

2. Plug the power cord into an electrical outlet.

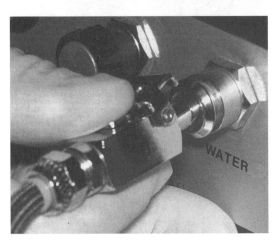

3. Connect the blue hose to the water outlet on the dental unit. Turn on the dental unit and open the water control knob. <u>If using a unit with a independent fluid reservoir</u>, attach the reservoir bottle to the ultrasonic unit.

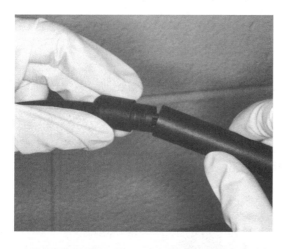

4. Connect a sterilized handpiece to the handpiece tubing. Place barrier coverings over the power unit control knobs and wrap the handpiece tubing.

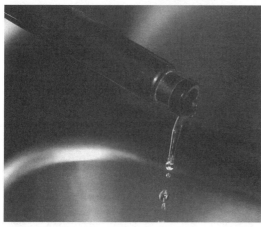

5. Flush the water tubing of stagnant water by holding the handpiece over a sink and stepping on the foot pedal to activate a steady stream of fluid. At the start of each day, flush for <u>2 minutes</u>. Between patients, flush for <u>30 seconds</u>.

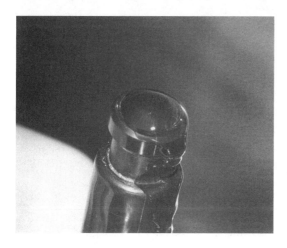

6. Hold the handpiece upright, step on the foot control, and fill the handpiece completely with fluid. Keeping the handpiece in an upright position, release the foot pedal. This step expels air bubbles from the handpiece that could cause overheating. <u>Repeat this procedure whenever you change instrument inserts</u>.

7. Insert a sterilized instrument insert into the handpiece, pushing until the insert snaps into place.

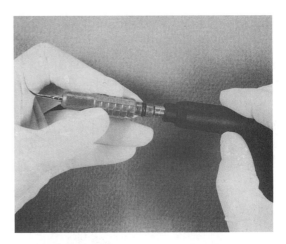

8. Adjust power and water controls while holding the handpiece over the sink. For the most efficient **calculus removal**, adjust the water spray to create a light mist or "halo" effect at the working-end.

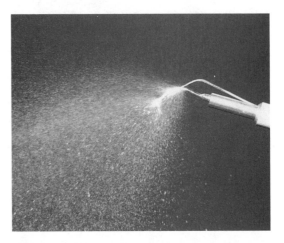

9. At the <u>lowest power setting</u>, the water flow can be adjusted to produce a rapid drip at the working-end. Power and water to the insert can be adjusted in this manner to **reduce patient sensitivity** and for **deplaquing**.

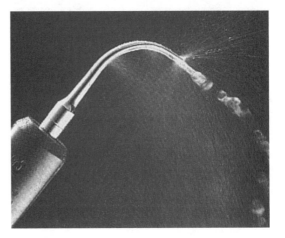

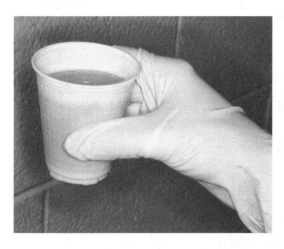

10. Ask your patient to rinse with an antimicrobial solution for 30 seconds. Or, if appropriate, complete a pre-procedural subgingival irrigation of the <u>treatment area</u> prior to instrumentation.

11. Ask the patient to turn to the side. Establish an intra- or extraoral finger rest. Hold the working-end off of the tooth surface as you step on the foot pedal to activate the instrument tip.

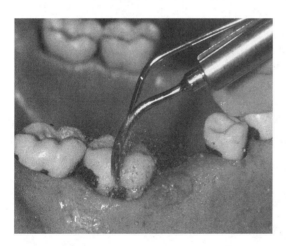

12. Adapt the <u>activated</u> working-end to the tooth surface. Position the tip in a manner similar to that of a periodontal probe. Use light stroke pressure in a tapping motion against a calculus deposit or in sweeping, brush-like motion against the tooth surface.

Suction. Use a high-volume suction tip or ask your patient to hold a saliva ejector. Position the suction tip or saliva ejector on the side of the mouth where the fluid will pool. Deactivate the ultrasonic tip occasionally to keep excessive amounts of fluid from pooling in the mouth. Cup lips and cheeks to deflect fluid.

Skill Activities. Turn to page 502 for Skill Building Activities.

Section 2: Piezoelectric Ultrasonic Devices

There are many brands of piezoelectric ultrasonic units on the market; fortunately, most are operated in a similar manner.

Brand Name Examples of Piezoelectric Equipment

Amadent—all models   Spartan Piezoelectric
EMS miniPiezon, EMS Piezon Master   Ultra Scaler
PDT Sensor Sc/RP   Young PS
Pro-Dentec Pro-Select

Components of Piezoelectric Ultrasonic Devices

Portable unit. Piezoelectric ultrasonic devices are housed in a portable unit that contains an electronic generator and a water control system. At least two "cables" are attached to the portable unit: (1) a cable attached to a foot pedal, and (2) tubing to which the handpiece attaches. The unit may have either a fluid reservoir or a hose used to connect the unit to an external water supply. The ultrasonic device also has a power cord that is plugged into an electrical outlet.

Foot Pedal. A foot pedal is used to activate power and fluid flow to the instrument tip. Some brands have a foot pedal with a two-step control mechanism. Use light foot pressure to depress the pedal to the first level for fluid irrigation only. Use heavier foot pressure to depress the pedal to the second level for ultrasonic action and irrigation.

Handpiece. Some piezoelectric units have handpieces that can be removed from the tubing for sterilization, others have permanently attached handpieces that must be surface disinfected. For purposes of infection control, units with detachable handpieces are preferred.

Instrument Tips. Instrument tips screw directly onto the handpiece with the use of a special tool. Tips are not interchangeable from manufacturer to manufacturer. The electric generator produces an alternating, high voltage in the handpiece. This voltage produces an electric field in the handpiece that causes the piezo crystals to expand and contract along their diameter and in turn causes the instrument tip to vibrate.

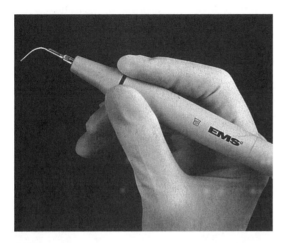

The EMS handpiece with screw-on instrument tip.

Fluid. The primary purpose of water in the piezo system is to cool the tip-to-tooth interface and to flush the sulcus. Some systems, such as the EMS Piezon Master, can be used with antimicrobial solutions instead of water for enhanced elimination of bacteria.

Tip Vibration Frequency. Tip vibration frequency of the working-end of a piezoelectric instrument ranges from 24,000 to 45,000 cycles per second.

Tip Motion. The active tip area ranges from 2.5-3.5 millimeters for both the 25 kHz and 30 kHz instrument tips. The active tip area of a piezoelectric instrument tip typically vibrates in a controlled linear pattern.

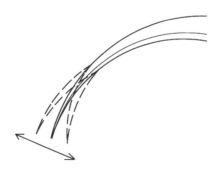

In most cases, the active tip area of a piezoelectric instrument tip vibrates in a linear pattern. There are a few piezoelectric instrument tips that vibrate in an elliptical pattern.

Step-by-Step Technique: Piezoelectric

Example: EMS piezoelectric ultrasonic device
[Reference—EMS *Instructional Manual EMS Master 400 North American Instructions.* Richardson, TX: Electro Medical Systems.]

1. Place the ultrasonic power unit on a counter or cart so that you have easy access to the device at the dental chair.

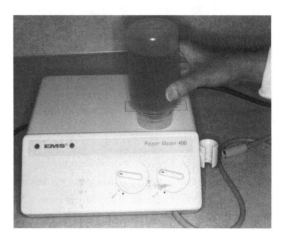

2. Install fluid reservoir according to the directions listed under #3 below. Or <u>if your unit does not have a reservoir</u>, plug the unit water line connection into the water outlet on the dental unit.

3. **Installing the fluid reservoir:**
   a. Place the handpiece cord in its holder before installing the fluid reservoir. The handpiece holder is equipped with a red on/off button that automatically deactivates the unit when the handpiece is not in use.
   b. Set the "water" control knob to its lowest setting. Fill the fluid reservoir with distilled water or other fluid. Screw on the reservoir cap without forcing. Make sure that the flat red gasket is completely seated in the cap.
   c. Attach the fluid reservoir by seating it on its base and turning it one quarter-turn clockwise until it just meets with resistance. The fluid bottle will need 20-30 seconds to pressurize before fluid can be delivered to the handpiece.

4. **Connect handpiece:**
   a. Before connecting the handpiece, "flick" the handpiece cord to expel any fluid or use compressed air to dry the cord's plastic connector if it is wet. Fluid in the connection cord may prevent the unit from operating.
   b. Align the four internal connectors (power and water) and gently insert the handpiece until it is firmly seated in the plastic connector. Do not force the

connection. If the handpiece does not easily connect, check the alignment of the power and water connectors and retry.

c. Do NOT twist or turn the handpiece while connecting or disconnecting it from the cord.

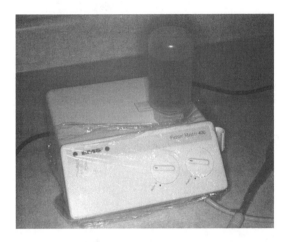

5. Cover power unit and handpiece hose with barriers.

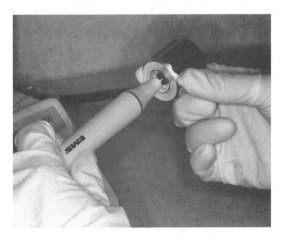

6. Attach instrument tip, hand tightening in a clockwise motion.

Next, tighten the instrument tip with the round torque tool. Insert the tool with the flat, closed end going on first. Turn the tool in a clockwise direction a half to one full turn after resistance is felt. The torque tool must be used to complete the tightening process.

7. **Flushing unit at start and end of day.**
   a. Flush the unit for 2 minutes with water at the beginning and end of each day. Flush for 30 seconds between patients.
   b. For flushing, set the water control to maximum and fill the reservoir with distilled water. Then with an empty reservoir (water control at maximum), flush the unit with air until all fluid is expelled.

8. Adjust the power control while holding the handpiece over the sink. Begin with the low power setting (9 o'clock on dial) and adjust the setting according to patient sensitivity and the tenacity of the calculus deposits.

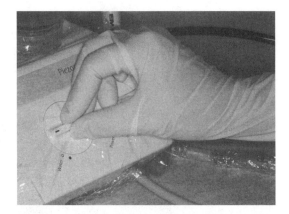

9. Use the water control knob to adjust the fluid spray on the instrument tip to a fine spray. When using precision-thin tips, increase the irrigant setting to at least the 11 o'clock setting.

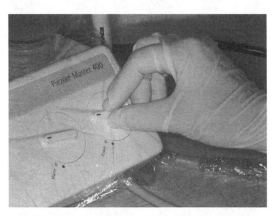

10. Ask your patient to rinse with an antimicrobial solution for 30 seconds. If appropriate, complete a pre-procedural subgingival irrigation of the <u>treatment area</u> prior to instrumentation.

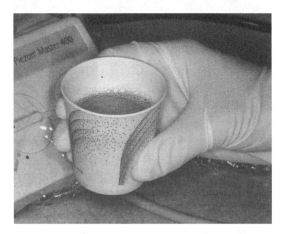

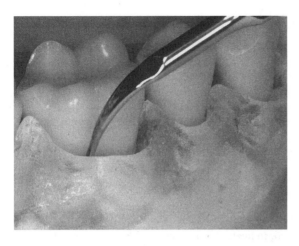

11. Fill the periodontal pocket with fluid. Adapt the <u>activated</u> working-end to the tooth surface. Position the tip in a manner similar to that of a periodontal probe.

Foot Pedal Operation. Use light foot pressure to depress the pedal to the first level for fluid irrigation only. Use heavier foot pressure to depress the pedal to the second level for ultrasonic action plus irrigation.

12. Use a high-volume suction tip or ask your patient to hold a saliva ejector. Position the suction tip or saliva ejector on the side of the mouth where the fluid will pool. Deactivate the ultrasonic tip occasionally to keep excessive amounts of fluid from pooling in the mouth. Cup lips and cheeks to contain the fluid.
13. After completion of appointment, put on utility gloves. Flush the unit with distilled water for 30 seconds between patients.

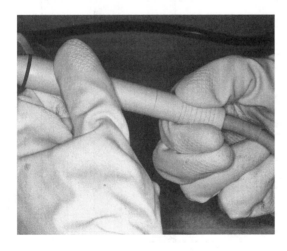

14. Uncouple the handpiece from handpiece hose. Grip the larger, hard ribbed end of the handpiece hose and pull straight out (do NOT twist).

Skill Activities. Turn to page 502 for Skill Building Activities.

Skill Evaluation #1: Magnetostrictive Ultrasonic Equipment

Student: _____   Area 1 = _____

Evaluator: _____   Area 2 = _____

Date: _____   Area 3 = _____

DIRECTIONS: For each area, use **Column S** for student self-evaluation and **Column I** for instructor evaluation. For each skill evaluated, indicate the skill level as: **S** (satisfactory), **I** (improvement needed), or **U** (unsatisfactory).

CRITERIA:	Area 1 S	Area 1 I	Area 2 S	Area 2 I	Area 3 S	Area 3 I
Connects unit to electrical outlet and dental unit water source						
Covers unit and upper portion of handpiece tubing with barriers						
Attaches sterilized handpiece and flushes for 2 minutes						
Holds handpiece in an upright position and fills with water						
Selects appropriate instrument tip for instrumentation task						
Places sterilized insert securely into water-filled handpiece						
Adjusts power and water to appropriate settings						
Uses protective attire for self and patient						
Provides patient with pre-procedural rinse or irrigation						
Places saliva ejector on side of mouth where water will pool						
Establishes appropriate extra- or intraoral fulcrum						
Correctly adapts tip at a 0°-15° angle to tooth surface						
Uses digital activation and light stroke pressure						
Uses overlapping strokes, keeping tip moving at all times						
Demonstrates tapping and sweeping strokes						
Cups patient's lip or cheek to deflect fluid and deactivates tip occasionally to prevent excessive pooling of fluid in mouth						
Demonstrates how to change inserts to prevent air bubbles						
Prepares equipment for storage; handpiece & tips for autoclaving						

Skill Evaluation #2: Piezoelectric Ultrasonic Equipment

Student: _____   Area 1 = _____

Evaluator: _____   Area 2 = _____

Date: _____   Area 3 = _____

DIRECTIONS: For each area, use **Column S** for student self-evaluation and **Column I** for instructor evaluation. For each skill evaluated, indicate the skill level as: **S** (satisfactory), **I** (improvement needed), or **U** (unsatisfactory).

CRITERIA:	Area 1		Area 2		Area 3	
	S	**I**	**S**	**I**	**S**	**I**
Connects unit to electrical outlet and water source						
Covers unit and upper portion of handpiece tubing with barriers						
Attaches sterilized handpiece						
Selects appropriate instrument tip for instrumentation task						
Places sterilized tip securely using attachment tools						
Flushes unit with water for 2 minutes						
Adjusts power and water to appropriate settings						
Uses protective attire for self and patient						
Provides patient with pre-procedural rinse or irrigation						
Places saliva ejector on side of mouth where water will pool						
Uses correct patient and clinician positioning						
Places saliva ejector on side of mouth where water will pool						
Establishes appropriate extra- or intraoral fulcrum						
Correctly adapts tip at a 0°–15° angle to tooth surface						
Uses digital activation and light stroke pressure						
Uses overlapping strokes, keeping tip moving at all times						
Demonstrates tapping and sweeping strokes						
Cups patient's lip or cheek to deflect fluid and deactivates tip occasionally to prevent excessive pooling of fluid in mouth						
Demonstrates how to change tips						
Prepares equipment for storage; handpiece & tips for autoclaving						

Skill Evaluation: Ultrasonic Equipment

Student: _____

Evaluator Comments:

_____

_____

_____

_____

_____

_____

_____

_____

_____

_____

_____

_____

_____

_____

_____

_____

Box for sketches pertaining to written comments.

23
MODULE

Sonic Instruments

This module contains step-by-step instructions for the use of sonic instruments. Many similarities exist in the basic instrumentation concepts applied to ultrasonic and sonic instrumentation. <u>You should complete Module 21 and be thoroughly familiar with the concepts of ultrasonic instrumentation before attempting this module</u>.

Required Equipment:

- sonic handpiece and instrument tips
- dental mirror
- personal protective equipment for clinician and patient
- antimicrobial solution for patient
- high-volume suction tip or saliva ejector

Section 1: Introduction to Sonic Instruments

Sonic devices are mechanized instruments comprised of an air-driven handpiece and removable instrument tips. <u>Sonic handpieces use air pressure to create mechanical vibrations that in turn cause the instrument tip to vibrate</u>. The instrument tip of a sonic device vibrates between 3000 to 8000 cycles per second (3-8 kHz).

Sonic devices have a limited ability to remove tenacious calculus deposits but function well for removal of newly formed and light calculus deposits. Sonic instruments are less efficient in removing calculus deposits than ultrasonic instruments because the sonic instrument tip vibrates at a slower rate. While an ultrasonic instrument tip vibrates back and forth at a rate of 18,000 to 45,000 strokes per second, a sonic instrument tip only vibrates back and forth at a rate of 3000 to 8000 strokes per second. The slower rate of vibration of the sonic instrument tip results in fewer instrumentation strokes per second for calculus removal.

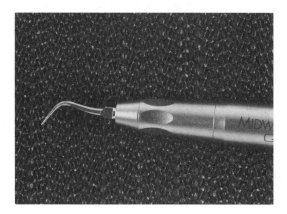

Sonic handpiece and instrument tip.

Sonic Equipment

Handpiece. The sonic handpiece attaches to the dental unit's slow-speed handpiece line. Like a conventional dental low-speed handpiece, the sonic handpiece operates on air pressure. The rheostat foot pedal attached to the dental unit is used to activate the sonic handpiece.

Instrument Tips. Instrument tips screw directly onto the handpiece with the use of a special tool. Tips are not interchangeable from manufacturer to manufacturer. At this time, most sonic units are limited to standard size instrument tip designs. For this reason, sonic instruments are restricted to removal of *supra*gingival or subgingival deposits if tissue distention permits *easy* insertion of the tip. Instrument tips are active on all four sides.

Water. Strictly speaking water cooling is not necessary with most brands of sonic handpieces; water cooling is indicated, however, to obtain the benefits of the flushing action of the water lavage. Sonic instruments cannot be used with antimicrobial solutions since they connect directly to the dental unit and have no ability to accommodate a fluid reservoir. The water coolant flows directly through the working-end. Some brands have a small diameter flow tube that blocks easily and must be routinely cleaned with an orthodontic wire.

Tip Vibration Frequency. Tip vibration frequency of the working-end of a sonic instrument ranges from 3000 to 8000 cycles per second (24-45 kHz). Sonic devices operate at frequencies within the audible range (ultrasonic devices operate at frequencies above the audible range). Some clinicians and patients find the noise generated by the sonic tip to be annoying.

Tip Motion. The active tip area ranges from 2.5-3.5 millimeters for both the 25 kHz and 30 kHz instrument tips. The sonic instrument tip typically vibrates in an orbital motion. Metal and plastic tips are available for some sonic handpieces; studies indicate that patients report more pain sensitivity to plastic than to metal sonic tips. Specialized sonic tips covered with plastic sleeves can be used for debridement of titanium implants.

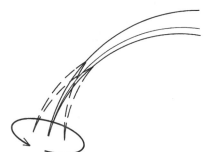

Sonic instrument tips vibrate in an orbital pattern.

Tip Frequency. Tip frequency is pre-set and cannot be adjusted by the clinician.

Power Setting. Sonic devices have pre-set power levels that cannot be adjusted by the clinician.

Water Setting. The clinician should make sure that the water control knob *on the dental unit* is open and that the flow tube in the instrument tip is not blocked. The sonic device, itself, has no mechanism for adjusting the water flow.

Equipment Cost. The average cost of a sonic handpiece is about half that of an ultrasonic unit.

Instrument Tips. Instrument tips for sonic devices are NOT interchangeable from manufacturer to manufacturer (tips for one brand will not fit another brand). At this time, the selection of instrument tip designs for sonic handpieces is limited. For this reason, many sonic mechanized instruments are restricted to the removal of supragingival calculus deposits. Some sonic instrument tip designs may be used subgingivally if tissue distention permits easy insertion.

Brand Name Examples of Sonic Equipment

Adec Corsair II	Micro-Motors Micro ICS Scaler
DentalEZ Titan SW	Midwest Quixonic
Kavo Sonicflex Lux	Scale-aire
Mar-a-Mar Dental K-2 Auto-Scaler	Scalerite
Medidenta Scalerite	Titan-S

Treatment Considerations

The treatment considerations for sonic instrumentation are the same as those for ultrasonic instrumentation. Refer to Module 21, *Treatment Considerations* section, for a discussion of contraindications for use of mechanized instruments, biofilm contamination, prevention of bacteremias, aerosol production, and universal precautions.

Section 2: Step-by-Step Technique

Example: Midwest Quixonic sonic handpiece

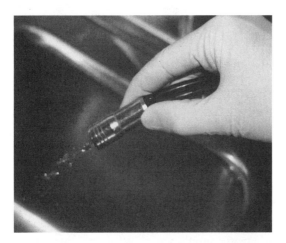

1. Position the dental unit water switch to the ON position. Hold the slow-speed handpiece line over a sink. Step on the rheostat to activate a stream of running water. Flush the handpiece line for 2 minutes at the start of the day and for 30 seconds between patients.

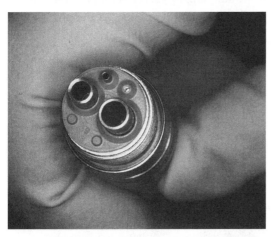

2. Turn the unit water switch to the OFF position. Connect a sterilized sonic handpiece to the slow-speed handpiece line.

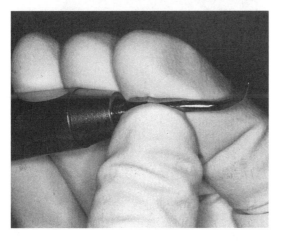

3. Select a sterilized instrument tip and place the threaded end into the handpiece. Hand-tighten the tip by turning it in a clockwise direction until fully seated.

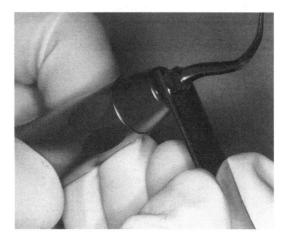

4. Use the wrench to securely tighten the tip. Do not use excessive force with the wrench.

5. **Adjust Water Flow Rate.**
    a. With the water switch in the OFF position, adjust the air pressure to 40-to-50 pounds per square inch (psi).
    b. Return the water switch to the ON position. With the handpiece operating at 45 psi, slowly open the dental unit's water supply valve. While holding the handpiece over a sink, adjust the flow rate until a fine mist surrounds the tip.

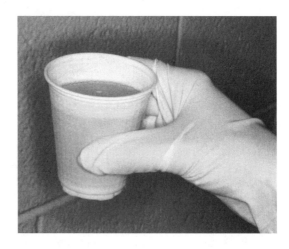

6. Ask patient to rinse with an antimicrobial solution for 30 seconds.

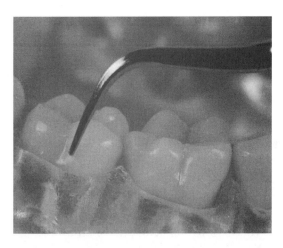

7. Establish an extra- or intraoral finger rest. Hold the tip off of the tooth surface as you step on the rheostat to activate the tip.

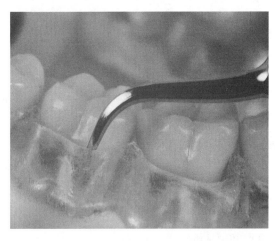

8. Adapt the activated instrument tip to the tooth surface. Position the tip so that the length of the tip is adapted to the tooth surface, in a manner similar to that of a calibrated periodontal probe.

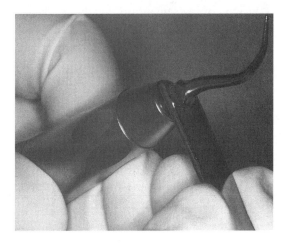

9. To change tips or remove a tip at the completion of the appointment, turn the instrument tip in a counterclockwise direction with the wrench.

Section 3: Activities and Evaluation

Skill Building Activities for Ultrasonic and Sonic Instruments

Skill Building Activity on Extracted Teeth

Materials and Equipment: extracted teeth with calculus deposits and ultrasonic and/or sonic equipment. If extracted teeth are not available, you might try using typodont teeth with synthetic calculus as a substitute. Complete this activity with each type of mechanized equipment available in your clinic (magnetostrictive ultrasonic, piezoelectric ultrasonic, and/or sonic).

Hold an extracted tooth over a sink and practice removing the calculus with a mechanized instrument tip. Remember to use either a **tapping** or a **sweeping** stroke with the instrument tip.

What happens if you use the point of the instrument directly against the root surface?

Compare calculus removal using the (1) point, (2) back, and (3) a lateral surface of the instrument tip against the deposit. Which is most efficient at removing calculus deposits? If available, compare ultrasonic and sonic instruments. Which is most efficient at removing large deposits?

Compare a tapping stroke to a sweeping stroke for calculus removal. Which motion is the most effective at removing a large calculus deposit?

Skill Building Activity: Mechanized Instrument Tips

Obtain samples of each of the different designs of instrument tips available for the mechanized equipment in your clinic. How would each tip be used (calculus type, calculus location?)?

Skill Evaluation: Sonic Equipment

Student: _____   Area 1 = _____

Evaluator: _____   Area 2 = _____

Date: _____   Area 3 = _____

DIRECTIONS: For each area, use **Column S** for student self-evaluation and **Column I** for instructor evaluation. For each skill evaluated, indicate the skill level as: **S** (satisfactory), **I** (improvement needed), or **U** (unsatisfactory).

CRITERIA:	Area 1		Area 2		Area 3	
	S	I	S	I	S	I
Flushes slow-speed handpiece line for 2 minutes						
Connects sterilized sonic handpiece to the slow-speed handpiece line						
Selects appropriate instrument tip for instrumentation task						
Attaches sterilized instrument tip and hand-tightens tip						
Uses wrench to fully tighten the tip						
Adjusts water flow rate until a fine mist ejects from the tip						
Uses protective attire for self and patient						
Provides patient with pre-procedural rinse						
Uses correct patient and clinician positioning						
Places saliva ejector on side of mouth where water will pool						
Establishes appropriate extra- or intraoral fulcrum						
Correctly adapts tip at a 0°-15° angle to tooth surface						
Uses digital activation and light stroke pressure						
Uses overlapping strokes, keeping tip moving at all times						
Demonstrates tapping and sweeping strokes						
Cups patient's lip or cheek to deflect fluid and deactivates tip occasionally to prevent excessive pooling of fluid in mouth						
Demonstrates how to change tips						
Prepares handpiece & tips for autoclaving						

Skill Evaluation: Sonic Equipment

Student: _____

Evaluator Comments:

_____

_____

_____

_____

_____

_____

_____

_____

_____

_____

_____

_____

_____

_____

_____

_____

Box for sketches pertaining to written comments.

24
MODULE

Concepts in
Periodontal Debridement

This module presents some of the recent scientific knowledge relating to instrumentation and the changes in instrumentation terminology prompted by those research findings.

Key Terms:

Attached plaque
Unattached plaque
Closed debridement
Surgical debridement
Scaling and root planing
Periodontal debridement

Deplaquing
Bacterial byproducts
Endotoxin
Plaque retentive factors
Pathologically deepened sulcus
Sulcus with increased depth

Section 1: Periodontal Debridement

A New Model for Instrumentation

Twenty years ago basic scientific knowledge about the nature of periodontal disease was quite limited. Researchers believed that calculus deposits were the main cause of periodontal disease and that endotoxins from bacterial plaque were absorbed into the root surface creating tissue inflammation. Today, research investigations combined with long-term clinical trial results indicate that periodontal diseases are bacterial infections. This knowledge requires dental healthcare providers to shift their thinking away from the mechanical "smoothing of tooth surfaces" to target the real cause of periodontal disease, the pathogenic bacteria.

Research findings that have caused this change in thinking are:

1. **Etiology.**
   Then. Before the 1960's, mechanical irritants, such as calculus deposits, were thought to be the cause of periodontal disease. Treatment for periodontal disease was a procedure called <u>scaling</u>, the thorough removal of calculus deposits.
   Now. Current theory recognizes that periodontal disease occurs when bacterial pathogens overwhelm the host's immune response.[1-4] Modern periodontal instrumentation focuses on the control of pathogenic bacteria and in obtaining a favorable tissue response.
2. **Calculus Removal.**
   Then. It was thought that complete calculus removal is necessary for healing of the periodontal tissues to occur and that it is possible for a competent clinician to remove all subgingival calculus deposits.
   Now. Removal of all calculus deposits from periodontally involved root surfaces is not a realistic goal regardless of the skill of the clinician.[5, 6] Instead, the clinician should try to remove all clinically detectable deposits. For the majority of patients, healing of the periodontal tissues occurs despite calculus remaining after instrumentation.[7]
3. **Bacterial Endotoxins.**
   Then. In the past, endotoxins from gram-negative bacteria were believed to be

deeply embedded in the cementum. A procedure called <u>root planing</u> was used to aggressively remove the contaminated cementum. Root planing was performed until "the root surfaces were as smooth as glass". Over time root planing resulted in a significant loss or complete removal of cementum, hourglass-shaped roots, root sensitivity, and occasionally, pulp exposures.

Now. Toxins are loosely associated with the outer layers of the cementum and are easily removed with brushes, light instrumentation strokes, and ultrasonic acoustic turbulence.[8-13] Extensive root planing to produce glassy root surfaces in all areas is not appropriate; conservation of cementum is indicated.[7, 12, 14-18]

4. **Treatment of Pocket Environment.**

   Then. Subgingival instrumentation was limited to the root surface.

   Now. Ideally, instrumentation should be directed at the entire pocket environment (root surface, pocket space, and soft tissue wall). Two types of bacterial plaque exist within the pocket environment. <u>Attached</u> plaque (also known as <u>adherent bacterial plaque</u>) plays an important role in periodontal disease and should be removed. <u>Unattached plaque</u> (also known as <u>loosely adherent plaque</u>) is found within the pocket space and in contact with the soft tissue wall. Research investigations suggest that unattached plaque may play a more significant role in periodontal disease than attached plaque.[19, 20] Ultrasonic instrumentation is the method of choice for the disruption of unattached plaque. The acoustic turbulence produced by ultrasonic instruments has been shown to have an antimicrobial effect on subgingival bacteria within the environment of the pocket and even into the ulcerated lining of the tissue wall.[21, 22] In addition, fluid lavage from the ultrasonic tip washes unattached plaque from the pocket.

5. **Detection of Residual Calculus Deposits.**

   Then. A skilled clinician should be able to use an explorer to detect all residual calculus deposits (minute spicules of calculus) remaining on the root surface.

   Now. In a clinical study by Sherman, et al., skilled clinicians were wrong 50% of the time in trying to detect the presence of residual calculus deposits remaining on root surfaces after instrumentation.[23]

6. **Closed Debridement.**

   Then. Periodontal pockets deeper than 5 mm must be treated with surgical debridement (periodontal surgery). <u>Closed debridement</u> (periodontal instrumentation within a pocket) was thought to be too technically demanding to be successful in deep pockets.

   Now. Closed debridement is as successful as surgical debridement for treatment of periodontal disease at all levels of severity.[7, 24-31]

7. **Ultrasonic Instrumentation.**
   Then. Ultrasonic instrumentation was limited to <u>supragingival</u> use and was followed by hand instrumentation.
   Now. Ultrasonic instrumentation is as effective as hand instrumentation and in fact, has several advantages over hand instrumentation (many mechanisms of action, instrument tip design, and instrumentation technique). Ultrasonic instrumentation will detoxify root surfaces. [12] Refer to Module 21 for more information on the advantages of ultrasonic instrumentation.

8. **Extent of Subgingival Instrumentation.**
   Then. All root surfaces within a periodontal pocket must be aggressively root planed.
   Now. Some root surfaces may need to be root planed. Periodontal disease results when an imbalance exists between the host's immune response and pathogenic bacteria plus other risk factors. Different individuals (hosts) vary in their ability to tolerate periodontal pathogens. We see the same difference in two individuals' susceptibility to the common cold. Two students are seated in a classroom and both are exposed to an individual who is coughing and sneezing. Yet, only one of the two students actually "catches" the cold (perhaps because he or she was awake all night studying for an exam). Some individuals can tolerate a moderate amount of bacterial plaque and yet never experience periodontal destruction. Other individuals experience periodontal destruction in the presence of light bacterial plaque. Other host factors, such as medications, smoking, neutrophil deficiencies, and systemic illness, can effect the host's susceptibility to the periodontal pathogens.[3] Since individuals differ in their susceptibility to periodontal pathogens, the amount of plaque and calculus that individuals can tolerate also varies. For this reason, the extent of instrumentation necessary to achieve tissue health varies from patient to patient. Intentional removal of cementum on all root surfaces is not indicated. When the tissue adjacent to a particular tooth surface does not respond to instrumentation, the removal of cementum <u>on that surface</u> may be indicated.

Endpoint of Instrumentation

A patient comes to the dental office with inflamed bleeding tissue and exhibits generalized plaque, 4-5 mm clinical attachment loss, and moderate subgingival calculus deposits. How do you know when your instrumentation on this patient is completed? In the past, it was easier for a clinician to say when he or she "was done" with instrumentation. That is, when the calculus had been removed and the root surfaces were glassy smooth, instrumentation was complete. Today, with tissue health as the goal, it is not quite so easy to say exactly when the endpoint of instrumentation has been reached. Tissue healing does not occur overnight, in fact, it is not really possible to assess tissue response for at least a month after the completion of the initial series of appointments with the patient.

The patient should be scheduled for a re-evaluation appointment 4 to 6 weeks after completion of the initial instrumentation. A complete periodontal assessment should be done at this time, including probing depths, clinical attachment levels, and bleeding upon probing.

Ideally, the clinical level of attachment has stayed the same or even decreased, and bone levels are stable. In evaluating the patient, it is important to differentiate between a "diseased" periodontal pocket and a "healthy" periodontal pocket. If you do not understand the distinction between these two conditions, then you may mistake health for disease. At the re-evaluation appointment if an area experiences an increased loss of attachment, the tissue is not healthy. If, however, the clinical attachment level of the pocket remains the same or decreases, then the tissue is healthy. In this case, the pocket itself is just a "monument" to past disease destruction, only surgery could reduce the depth of this pocket to 3 mm or less. In fact, the term "periodontal pocket" is more correctly referred to as a "**pathologically deepened sulcus**". A "healthy" periodontal pocket with clinical attachment levels that remain the same or decrease is termed a **sulcus with increased depth**. A sulcus with increased depth is a sign of success in the struggle to stop the progress of periodontal disease.

Non-responsive sites (sites that show continued loss of attachment) should be carefully re-evaluated with an explorer for the presence of residual calculus deposits or roughness. In addition to deeper attachment levels, non-responsive sites also may exhibit the clinical signs of inflammation and/or bleeding upon probing. If the root surface is rough, root planing of the site may be indicated. The non-responsive sites should be thoroughly deplaqued with an ultrasonic instrument (unless ultrasonic instrumentation is contraindicated for this patient). If the site is still not healed at the next re-evaluation appointment the clinician should try to determine what other factors might be contributing to the disease process (for example: host factors, dental factors). In your periodontics course, you will learn about these factors and about supportive therapies to help the patient.

The important thing to remember about instrumentation for the patient with periodontal disease is that the goal is to prepare the root surface so that it is acceptable to the tissue (and healing occurs). If a site is non-responsive, then it should be re-instrumented and re-evaluated.

Instrumentation Terminology

Scaling and root planing are the terms that have been used traditionally to describe the mechanical removal of calculus and cementum. As clinicians changed their way of thinking about the causes of periodontal disease, they began to search for new terminology that would more accurately describe current philosophies of instrumentation. The term "periodontal debridement" was first suggested as an alternative to the terms "scaling and root planing" in 1993.[17, 18]

Traditionally, **scaling** has been defined as the removal of bacterial plaque and calculus deposits from coronal & root surfaces. **Root planing** as traditionally defined, included the aggressive removal of cementum and the instrumenting of all root surfaces to a glassy smooth texture. Root planing is no longer recommended as routine procedure to be performed on all root surfaces. Some authors and clinicians have redefined the term "root planing" so that its meaning is similar to that of subgingival debridement. This approach of redefining the term root planing can be confusing, however, because it is difficult to determine which definition is being used by any one person.

Periodontal debridement is the removal or disruption of bacterial plaque, its byproducts, and plaque retentive calculus deposits from coronal surfaces, root surfaces, and within pocket space and tissue wall, as indicated, for the periodontal healing and repair. Calculus is removed only because it is a breeding ground for bacterial plaque. Conservation of cementum is a goal of periodontal debridement. The extent of instrumentation should be limited to that needed to obtain a favorable tissue response. Root surfaces only should be instrumented to a level that results in the resolution of tissue inflammation. The goal is returning the tissue to a healthy, non-inflamed state that can be maintained by the patient.

Trisha E. O'Hehir, one of the first individuals to suggest a change in instrumentation terminology, stresses that periodontal debridement is more than just another term for root planing. O'Hehir lists two primary distinctions of periodontal debridement: 1) debridement goes beyond treatment of the root surfaces, and 2) it has an objective goal (to stop the progression of disease and re-establish periodontal health).[32] Periodontal debridement as defined by O'Hehir includes treatment of the entire pocket environment: the root surface, pocket space, tissue wall, and underlying tissues. Another difference is that periodontal debridement recognizes the role of the patient's host response (susceptibility) to periodontal disease.

Supragingival debridement is the mechanical removal of bacterial plaque, its byproducts, and plaque retentive factors (such as calculus) from the clinical crowns of the teeth to assist the patient in maintaining periodontal health.

Subgingival debridement is the mechanical removal of bacterial plaque, its byproducts, and plaque retentive factors (such as calculus) apical to the gingival margin to assist the patient in maintaining periodontal health.

Surgical debridement is the use of a surgical procedure to gain access to the root surfaces for the purpose of removing plaque, its byproducts, and plaque retentive calculus deposits. In this procedure, a general dentist or periodontist makes incisions in the tissue and reflects the tissue to expose the roots of the teeth in the treatment area. After the roots have been instrumented, the tissue is sutured back in place.

Deplaquing is the disruption or removal of *subgingival* bacterial plaque and its byproducts from cemental surfaces and the pocket space following the completion of subgingival instrumentation. Ideally, an ultrasonic instrument is used to deplaque subgingival tooth surfaces, however, when ultrasonic instrumentation is contraindicated, a curet can be used for deplaquing.

Bacterial byproducts are substances produced or released by bacteria that irritate and produce changes in the periodontal tissues. These substances are cytotoxic to the tissues and must be removed for healing to occur. Bacterial byproducts include toxins, enzymes, bacterial antigens, waste products, and invasion factors.

Endotoxin is a component of the cell wall of gram-negative bacteria that is found in high concentrations in periodontal pockets and causes tissue destruction.

Plaque retentive factors are conditions in the mouth that foster the establishment and growth of bacterial plaque, such as calculus deposits and overhanging restorations.

A **pathologically deepened sulcus** is a more accurate term for a "periodontal pocket".

A **sulcus with increased depth** is a "healthy" periodontal pocket with clinical attachment levels that remain the same or decrease in depth.

Reference Sheet: Scaling Versus Debridement

Comparison of Scaling/Root Planing and Periodontal Debridement		
	Scaling and Root Planing	**Periodontal Debridement**
Focus	Complete calculus removal and glassy smooth root surfaces.	Removal of bacterial plaque, its byproducts, and plaque retentive calculus, with minimal iatrogenic damage to the tooth, to assist the patient in maintaining periodontal health.
Root Surfaces	Endotoxins believed to be deeply embedded in the surface of the cementum or tightly bound to cementum. Therefore, cementum must be removed. Cementum removal was intentional. Aggressive instrumentation removed significant amounts of cementum. Only the root surfaces must be treated.	Endotoxins are loosely associated and easily removed by washing or light instrumentation strokes. Conservation of cementum is a goal. Cementum removal is damaging to the periodontium. Thorough deplaquing of pocket environment is indicated. Unattached plaque can be flushed from the sulcus or pocket by ultrasonic instruments.
Method	Hand-activated instrumentation preferred.	A combination of hand-activated and ultrasonic instrumentation is preferred.
Endpoint of Instrumentation	Complete calculus removal and glassy smooth root surfaces.	Removal of all clinically detectable calculus, plaque and its byproducts.

Section 2: Activity and References

Skill Building Activity

Answer the following questions about the old and new models for instrumentation.

1. Explain the difference in the objectives of instrumentation today as compared to those of 20 years ago.
2. How has the role of ultrasonic instrumentation changed in the last 20 years?
3. How has the definition of successful treatment in regard to instrumentation changed in the last 20 years?
4. Twenty years ago subgingival instrumentation was limited to the root surfaces. How has the scope of subgingival instrumentation changed?

References

1. Genco, R.J., *Host responses in periodontal diseases: current concepts.* J Periodontol, 1992. **63**(4 Suppl): p. 338-55.
2. Christersson, L.A., et al., *Dental plaque and calculus: risk indicators for their formation.* J Dent Res, 1992. **71**(7): p. 1425-30.
3. Socransky, S.S., and A.D. Haffajee, *The bacterial etiology of destructive periodontal disease: current concepts.* J Periodontol, 1992. **63**(4 Suppl): p. 322-31.
4. Walters, C., *Periodontal debridement techniques. Using research results in the dental practice.* Dent Teamwork, 1996. **9**(3): p. 12-4.
5. Drisko, C.L., and W.J. Killoy, *Scaling and root planing: removal of calculus and subgingival organisms.* Curr Opin Dent, 1991. **1**(1): p. 74-80.
6. Kepic, T.J., T.J. O'Leary, and A.H. Kafrawy, *Total calculus removal: an attainable objective? [see comments].* J Periodontol, 1990. **61**(1): p. 16-20.
7. Greenstein, G., *Periodontal response to mechanical non-surgical therapy: a review.* J Periodontol, 1992. **63**(2): p. 118-30.
8. Hughes, F.J., and F.C. Smales, *Attachment and orientation of human periodontal ligament fibroblasts to lipopolysaccharide-coated and pathologically altered cementum in vitro.* Eur J Prosthodont Restor Dent, 1992. **1**(2): p. 63-8.
9. Cheetham, W.A., M. Wilson, and J.B. Kieser, *Root surface debridement—an in vitro assessment.* J Clin Periodontol, 1988. **15**(5): p. 288-92.

10. Hughes, F.J., and F.C. Smales, *Immunohistochemical investigation of the presence and distribution of cementum-associated lipopolysaccharides in periodontal disease.* J Periodontal Res, 1986. **21**(6): p. 660-7.

11. Moore, J., M. Wilson, and J.B. Kieser, *The distribution of bacterial lipopolysaccharide (endotoxin) in relation to periodontally involved root surfaces.* J Clin Periodontol, 1986. **13**(8): p. 748-51.

12. Smart, G.J., et al., *The assessment of ultrasonic root surface debridement by determination of residual endotoxin levels.* J Clin Periodontol, 1990. **17**(3): p. 174-8.

13. Chiew, S.Y., et al., *Assessment of ultrasonic debridement of calculus-associated periodontally-involved root surfaces by the limulus amoebocyte lysate assay. An in vitro study.* J Clin Periodontol, 1991. **18**(4): p. 240-4.

14. Nyman, S., et al., *Role of "diseased" root cementum in healing following treatment of periodontal disease. An experimental study in the dog.* J Periodontal Res, 1986. **21**(5): p. 496-503.

15. Nyman, S., et al., *Role of "diseased" root cementum in healing following treatment of periodontal disease. A clinical study.* J Clin Periodontol, 1988. **15**(7): p. 464-8.

16. Jeffcoat, M.K., M. McGuire, and M.G. Newman, *Evidence-based periodontal treatment. Highlights from the 1996 World Workshop in Periodontics.* J Am Dent Assoc, 1997. **128**(6): p. 713-24.

17. Woodall, I., N.S. Young, and T. O'Hehir, *Comprehensive Dental Hygiene Care. Periodontal debridement. Part 2.* RDH, 1993. **13**(10): p. 26, 28.

18. Woodall, I., et al., *Comprehensive Dental Hygiene Care. Periodontal debridement. Part 1.* Rdh, 1993. **13**(9): p. 26, 28, 32.

19. Fine, D.H., et al., *Studies in plaque pathogenicity. II. A technique for the specific detection of endotoxin in plaque samples using the limulus lysate assay.* J Periodontal Res, 1978. **13**(2): p. 127-33.

20. Fine, D.H., et al., *Studies in plaque pathogenicity. I. Plaque collection and limulus lysate screening of adherent and loosely adherent plaque.* J Periodontal Res, 1978. **13**(1): p. 17-23.

21. Walmsley, A.D., W.R. Laird, and A.R. Williams, *Dental plaque removal by cavitational activity during ultrasonic scaling.* J Clin Periodontol, 1988. **15**(9): p. 539-43.

22. Olsen, I., and S.S. Socransky, *Ultrasonic dispersion of pure cultures of plaque bacteria and plaque.* Scand J Dent Res, 1981. **89**(4): p. 307-12.

23. Sherman, P.R., et al., *The effectiveness of subgingival scaling and root planing. I. Clinical detection of residual calculus [see comments].* J Periodontol, 1990. **61**(1): p. 3-8.

24. Badersten, A., R. Nilveus, and J. Egelberg, *Effect of nonsurgical periodontal therapy. I. Moderately advanced periodontitis.* J Clin Periodontol, 1981. **8**(1): p. 57-72.

25. Badersten, A., R. Nilveus, and J. Egelberg, *Effect of nonsurgical periodontal therapy. II. Severely advanced periodontitis.* J Clin Periodontol, 1984. **11**(1): p. 63-76.

26. Badersten, A., R. Niveus, and J. Egelberg, *4-year observations of basic periodontal therapy.* J Clin Periodontol, 1987. **14**(8): p. 438-44.

27. Pihlstrom, B.L., et al., *Comparison of surgical and nonsurgical treatment of periodontal disease. A review of current studies and additional results after 61/2 years.* J Clin Periodontol, 1983. **10**(5): p. 524-41.

28. Lindhe, J., et al., *Long-term effect of surgical/non-surgical treatment of periodontal disease.* J Clin Periodontol, 1984. **11**(7): p. 448-58.

29. Knowles, J., et al., *Comparison of results following three modalities of periodontal therapy related to tooth type and initial pocket depth.* J Clin Periodontol, 1980. **7**(1): p. 32-47.

30. Low, S.B., and S.G. Ciancio, *Reviewing nonsurgical periodontal therapy.* J Am Dent Assoc, 1990. **121**(4): p. 467-70.

31. Ramfjord, S.P., et al., *Oral hygiene and maintenance of periodontal support.* J Periodontol, 1982. **53**(1): p. 26-30.

32. O'Hehir, T., *Debridement = scaling and root-planing plus..* RDH, 1999. **19**(5): p. 14.

25
MODULE

Advanced Fulcruming Techniques

This module explains advanced fulcruming techniques that supplement the standard intraoral fulcrum.

Key Terms:

Advanced fulcruming technique   Basic extraoral fulcrum
Advanced Intraoral fulcrum   Stabilized fulcrum

Section 1: Introduction

Fulcruming with your ring finger on a tooth provides stability while working in a patient's mouth with sharp instruments. Thus far, you have been using a **standard intraoral fulcrum** to establish a finger rest on a tooth surface as close as possible to the tooth being instrumented. There are times, however, when it is difficult to obtain parallelism with the lower shank or to adapt the cutting edge when using a standard intraoral fulcrum. In instances when a standard intraoral fulcrum doesn't seem to work well, an advanced fulcruming technique can improve access to the tooth surface. For example, when working within a deep periodontal pocket, sometimes it is difficult to position the lower shank parallel to the root surface being treated. This is especially true for the maxillary molars. In such instances, advanced fulcruming techniques are useful in obtaining parallelism.

The Standard Intraoral Fulcrum	
Technique	Tip of ring finger rests on a stable tooth surface
Location	On the same arch as the treatment area, near the tooth being instrumented
Advantages	• Provides the most stable, secure support for hand • Provides leverage and power for instrumentation • Provides excellent tactile transfer to the fingers • Allows hand and instrument to work together effectively • Permits precise stroke control • Allows forceful stroke pressure with the least amount of stress to the hand and fingers • Decreases the likelihood of injury to the patient if he or she moves unexpectedly during instrumentation
Disadvantages	• May be difficult to obtain parallelism of the lower shank to the tooth surface for access to deep pockets • May not be practical for use in edentulous areas

An **advanced fulcrum** is a fulcruming technique that is used instead of the basic intraoral finger rest. Advanced fulcrums require greater clinician skill and are helpful in working in areas of limited access. Advanced fulcruming techniques can allow you to gain access to a deep pocket and increase the power of the instrumentation stroke.

Advanced fulcrums should be used selectively in areas of limited access, and/or in order to maintain neutral body position. Advanced fulcruming techniques are not intended to replace the intraoral fulcrum since it places the least amount of strain on the clinician's muscles. An advanced fulcrum should be used if an intraoral fulcrum is not effective or possible.

Before attempting advanced fulcruming techniques, you should have mastered the fundamentals of neutral position and standard fulcruming technique. Bad habits with fundamental techniques cannot be corrected by the use of advanced fulcrums. In fact, a clinician with poor fundamental techniques will compound his or her problems by attempting to use advanced fulcrums. Unorthodox methods of instrumentation may serve as a quick fix for achieving an end-product, but usually at the expense of the clinician's musculoskeletal system. Before attempting advanced fulcruming techniques, you should self-evaluate your skill level with a standard intraoral fulcrum and request a critique from an instructor.

Assessment of Advanced Fulcruming Techniques

Advanced Fulcruming Techniques	
Advantages	**Disadvantages**
• Easier access to maxillary second and third molars • Easier access to deep pockets on molar teeth • Improved parallelism of the lower shank to molar teeth • Facilitate neutral wrist position for molar teeth	• Require a greater degree of muscle coordination and instrumentation skill to achieve calculus removal • Greater risk for instrument stick if using finger-on-finger fulcrum • Reduce tactile information to the fingers • May cause more muscle strain to hand and fingers • Not well tolerated by patient's with limited opening or TMJ problems

Reference Sheet: Advanced Fulcruming Techniques

Advanced Fulcruming Techniques		
Types	**Description**	**Efficacy**
Modified Intraoral	Intraoral fulcrum with an altered point of contact between the middle and ring fingers in the grasp	Very effective
Piggy-Backed	Intraoral fulcrum in which the middle finger is stacked on top of the ring finger	Effective
Cross-Arch	Intraoral fulcrum in which the finger rest is established on opposite side of arch from the treatment area	Moderately effective
Opposite Arch	Intraoral fulcrum in which the finger rest is established on opposite arch from the treatment area	Moderately effective
Finger-on-Finger	Intraoral fulcrum in which the finger of the non-dominant hand serves as the resting point for the dominant hand	Very effective
Basic Extraoral	Extraoral fulcrum in which the dominant hand rests against the patient's chin or cheek	Least effective
Stabilized	Intraoral or extraoral fulcrum in which a finger of the non-dominant hand is used to concentrate lateral pressure against the tooth surface and help control the instrument stroke	Very effective

Section 2: Advanced Intraoral Fulcrums

Modified Intraoral Fulcrum

The **modified intraoral fulcrum** is achieved by combining an <u>altered</u> modified pen grasp with a standard intraoral fulcrum. This technique is particularly useful when instrumenting the maxillary teeth. It involves altering the point of contact between the middle and ring fingers in the grasp. In a standard modified pen grasp, the middle and ring fingers contact one another near the tips of the fingers. For the modified intraoral fulcrum, the middle and ring fingers contact one another near the middle knuckle region of the fingers. The modified intraoral fulcrum should not be confused with a split fulcrum. In a split fulcrum, there is no contact between the middle and ring fingers.

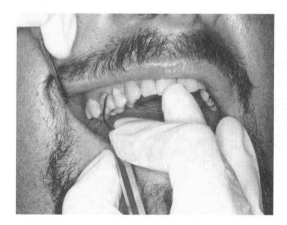

The **modified intraoral fulcrum** alters the point of contact between the middle and ring fingers in the grasp.

Advantages:
- Provides good stable support for the clinician's hand while improving access to difficult to reach proximal root surfaces of maxillary molars.
- Provides leverage, strength, and good stroke control during instrumentation
- Provides good tactile sensitivity to clinician's fingers
- Improves access to deep pockets on maxillary teeth and facilitates parallelism of lower shank to proximal root surfaces

Disadvantage:
Requires more muscle control than a standard intraoral fulcrum

Piggy-Backed Fulcrum

The **piggy-backed fulcrum** is accomplished by stacking the middle finger on top of the ring finger in a piggy-back style. This technique elevates the index finger and thumb and is particularly useful in obtaining better access to the mandibular posterior teeth, especially the aspects away from the clinician. (For right-handed clinicians the aspects away are the mandibular right posteriors, lingual aspect and mandibular left posteriors, facial aspect. For left-handed clinicians, these are the mandibular left posteriors, lingual aspect and the mandibular right posteriors, facial aspect.)

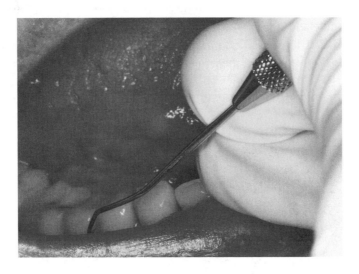

For the **piggy-backed fulcrum** the middle finger rests on top of the ring finger.

Advantages:
- Improves access to the mandibular posterior aspects away from the clinician
- Enhances the whole hand working together as a unit

Disadvantage:
Patients with limited opening may not be able to accommodate this fulcrum

Cross-Arch Fulcrum

The **cross-arch fulcrum** is accomplished by resting the ring finger on a tooth on the opposite side of the arch from the teeth being instrumented (for example, resting on the left side of the mandible to instrument a mandibular right molar).

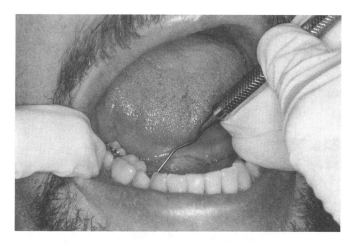

This photograph shows a **cross-arch fulcrum** on the mandibular left premolars used to instrument the lingual aspect of the mandibular right posterior sextant.

Advantage:
Allows improved access to the lingual aspect of mandibular posterior teeth

Disadvantages:
Usually requires the clinician to grasp near the midpoint of the handle and to rest the middle finger on the handle (rather than on the instrument shank); this grasp makes stroke control more difficult and decreases tactile information to the clinician's fingers

---

Opposite Arch Fulcrum

The **opposite arch fulcrum** is an advanced fulcrum used to improve access to deep pockets and to facilitate parallelism to proximal root surfaces. It is accomplished by resting the ring finger on the opposite arch from the treatment area (for example, resting on the mandibular arch to instrument maxillary teeth).

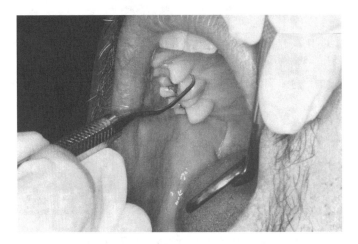

In this example, an **opposite arch fulcrum** is being used on the mandibular anterior teeth for instrumentation of the maxillary right first molar.

Advantage:
Facilitates access to deep pockets, especially on maxillary posterior teeth

Disadvantages:
- Requires the clinician to grasp near the midpoint of the handle and to rest the middle finger on the handle (rather than on the instrument shank); this grasp makes stroke control more difficult and decreases tactile information to the clinician's fingers
- May be uncomfortable for patients with TMJ problems. The pressure of the fulcrum resting on the mandibular teeth places a strain on the muscles associated with TMJ disorders

Finger-on-Finger Fulcrum

The **finger-on-finger fulcrum** is accomplished by resting the ring finger of the dominant hand on the index finger of the <u>non</u>-dominant hand. This positioning allows the clinician to fulcrum in line with the long axis of the tooth to improve parallelism of the lower shank to the tooth surface.

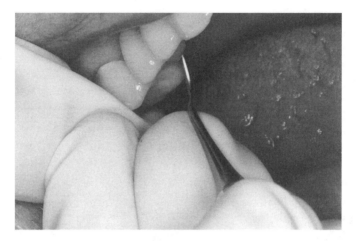

A close-up view of a **finger-on-finger fulcrum** used by a right-handed clinician while instrumenting the maxillary right posteriors, lingual aspect. The fulcrum finger of the right hand rests on the index finger of the left hand.

Advantages:
- Provides stable rest for fulcrum finger
- Improves access to deep pockets

Disadvantages:
- Possibility of an instrument stick to finger of non-dominant hand if the clinician slips while making an instrumentation stroke
- Non-dominant hand cannot be used for retraction or to hold the mirror

Finger-on-finger fulcrum demonstrated by a right-handed clinician for the maxillary right molars, lingual aspect. The clinician's right fulcrum finger is resting on the index finger of the left hand.

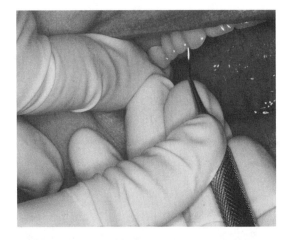

Finger-on-finger fulcrum demonstrated by a right-handed clinician for the mandibular left posteriors, facial aspect.

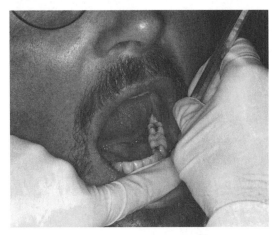

A close-up of a **finger-on-finger fulcrum** while instrumenting the mandibular left posteriors, facial aspect. The right-handed clinician rests the ring finger of her right hand on her left index finger.

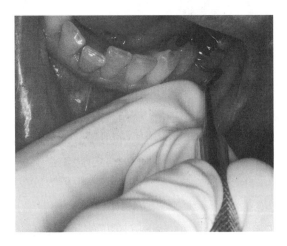

Section 3: Basic Extraoral Fulcrums

The **basic extraoral fulcrum** involves resting the fingers or palm of the hand against the patient's chin or cheeks.

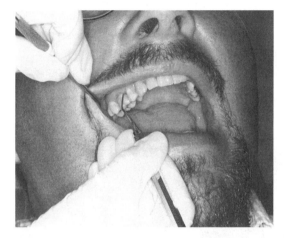

Basic extraoral fulcrum using knuckle-rest technique. For this technique, the clinician rests the knuckles against the patient's chin or cheek.

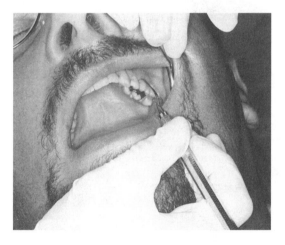

Basic extraoral fulcrum using the chin-cup technique. For this technique the clinician cups the patient's chin with the palm of the hand.

Advantages:
- Facilitates instrumentation of the proximal root surfaces of maxillary molars

Disadvantages:
- Requires the clinician to grasp near the midpoint of the handle and to rest the middle finger on the handle (rather than on the instrument shank); this grasp makes stroke control more difficult and decreases tactile information
- Least effective of all fulcruming techniques; the technique of last resort

Section 4: Stabilized Fulcrums

A **stabilized fulcrum** is accomplished by using the thumb or index finger of the non-dominant hand against the instrument shank. The finger of the non-dominant hand is placed against the instrument shank to (1) concentrate stroke pressure against the tooth surface and (2) help control the working-end throughout the instrumentation stroke. The stabilized fulcrum can be combined with a basic intraoral fulcrum or used with other advanced fulcruming techniques such as the opposite arch fulcrum or an extraoral fulcrum. This technique is especially useful on proximal surfaces where the calculus is tenacious and the tissue is fragile.

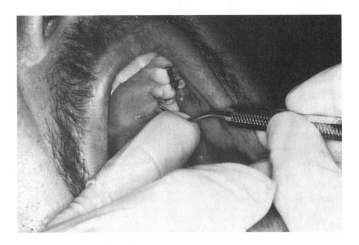

Stabilized Fulcrum. In this example demonstrated by a right-handed clinician, the index finger of the left hand is placed behind the shank to press the cutting edge forward against the distal surface of the molar.

Advantages:
- Concentrates stroke pressure for removal of tenacious subgingival deposits
- Creates a well controlled instrumentation stroke
- Reduces muscle strain and workload for the dominant hand

Disadvantage:
The non-dominant hand is not available to hold the mirror for retraction or indirect vision

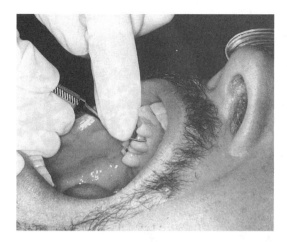

Example 1. A stabilized fulcrum demonstrated by a right-handed clinician for the maxillary right posteriors, lingual aspect. The clinician is using an opposite arch fulcrum and the left index finger against the instrument shank.

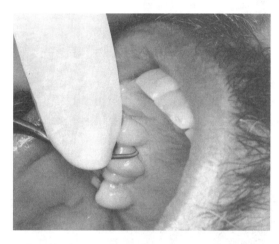

Example 1—close up view. The index finger of the non-dominant hand is used to press against the front side of the shank, concentrating pressure with the cutting edge <u>back against the mesial surface</u> of the first molar.

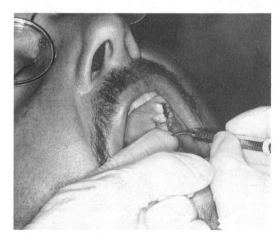

Example 2. A stabilized fulcrum demonstrated by a right-handed clinician for the maxillary left posteriors, lingual aspect. In this instance, the clinician is instrumenting the distal surface of the first molar. The clinician is using an opposite arch fulcrum.

Example 2—close up view. The clinician positions his left index finger behind the shank to concentrate lateral pressure <u>forward against the distal surface</u> of the first molar.

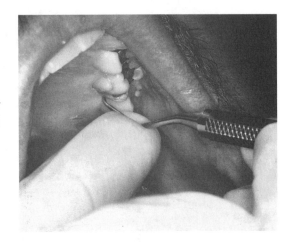

Example 3. A stabilized fulcrum demonstrated by a right-handed clinician to instrument the facial surface of a mandibular anterior tooth. The clinician is seated behind the patient and using an intraoral fulcrum. The left index finger is on the instrument shank and the left thumb is retracting the lip.

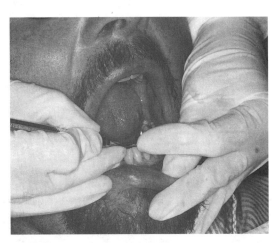

Example 3—close up view. The right-handed clinician positions his left index finger on the shank to stabilize a short horizontal stroke. The stabilized fulcrum helps to control the instrumentation stroke by concentrating pressure precisely on the cutting edge.

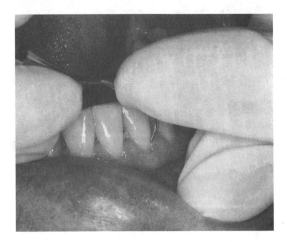

Skill Evaluation: Advanced Fulcruming Techniques

Student: _____

Evaluator: _____

Date: _____

DIRECTIONS: For each grasp, use **Column S** for student self-evaluation and **Column I** for instructor evaluation. For each advanced fulcruming technique evaluated, indicate the skill level as: **S** (satisfactory), **I** (improvement needed), or **U** (unsatisfactory).

CRITERIA:	S	I
States the advantages and disadvantages of a standard intraoral fulcrum		
States the advantages and disadvantages of advanced fulcruming techniques		
Demonstrates a modified intraoral fulcrum for instrumentation of an appropriate treatment area		
Demonstrates a piggy-backed fulcrum for instrumentation of an appropriate treatment area		
Demonstrates a cross-arch fulcrum for instrumentation of an appropriate treatment area		
Demonstrates an opposite arch fulcrum for instrumentation of an appropriate treatment area		
Demonstrates a finger-on-finger fulcrum for instrumentation of an appropriate treatment area		
Demonstrates an extraoral fulcrum using the knuckle-rest technique for instrumentation of an appropriate treatment area		
Demonstrates an extraoral fulcrum using the chin-cup technique for instrumentation of an appropriate treatment area		
Demonstrates a stabilized fulcrum for instrumentation of the distal surface of a maxillary first molar		
Demonstrates a stabilized fulcrum for instrumentation of the mesial surface of a maxillary first molar		

Skill Evaluation: Advanced Fulcruming Techniques

Student: _____

Evaluator Comments:

_____

_____

_____

_____

_____

_____

_____

_____

_____

_____

_____

_____

_____

_____

_____

_____

Box for sketches pertaining to written comments.

26
MODULE

Debridement of Dental Implants

This module will introduce you to the special instruments used to debride dental implants.

Required Equipment:

- dental mirror
- plastic implant instruments
- a typodont with a dental implant prosthesis and/or a patient with dental implants
- protective attire for the clinician and patient

Key Terms:

Dental implant
Endosseous dental implant
Subperiosteal dental implant

Transosteal implant
Plastic instrument

Section 1: Introduction

A **dental implant** is a nonbiologic device surgically inserted into or onto the jawbone to replace a missing tooth or act as an abutment to provide support for a fixed bridge or denture. The three types of dental implants are endosseous, subperiosteal, and transosteal.

- An **endosseous implant** is a type of dental implant that is placed into the alveolar and/or basal bone and protrudes through the mucoperiosteum. It is the most widely used type of dental implant.
- A **subperiosteal** implant is a type of dental implant that placed on the surface of the bone beneath the periosteum.
- A **transosteal implant** is a type of dental implant that is placed through the alveolar bone.

Endosseous Implant. The implant fixture is placed into the bone and serves as the anchor for the dental implant. Later, a titanium abutment post is attached to the implant fixture. The titanium abutment is extremely biocompatible and not rejected by the body.

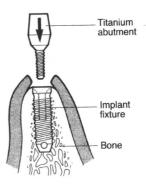

The abutment post is used to connect the implant fixture to a prosthetic crown or denture.

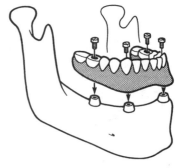

Section 2: Technique

Guidelines for Debridement of Dental Implants

Special instruments made of plastic are used for the debridement of dental implants. The use of stainless steel and carbon steel instruments and ultrasonic or sonic devices with metal tips is <u>not recommended</u> with implants. Calculus is removed readily from dental implants since there is no interlocking or penetration of calculus deposits with the implant surface. Light lateral pressure with a plastic instrument is recommended; care must be taken not to scratch the surface of the implant. Scratches in the surface of the implant would favor plaque accumulation and calculus formation.

Guidelines for Instrumentation of Dental Implants

1. Plastic instruments are recommended. Metal instruments and ultrasonic or sonic devices with metal tips are not recommended.

2. Instrumentation should be restricted to *supra*gingival deposit removal.

3. Strokes should be short, controlled and activated with light pressure. Calculus does not adhere to titanium as tenaciously as on natural teeth.

Types of Plastic Instruments

Instruments used for assessment and debridement of implant teeth should be made of a material that is softer than the implant material. Plastic instruments are most commonly used. Plastic instruments are available in a variety of designs, some of which have working-ends that are similar to conventional periodontal probes, sickle scalers, and universal curets. Plastic instruments are safe for use on all types of implants without damage to the abutment surface.

A separate category of implant instruments is comprised of instruments made of plastic materials containing graphite fillers. These instruments work well on the implant **superstructure** (denture, or prosthetic crown); but can scratch certain types of abutments. For this reason, plastic instruments containing graphite fillers should be limited to use on the implant superstructure and not used directly on the implant abutment.

Working-End Design

Instrument working ends can be classified into one of four design types: (1) wrench-shaped, (2) crescent-shaped, (3) hoe-like, and (4) those with working-ends that are similar to those of conventional metal periodontal instruments (probe, sickle scaler, curet). It is recommended that an instrument kit contain all four of these working-end design types.

Examples of plastic instruments with wrench-shaped, crescent-shaped, and hoe-like working-ends.

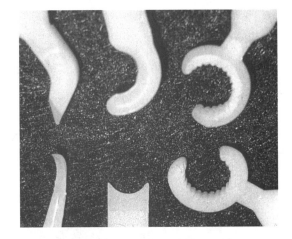

Examples of plastic instruments with curet-like working-ends.

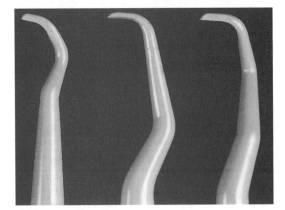

Techniques for Use

Wrench-shaped, crescent-shaped, and hoe-like plastic instruments are used to clean the titanium abutment posts of a prosthetic denture.

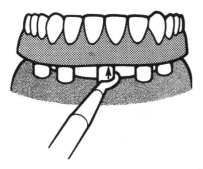

The wrench-shaped working-end wraps around the abutment. This working-end should be used with vertical instrumentation strokes.

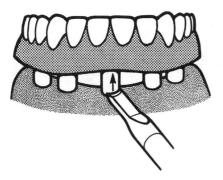

The crescent-shaped working-end is used to clean the surface of the abutment using vertical strokes.

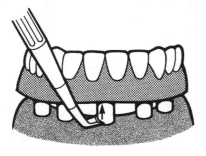

The contra-angled crescent-shaped working-end is used to clean the surface of the abutment using vertical strokes.

The hoe-like working-end is used for cleaning the apical portion (underside) of the prosthetic framework. Instrumentation strokes should be in a facial-to-lingual direction.

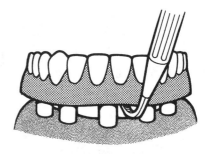

Sickle- or curet-shaped working-ends adapt well to abutment posts and single implant crowns. (Photo courtesy of Hu-Friedy Mfg. Co., Inc.)

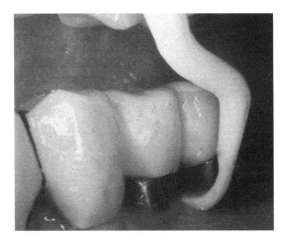

Plastic periodontal probes are used to assess the tissues surrounding a dental implant.

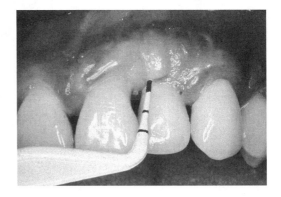

Skill Evaluation: Debridement of Dental Implants

Student: _____   Area 1 = _____

Evaluator: _____   Area 2 = _____

Date: _____   Area 3 = _____

                                Area 4 = _____

DIRECTIONS: For each area, use **Column S** for student self-evaluation and **Column I** for instructor evaluation. For each skill evaluated, indicate the skill level as: **S** (satisfactory), **I** (improvement needed), or **U** (unsatisfactory).

CRITERIA:	Area 1		Area 2		Area 3		Area 4	
	S	I	S	I	S	I	S	I
States special guidelines for instrumentation of dental implants								
Positioned correctly in relation to the patient, equipment, and treatment area								
Uses correct patient head position								
Ring finger acts as "support beam"; finger rest is on a stable tooth surface								
Uses mirror appropriately								
Selects appropriate instrument for the instrumentation task								
Maintains correct adaptation and angulation								
Uses controlled work strokes								
Applies stroke pressure in a coronal direction only								
Restricts instrumentation to supragingival deposit removal								
Uses appropriate motion activation								

Skill Evaluation: Debridement of Dental Implants

Student: _____

Evaluator Comments:

_____

_____

_____

_____

_____

_____

_____

_____

_____

_____

_____

_____

_____

_____

_____

_____

_____

Box for sketches pertaining to written comments.

Index

539